Advanced Heart Failure: From Pathophysiology to Clinical Management

Editors

GIUSEPPE PACILEO
FRANCESCO GRIGIONI
DANIELE MASARONE
LUCIANO POTENA

HEART FAILURE CLINICS

www.heartfailure.theclinics.com

Consulting Editor
EDUARDO BOSSONE

Founding Editor
JAGAT NARULA

October 2021 • Volume 17 • Number 4

ELSEVIER

1600 John F. Kennedy Boulevard • Suite 1800 • Philadelphia, Pennsylvania, 19103-2899

http://www.theclinics.com

HEART FAILURE CLINICS Volume 17, Number 4
October 2021 ISSN 1551-7136, ISBN-13: 978-0-323-89716-7

Editor: Joanna Collett
Developmental Editor: Jessica Cañaberal

Heart Failure Clinics (ISSN 1551-7136) is published quarterly by Elsevier Inc., 360 Park Avenue South, New York, NY 10010-1710. Months of publication are January, April, July, and October. Business and editorial offices: 1600 John F. Kennedy Boulevard, Suite 1800, Philadelphia, PA 19103-2899. Periodicals postage paid at New York, NY, and additional mailing offices. Subscription prices are USD 277.00 per year for US individuals, USD 661.00 per year for US institutions, USD 100.00 per year for US students and residents, USD 300.00 per year for Canadian individuals, USD 684.00 per year for Canadian institutions, USD 315.00 per year for international individuals, USD 684.00 per year for international institutions, and USD 100.00 per year for Canadian and foreign students/residents. To receive student and resident rate, orders must be accompanied by name of affiliated institution, date of term, and the *signature* of program/residency coordinator on institution letterhead. Orders will be billed at individual rate until proof of status is received. Foreign air speed delivery is included in all *Clinics* subscription prices. All prices are subject to change without notice. **POSTMASTER:** Send address changes to *Heart Failure Clinics*, Elsevier Health Sciences Division, Subscription Customer Service, 3251 Riverport Lane, Maryland Heights, MO 63043. **Customer Service: 1-800-654-2452 (US and Canada). From outside of the US and Canada, call 314-447-8871. Fax: 314-447-8029. For print support, E-mail: JournalsCustomerService-usa@elsevier.com. For online support, E-mail: JournalsOnlineSupport-usa@elsevier.com.**

Reprints. For copies of 100 or more of articles in this publication, please contact the Commercial Reprints Department, Elsevier Inc., 360 Park Avenue South, New York, NY 10010-1710. Tel.: 212-633-3874; Fax: 212-633-3820; E-mail: reprints@elsevier.com.

Heart Failure Clinics is covered in *MEDLINE/PubMed (Index Medicus).*

Contributors

CONSULTING EDITOR

EDUARDO BOSSONE, MD, PhD, FCCP, FESC, FACC
Director, Division of Cardiology, AORN Antonio Cardarelli Hospital, Naples, Italy

EDITORS

GIUSEPPE PACILEO, MD
Heart Failure Unit, Department of Cardiology, AORN dei Colli, Monaldi Hospital, Naples, Italy

FRANCESCO GRIGIONI, MD, PhD
Department of Cardiology, Policlinico Universitario Campus Bio-Medico, Roma, Italy

DANIELE MASARONE, MD, PhD
Heart Failure Unit, Department of Cardiology, AORN dei Colli, Monaldi Hospital, Naples, Italy

LUCIANO POTENA, MD, PhD
Medical Director, Heart Failure and Heart Transplant Program, UO Cardiologia Dipartimento Cardio-Toraco-Vascolare IRCCS Policlinico di Sant'Orsola Padiglione, Bologna, Italy

AUTHORS

WILLIAM T. ABRAHAM, MD, FACP, FACC, FAHA, FESC, FRCP
Professor of Medicine, Physiology, and Cell Biology, College of Medicine, Distinguished Professor, Division of Cardiovascular Medicine, The Ohio State University, Columbus, Ohio, USA

MARIANNA ADAMO, MD
Cardiology Unit, Department of Medical and Surgical Specialties, Radiological Sciences, and Public Health, University of Brescia, Brescia, Italy

PIERGIUSEPPE AGOSTONI, MD, PhD
Centro Cardiologico Monzino, IRCCS, Department of Clinical Sciences and Community Health, University of Milan, Milan, Italy

ERNESTO AMMENDOLA, MD
Heart Failure Unit, AORN dei Colli, Monaldi Hospital, Naples, Italy

MATTIA ARRIGO, MD
Department of Internal Medicine, Triemli Hospital Zürich, Zürich, Switzerland

RAED ASER, MD
Department of Cardiac Surgery, University Hospital of Zürich, Zürich, Switzerland

EDUARDO BARGE-CABALLERO, MD, PhD
Heart Failure and Heart Transplant Unit, Cardiology Department, Complexo Hospitalario Universitario A Coruña (CHUAC), A Coruña, Spain; Instituto Investigación Biomedica A Coruña (INIBIC); Centro de Investigación Biomedica en Red Cardiovascular (CIBERCV)

ELENA BIAGINI, MD PhD
Cardiology Unit, St. Orsola Hospital, IRCCS
Azienda Ospedaliero-Universitaria di Bologna,
Bologna, Italy

JAN BIEGUS, MD, PhD
Department of Heart Diseases, Medical
University, Centre for Heart Diseases,
University Hospital, Wroclaw, Poland

ANDREA BONELLI, MD
Cardiology Unit, Department of Medical and
Surgical Specialties, Radiological Sciences,
and Public Health, University of Brescia,
Brescia, Italy

**NATALE DANIELE BRUNETTI, MD, PhD,
FESC**
Cardiology Unit, Department of Medical and
Surgical Sciences, University of Foggia,
Foggia, Italy

MARTINA CAIAZZA, MD
Inherited and Rare Cardiovascular Diseases
Unit, Department of Translational Medical
Sciences, University of Campania "Luigi
Vanvitelli," Monaldi Hospital, Naples, Italy

ANGELO CAIAZZO, MD
Heart Transplant Unit, Department of Cardiac
Surgery and Transplant, AORN dei Colli,
Monaldi Hospital, Naples, Italy

PAOLO CALABRÒ, MD, PhD
Inherited and Rare Cardiovascular Diseases
Unit, Department of Translational Medical
Sciences, University of Campania "Luigi
Vanvitelli," Monaldi Hospital, Naples, Italy

VALERIA CAMMALLERI, MD, PhD
Department of Cardiology, Policlinico
Universitario Campus Bio-Medico, Department
of Cardiology, Policlinico Universitario Tor
Vergata, Roma, Italy

ANGELO GIUSEPPE CAPONETTI, MD
Cardiology Unit, St. Orsola Hospital, IRCCS
Azienda Ospedaliero-Universitaria di Bologna,
Department of Experimental, Diagnostic and
Specialty Medicine (DIMES), University of
Bologna, Bologna, Italy

VALENTINA CARUBELLI, PhD
Cardiology Unit, Department of Medical and
Surgical Specialties, Radiological Sciences,

and Public Health, University of Brescia,
Brescia, Italy

ARTURO CESARO, MD
Inherited and Rare Cardiovascular Diseases
Unit, Department of Translational Medical
Sciences, University of Campania "Luigi
Vanvitelli," Monaldi Hospital, Naples, Italy

GIULIANA CIMINO, MD
Cardiology Unit, Department of Medical and
Surgical Specialties, Radiological Sciences,
and Public Health, University of Brescia,
Brescia, Italy

ANNAPAOLA CIRILLO, MD
Inherited and Rare Cardiovascular Diseases
Unit, Department of Translational Medical
Sciences, University of Campania "Luigi
Vanvitelli," Monaldi Hospital, Naples, Italy

VALENTINO COLLINI, MD
Cardiovascular Department, Azienda Sanitaria
Universitaria Integrata, Trieste, Italy

MARIA DELIA CORBO, MD
Cardiology Unit, Department of Medical and
Surgical Sciences, University of Foggia,
Foggia, Italy

MICHELE CORREALE, MD, PhD
Cardiology Unit, Department of Medical and
Surgical Sciences, University of Foggia,
Foggia, Italy

**MARIA GENEROSA CRESPO-LEIRO, MD,
PhD**
Heart Failure and Heart Transplant Unit,
Cardiology Department, Complexo
Hospitalario Universitario A Coruña (CHUAC),
A Coruña, Spain; Instituto Investigación
Biomedica A Coruña (INIBIC); Centro de
Investigación Biomedica en Red
Cardiovascular (CIBERCV); Universidade da
Coruña (UDC)

SIMONE PASQUALE CRISPINO, MD
Unit of Cardiovascular Science, Campus Bio-
Medico University of Rome, Rome, Italy

FRANCESCO DI FRAIA, MD
Inherited and Rare Cardiovascular Diseases
Unit, Department of Translational Medical
Sciences, University of Campania "Luigi
Vanvitelli," Monaldi Hospital, Naples, Italy

VITTORIA ERRIGO, MD
Heart Failure Unit, Department of Cardiology,
AORN dei Colli, Monaldi Hospital, Naples, Italy

AUGUSTO ESPOSITO, MD
Inherited and Rare Cardiovascular Diseases
Unit, Department of Translational Medical
Sciences, University of Campania "Luigi
Vanvitelli," Monaldi Hospital, Naples, Italy

ANDREAS J. FLAMMER, MD
Department of Cardiology, University Hospital
of Zürich, Zürich, Switzerland

MICHELLE FRANK, MD
Department of Cardiology, University Hospital
of Zürich, Zürich, Switzerland

MARIA FRIGERIO, MD
2nd Section of Cardiology, Heart Failure and
Transplant Unit, DeGasperis CardioCenter,
Niguarda Great Metropolitan Hospital, Milan,
Italy

ADELAIDE FUSCO, MD
Inherited and Rare Cardiovascular Diseases
Unit, Department of Translational Medical
Sciences, University of Campania "Luigi
Vanvitelli," Monaldi Hospital, Naples, Italy

CHRISTIAN GAGLIARDI, MD, PhD
Cardiology Unit, St. Orsola Hospital, IRCCS
Azienda Ospedaliero-Universitaria di Bologna,
Bologna, Italy

RITA GRAVINO, MD
Heart Failure Unit, Department of Cardiology,
AORN dei Colli, Monaldi Hospital, Naples, Italy

FRANCESCO GRIGIONI, MD, PhD
Department of Cardiology, Policlinico
Universitario Campus Bio-Medico, Roma, Italy

FEDERICA GUIDETTI, MD
Department of Cardiology, University Hospital
of Zürich, Zürich, Switzerland

MASSIMO IACOVIELLO, MD, PhD
Cardiology Unit, Department of Medical and
Surgical Sciences, University of Foggia,
Foggia, Italy

RICCARDO MARIA INCIARDI, MD
Cardiology Unit, Department of Medical and
Surgical Specialties, Radiological Sciences,

and Public Health, University of Brescia,
Brescia, Italy

KRYSTIAN JOSIAK, MD
Department of Heart Diseases, Medical
University, Centre for Heart Diseases,
University Hospital, Wroclaw, Poland

MICHELLE M. KITTLESON, MD, PhD
Department of Cardiology, Smidt Heart
Institute, Cedars-Sinai, Los Angeles, California,
USA

KATARZYNA KULEJ
Department of Heart Diseases, Medical
University, Centre for Heart Diseases,
University Hospital, Wroclaw, Poland

GIUSEPPE LIMONGELLI, MD, PhD, FESC
Inherited and Rare Cardiovascular Diseases
Unit, Department of Translational Medical
Sciences, University of Campania "Luigi
Vanvitelli," Monaldi Hospital, Naples, Italy;
Institute of Cardiovascular Sciences, University
College of London and St. Bartholomew's
Hospital, London, United Kingdom; Member of
the European Reference Network for Rare, Low
Prevalence and Complex Diseases of the
Heart-ERN GUARD-Heart, Italy

MICHELE LIONCINO, MD
Inherited and Rare Cardiovascular Diseases
Unit, Department of Translational Medical
Sciences, University of Campania "Luigi
Vanvitelli," Monaldi Hospital, Naples, Italy

CARLO MARIO LOMBARDI, MD
Professor, Cardiology Unit, Department of
Medical and Surgical Specialties, Radiological
Sciences, and Public Health, University of
Brescia, Brescia, Italy

SIMONE LONGHI, MD, PhD
Cardiology Unit, St. Orsola Hospital, IRCCS
Azienda Ospedaliero-Universitaria di Bologna,
Bologna, Italy

MARIA LUIGIA MARTUCCI, MD
Heart Failure Unit, Department of Cardiology,
AORN dei Colli, Monaldi Hospital, Naples, Italy

DANIELE MASARONE, MD, PhD
Heart Failure Unit, Department of Cardiology,
AORN dei Colli, Monaldi Hospital, Naples, Italy

ALFREDO MAURIELLO, MD
Inherited and Rare Cardiovascular Diseases
Unit, Department of Translational Medical
Sciences, University of Campania "Luigi
Vanvitelli," Monaldi Hospital, Naples, Italy

SIMONA MEGA, MD
Department of Cardiology, Policlinico
Universitario Campus Bio-Medico, Roma, Italy

ENRICO MELILLO, MD
Heart Failure Unit, Department of Cardiology,
AORN dei Colli, Monaldi Hospital, Naples, Italy

MARCO METRA, MD
Professor, Cardiology Unit, Department of
Medical and Surgical Specialties, Radiological
Sciences, and Public Health, University of
Brescia, Brescia, Italy

FRAN MIKULICIC, MD
Department of Cardiology, University Hospital
of Zürich, Zürich, Switzerland

EMANUELE MONDA, MD
Inherited and Rare Cardiovascular Diseases
Unit, Department of Translational Medical
Sciences, University of Campania "Luigi
Vanvitelli," Monaldi Hospital, Naples, Italy

PIOTR NIEWINSKI, MD
Department of Heart Diseases, Medical
University, Centre for Heart Diseases,
University Hospital, Wroclaw, Poland

KRZYSZTOF NOWAK, MD
Department of Heart Diseases, Medical
University, Centre for Heart Diseases,
University Hospital, Wroclaw, Poland

JAE K. OH, MD
Department of Cardiovascular Medicine, Mayo
Clinic, Rochester, Minnesota, USA

GERHARD PÖLZL, MD
Department of Internal Medicine III, Cardiology
and Angiology, Medical University of
Innsbruck, Innsbruck, Austria

GIUSEPPE PACILEO, MD
Heart Failure Unit, Department of Cardiology,
AORN dei Colli, Monaldi Hospital, Naples, Italy

ROBERTA PACILEO, MD
Inherited and Rare Cardiovascular Diseases
Unit, Department of Translational Medical
Sciences, University of Campania "Luigi
Vanvitelli," Heart Failure Unit, AORN dei Colli,
Monaldi Hospital, Naples, Italy

MATTEO PAGNESI, MD
Cardiology Unit, Department of Medical and
Surgical Specialties, Radiological Sciences,
and Public Health, University of Brescia,
Brescia, Italy

PIERPAOLO PELLICORI, PhD
Robertson Institute of Biostatistics and Clinical
Trials Unit, University of Glasgow, Glasgow,
United Kingdom

ANDREA PETRAIO, MD
Heart Transplant Unit, Department of Cardiac
Surgery and Transplant, AORN dei Colli,
Monaldi Hospital, Naples, Italy

BARBARA PONIKOWSKA
Student Scientific Organization, Department of
Heart Diseases, Wroclaw Medical University,
Wroclaw, Poland

PIOTR PONIKOWSKI, MD, PhD, FESC
Department of Heart Diseases, Medical
University, Centre for Heart Diseases,
University Hospital, Wroclaw, Poland

LUCIANO POTENA, MD, PhD
Medical Director, Heart Failure and Heart
Transplant Program, UO Cardiologia
Dipartimento Cardio-Toraco-Vascolare IRCCS
Policlinico di Sant'Orsola Padiglione, Bologna,
Italy

PAOLA PRESTINENZI, MD
Heart Failure and Transplant Program, IRCCS
Policlinico di Sant'Orsola, Bologna, Italy

ALICE RAVERA, MD
Cardiology Unit, Department of Medical and
Surgical Specialties, Radiological Sciences,
and Public Health, University of Brescia,
Brescia, Italy

MARTA RUBINO, MD
Inherited and Rare Cardiovascular Diseases
Unit, Department of Translational Medical

Sciences, University of Campania "Luigi Vanvitelli," Monaldi Hospital, Naples, Italy

FRANK RUSCHITZKA, MD
Department of Cardiology, University Hospital of Zürich, Zürich, Switzerland

MARIA GIOVANNA RUSSO, MD, PhD
Inherited and Rare Cardiovascular Diseases Unit, Department of Translational Medical Sciences, University of Campania "Luigi Vanvitelli," Monaldi Hospital, Naples, Italy

GIULIA SATURI, MD
Cardiology Unit, St. Orsola Hospital, IRCCS Azienda Ospedaliero-Universitaria di Bologna, Department of Experimental, Diagnostic and Specialty Medicine (DIMES), University of Bologna, Bologna, Italy

ANDREA SEGRETI, MD
Unit of Cardiovascular Science, Campus Bio-Medico University of Rome, Rome, Italy

GIANFRANCO SINAGRA, MD
Cardiovascular Department, Azienda Sanitaria Universitaria Integrata, Trieste, Italy

MATEUSZ SOKOLSKI, MD
Department of Heart Diseases, Wroclaw Medical University, Wroclaw, Poland

DAVIDE STOLFO, MD
Cardiovascular Department, Azienda Sanitaria Universitaria Integrata, Trieste, Italy

VIVIANA TESSITORE, MD
Inherited and Rare Cardiovascular Diseases Unit, Department of Translational Medical Sciences, University of Campania "Luigi Vanvitelli," Monaldi Hospital, Naples, Italy

DANIELA TOMASONI, MD
Cardiology Unit, Department of Medical and Surgical Specialties, Radiological Sciences,

and Public Health, University of Brescia, Brescia, Italy

GIAN PAOLO USSIA, MD
Department of Cardiology, Policlinico Universitario Campus Bio-Medico, Roma, Italy

FABIO VALENTE, MD
Heart Failure Unit, AORN dei Colli, Monaldi Hospital, Naples, Italy

ROSSELLA VASTARELLA, MD
Heart Failure Unit, AORN dei Colli, Monaldi Hospital, Naples, Italy

GIUSEPPE VEROLINO, MD
Unit of Cardiovascular Science, Campus Bio-Medico University of Rome, Rome, Italy

MARINA VERRENGIA, MD
Heart Failure Unit, AORN dei Colli, Monaldi Hospital, Naples, Italy

FEDERICA VERRILLO, MD
Inherited and Rare Cardiovascular Diseases Unit, Department of Translational Medical Sciences, University of Campania "Luigi Vanvitelli," Monaldi Hospital, Naples, Italy

ENRICA VITALE, MD
Cardiology Unit, Department of Medical and Surgical Sciences, University of Foggia, Foggia, Italy

MARKUS J. WILHELM, MD
Department of Cardiac Surgery, University Hospital of Zürich, Zürich, Switzerland

STEPHAN WINNIK, MD, PhD
Department of Cardiology, University Hospital of Zürich, Zürich, Switzerland

ROBERT ZYMLINSKI, MD, PhD
Department of Heart Diseases, Medical University, Centre for Heart Diseases, University Hospital, Wroclaw, Poland

Contents

Understanding of heart failure (HF) has evolved from a simple hemodynamic problem through a neurohormonally and proinflammatory-driven syndrome to a complex multiorgan dysfunction accompanied by inadequate energy handling. This article discusses the most important clinical aspects of advanced HF pathophysiology. It presents the concept of neurohormonal activation and its deleterious effect on cardiovascular system and reflex control. The current theories regarding the role of inflammation, cytokine activation, and myocardial remodeling in HF progression are presented. Advanced HF is a multiorgan syndrome with interplay between cardiovascular system and other organs. The role of iron deficiency is also discussed.

Advanced heart failure (HF) is characterized by a progressive worsening of symptoms disabling for daily life, refractory to all therapies, and with high mortality. These patients may be candidates for life-prolonging therapies, such as heart transplantation (HT) or long-term (LT) mechanical circulatory support (MCS) or must just require palliative therapies. The 1-year survival after HT and/or LT-MCS is approaching 80% to 90%, being patient selection and timely referral to advanced HF centers critical for optimal outcomes. There is no single symptom, sign, or test that can identify these patients and different classifications are complementary and helpful for clinical decision-making.

Advanced heart failure, an end-stage disease characterized by high mortality and morbidity despite standard medical therapy, requires various therapeutic strategies like heart transplant and long-term mechanical circulatory support. Echocardiography is the main imaging technique to identify transitions to advanced stages of disease and guide risk stratification and therapeutic decision-making processes. Progressive development of advanced echocardiographic techniques allows more comprehensive assessment of the hemodynamic and structural profiles of patients with advanced heart failure, and its use in clinical practice continues to expand. This article provides an overview of basic and emerging echocardiographic tools to assess patients with advanced heart failure.

Therapy based on disease-modifier drugs is among the required criteria to diagnose advanced heart failure (AdvHF). Nevertheless, several conditions, such as hospitalization, hypotension, renal dysfunction, electrolyte abnormalities, medical inertia, and patients' adherence, can make the maintenance of optimal medical therapy in patients with AdvHF challenging. Moreover, in recent years, new classes of drugs able have been shown to be able to further modify the natural history of heart failure with reduced ejection fraction, but they are still not widely adopted. This article discusses the optimal use of disease-modifier drugs in patients with AdvHF as well as the possible usefulness of the new therapeutic opportunities.

Heart failure (HF) is characterized by frequent hospital admissions due to acute decompensation and shortened life span with a progressive clinical course leading to an advanced stage where traditional therapies become ineffective. Due to aging of the population and improved therapies, only a small of proportion of patients with advanced HF are candidates for surgical treatments, such as mechanical circulatory support or heart transplantation. In most cases, prompt identification and management of congestion is paramount to improving symptoms and quality of life and avoiding progression to severe multiorgan dysfunction and death.

Patients with advanced heart failure suffer from severe and persistent symptoms, often not responding disease-modifying drugs, a marked limitation of functional capacity and poor quality of life that can ameliorate with inotropic drugs therapy. In small studies, pulsed infusions of classical inotropes (ie, dobutamine and milrinone) are associated with improvement in hemodynamic parameters and quality of life in patients with advanced heart failure. However, because of the adverse effects of these drugs, serious safety issues have been raised. Levosimendan is a calcium-sensitizing inodilators with a triple mechanism of action, whose infusion results in hemodynamic, neurohormonal, and inflammatory cytokine improvements in patients with chronic advanced HF. In addition, levosimendan has important pleiotropic effects, including protection of myocardial, renal, and liver cells from ischemia–reperfusion injury, and anti-inflammatory and antioxidant effects; these properties possibly make levosimendan an "organ protective" inodilator. In clinical trials and real-world evidence, infusion of levosimendan at fixed intervals is safe and effective in patients with advanced HF, alleviating clinical symptoms, reducing hospitalizations, and improving the quality of life. Therefore, the use of repeated doses of levosimendan could represent the therapy of choice as a bridge to transplant/left ventricular assist device implantation or as palliative therapy in patients with advanced heart failure.

Cardiac resynchronization therapy is a well-established treatment of heart failure with reduced left ventricular ejection fraction and a wide QRS complex. Cardiac contractility modulation therapy is an emerging electrical treatment indicated for use in patients with symptomatic heart failure caused by moderate-to-severe systolic left ventricular dysfunction (left ventricular ejection fraction ranging from 25% to 45%), with no indication for cardiac resynchronization therapy. Cardiac contractility modulation therapy improves functional status, exercise capacity, quality of life, and possibly prevents hospital admissions in indicated patients. An algorithm for patient selection for these two forms of electrical therapy for heart failure is presented.

In heart failure with reduced ejection fraction, the interventional landscape has recently expanded. New transcatheter approaches are emerging for both mitral and tricuspid secondary (functional) regurgitation. Transcatheter therapies for mitral and tricuspid valve require a more tailored approach than for the aortic valve, because of more heterogeneous clinical scenarios, anatomic features, and mechanisms of valvular lesions.

Left ventricular assist devices (LVADs) are indicated in inotrope-dependent heart failure (HF) patients with pure or predominant LV dysfunction. Survival benefit is less clear in ambulatory, advanced HF. Timing is crucial: early, unnecessary exposure to the risks of surgery, and device-related complications (infections, stroke, and bleeding) should be weighed against the probability of dying or developing irreversible right ventricular and/or end-organ dysfunction while deferring implant. The interplay between LVAD and heart transplantation depends largely on donor availability and allocation rules. Postoperatively, quality of life depends on patients' expectations and is influenced by complications. Patients' preferences, prognosis, and alternative options—including palliation—should be openly discussed and reviewed before and after the operation.

Patients with advanced heart failure (AdHF) have a reduced quality of life and poor prognosis. A heart transplant (HT) is an effective treatment for such patients. Still, because of a shortage of donor organs, the final decision to place a patient without contraindications on the HT waiting list is based on detailed risk-benefit analysis. Cardiopulmonary exercise tests (CPETs) play a pivotal role in guiding selection in patients with AdHF considered for an HT. Furthermore, several validated multivariable predicting scores obtained through various techniques, including the CPETs, are available and part of the decision-making process for HT listing.

challenge in the absence of a unique diagnostic algorithm universally recognized. Clinical trials conducted so far did not show a significant improvement of prognosis, but forthcoming therapies could provide innovative solutions.

Heart transplantation (HTx) is the treatment of choice in patients with late-stage advanced heart failure (Advanced HF). Survival rates 1, 5, and 10 years after transplantation are 87%, 77%, and 57%, respectively, and the average life expectancy is 9.16 years. However, because of the donor organ shortage, waiting times often exceed life expectancy, resulting in a waiting list mortality of around 20%. This review aims to provide an overview of current standard, recent advances, and future developments in the treatment of Advanced HF with a focus on long-term mechanical circulatory support and HTx.

HEART FAILURE CLINICS

Preface

Management of Advanced Heart Failure: The Science of Uncertainty and the Art of Probability

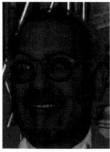

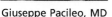

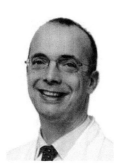

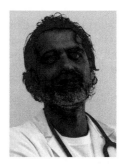

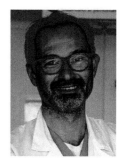

Giuseppe Pacileo, MD   Francesco Grigioni, MD, PhD   Daniele Masarone, MD, PhD   Luciano Potena, MD, PhD

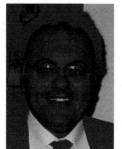

Eduardo Bossone, MD, PhD, FCCP, FESC, FACC,
Editors

Management of patients with advanced heart failure is one of the most challenging clinical scenarios for the clinical cardiologist.[1,2] To support clinicians in facing this challenge, we produced the current issue of *Heart Failure Clinics*.

We developed this project framework aiming to guide the reader along a multistep pathway that takes into consideration the multiple facets of diagnostic and therapeutic strategies of this complex scenario.

This journey could not begin without appropriate knowledge of the pathophysiology underlying the different clinical conditions.

Next, we move to the correct definition and epidemiological impact of advanced heart failure and the fundamental role of echocardiography,

the key diagnostic procedure that noninvasively plays a crucial role in this clinical setting.

We then discuss the optimal use of several drugs, such as "disease-modifying," diuretics, and inotropes, as well as the correct indication of new invasive procedures like cardiac contractility modulation and the percutaneous repair of the atrioventricular valves.

In keeping with the progression of this path of assistance, we provide criteria necessary to guarantee correct timing of left ventricular assist device implantation and heart transplant, as well as the role of right-sided cardiac catheterization.

To ensure a comprehensive overview, we also included some articles to help the reader manage advanced heart failure in specific subsets of patients, such as those with no dilated

Heart Failure Clin 17 (2021) xv–xvi
https://doi.org/10.1016/j.hfc.2021.06.003
1551-7136/21/© 2021 Published by Elsevier Inc.

cardiomyopathies, pediatric age, or heart failure with preserved ejection fraction.

The issue ends with an article illustrating new treatment perspectives, delineating a futuristic but feasible scenario.

Initially, we feared that the project was too demanding. However, there is no question that the collaboration of Italian and foreign opinion leaders in this field has been a great help and allowed us to accomplish our project with great enthusiasm.

Finally, we dedicate this issue to everyone close to us in our lives and those who collaborated with us in our daily work, without whom this project would have been impossible.

Giuseppe Pacileo, MD
Heart Failure Unit
Department of Cardiology
AORN dei Colli-Monaldi Hospital
Via Leonardo Bianchi 1
Naples, 80131 Italy

Francesco Grigioni, MD, PhD
University Campus Bio-Medico of Rome
Via Alvaro del Portillo 200
Rome, 00128 Italy

Daniele Masarone, MD, PhD
Heart Failure Unit
Department of Cardiology
AORN dei Colli-Monaldi Hospital
Via Leonardo Bianchi 1
Naples, 80131 Italy

Luciano Potena, MD, PhD
UO Cardiologia
Dipartimento Cardio-Toraco-Vascolare
IRCCS Policlinico di Sant'Orsola Padiglione
25 Via Massarenti 9
Bologna, 40138 Italy

Eduardo Bossone, MD, PhD, FCCP, FESC, FACC
Division of Cardiology
Cardarelli Hospital
Via A. Cardarelli, 9
80131 Naples, Italy

E-mail addresses:
gapacileo58@gmail.com (G. Pacileo)
f.griginoni@unicampus.it (F. Grigioni)
daniele.masarone@ospedalideicolli.it
(D. Masarone)
luciano.potena2@unibo.it (L. Potena)
ebossone@hotmail.com (E. Bossone)

REFERENCES

1. Crespo-Leiro MG, Metra M, Lund LH, et al. Advanced heart failure: a position statement of the Heart Failure Association of the European Society of Cardiology. Eur J Heart Fail 2018;20:1505–35.
2. Fang JC, Ewald GA, Allen LA, et al. Advanced (stage D) heart failure: a statement from the Heart Failure Society of America Guidelines Committee. J Card Fail 2015;21:519–34.

Pathophysiology of Advanced Heart Failure
What Knowledge Is Needed for Clinical Management?

Jan Biegus, MD, PhD[a,b], Piotr Niewinski, MD[a,b], Krystian Josiak, MD[a,b], Katarzyna Kulej[a,b], Barbara Ponikowska[c], Krzysztof Nowak, MD[a,b], Robert Zymlinski, MD, PhD[a,b], Piotr Ponikowski, MD, PhD, FESC[a,b],*

KEYWORDS

- Neurohormonal activation • Sympathetic drive • Cardiorespiratory reflex disbalance • Congestion
- Multiorgan dysfunction • Iron deficiency

KEY POINTS

- The pathophysiology of advanced heart failure (HF) can be characterized as a complex interplay of dysregulated mechanisms comprising impaired hemodynamics, neurohormonal and proinflammatory activation, dysfunctional cardiorespiratory reflex control, and inadequate energy handling, all of which ultimately lead to multiorgan dysfunction; at the later stage of HF, numerous comorbidities, whose underlying pathophysiologies often amplify HF progression, tend to dominate the clinical picture and therapeutic approach, and some of these mechanisms have been identified as therapeutic targets in HF.
- Blockade of the renin-angiotensin-aldosterone system (preferably with an angiotensin receptor-neprilysin inhibitor, but alternatively with angiotensin-converting enzyme inhibitors or angiotensin receptor blockers together with mineralocorticoid receptor antagonist) and sympathetic nervous system (with β-blockers) is now considered a fundamental element of pharmacologic therapy for all patients with advanced HF and reduced ejection fraction.
- Autonomic modulation (vagal nerve stimulation or baroreflex stimulation) in advanced HF tends to benefit functional variables (quality of life, New York Heart Association class, 6-minute walking distance), whereas improvement in the outcomes (total mortality, HF hospitalizations) still remains uncertain.
- Fluid overload with central and/or peripheral congestion characterize the clinical picture of advanced HF and is the main reason for hospital admission in these patients; distinction of different clinical patterns of congestion with different underlying mechanisms may improve the management of fluid overload in advanced HF.
- Recent clinical trials have shown that the following novel therapies targeting impaired pathophysiologic pathways in advanced HF seem to improve patients' outcomes: (1) vericiguat, a soluble guanylate cyclase stimulator; (2) omecamtiv mecarbil, a selective cardiac myosin activator; (3) sodium-glucose cotransporter 2 inhibitors; (4) ferric carboxymaltose, for patients with concomitant iron deficiency.
- Better understanding of the pathophysiology underlying HF progression may allow characterization of novel mechanisms that can be targeted in order to revert to a natural pathway of HF development and progression.

[a] Department of Heart Diseases, Wrocław Medical University, ul. Borowska 213, 50-556 Wrocław, Poland;
[b] Centre for Heart Diseases, Wrocław University Hospital, ul. Borowska 213, 50-556 Wrocław, Poland;
[c] Student Scientific Organization, Department of Heart Diseases, Wrocław Medical University, ul. Borowska 213, 50-556 Wrocław, Poland
* Corresponding author. Department of Heart Diseases, Wrocław Medical University, ul. Borowska 213, 50-556 Wrocław, Poland.
E-mail address: piotr.ponikowski@umed.wroc.pl

Heart Failure Clin 17 (2021) 519–531
https://doi.org/10.1016/j.hfc.2021.06.001
1551-7136/21/© 2021 The Authors. Published by Elsevier Inc.

The prognosis of patients with chronic heart failure (HF) has considerably improved, mainly because of implementation of evidence-based therapies. Because patients with HF live longer, many of them reach the late stage of the natural history of the disease, often referred to as advanced HF. Recent position paper from the Heart Failure Association of the European Society of Cardiology proposes a definition and classification of advanced HF and describes new diagnostic and treatment options for these patients.[1] Of note, the traditional approach to HF progression considers a unidirectional pathway in which the management can only stabilize patients at a certain stage of the disease (even for long time) with much less recognition that a reversal pathway is also possible, even at more advanced stages of the disease. However, it is now recognized that with comprehensive management comprising guideline-recommended HF therapies and treatment of comorbidities, some patients with HF may present improvement in symptoms, functional capacity and left ventricular function, and cardiac structure.[2,3] Better understanding of the pathophysiology underlying HF progression may allow clinicians to characterize mechanisms that can be targeted in order to potentially revert to a natural pathway of HF natural history. This article briefly summarizes the pathophysiologic mechanisms that are of particular importance at the later, advanced stage of HF and discusses them in the perspective of clinical management.

There is no evidence to support the assumption that pathophysiologic mechanisms operating at the advanced stage of HF substantially differ from those involved at the earlier stages of the disease. The difference seems to be mainly quantitative in the involvement of some pathologic pathways and systems rather than qualitative. Understanding of HF pathophysiology has evolved within recent decades, from a simple hemodynamic problem through neurohormonally and proinflammatory-driven syndrome, to a complex multiorgan dysfunction accompanied by inadequate energy handling. An additional important element to consider is the presence of numerous comorbidities, with underlying pathophysiologies often interfering and at the later stage of HF tending to dominate the clinical picture and therapeutic approach (**Box 1**).

NEUROHORMONAL AND PROINFLAMMATORY ACTIVATION IN ADVANCED HEART FAILURE

HF at the advanced stage is characterized by generalized activation of the neurohormonal and

---

> **Box 1**
> **The key mechanisms involved in pathophysiology and progression of advanced heart failure**
>
> Impaired central and peripheral hemodynamics:
> - Decreased cardiac output
> - Increased cardiac filing pressures (central venous pressure/pulmonary capillary wedge pressure)
> - Impaired peripheral perfusion (leading to organ dysfunction)
>
> Activation of the neurohormonal systems:
> - Renin-angiotensin-aldosterone system activation
> - Endothelin activation
> - Nonosmotic vasopressin release
> - Natriuretic peptide activation
> - Sympathetic nervous system activation
>
> Impaired cardiorespiratory reflex control:
> - Downregulated response from baroreceptors
> - Decreased vagal tone
> - Overactive peripheral chemoreceptors
> - Overactive muscle ergoreceptors
>
> Immune and proinflammatory pathways activation
>
> Activation of oxidative stress pathways
>
> Impaired intracellular calcium handling
>
> Inadequate energy handling
>
> Pathophysiologies of coexisting comorbid conditions (**Box 2**)

---

inflammatory systems with accompanied dysregulation of immune response and oxidative stress.[4–10] The degree of these abnormalities increases with disease severity and predicts poor outcomes.[6,7] Although they constitute separate pathophysiologic pathways, during HF development they often coexist and perpetuate detrimental effects on the cardiovascular system (and other systems), leading to the progression of the disease. Importantly, because of generalized character, activation of these systems can be seen at the molecular, cellular, and organ levels and is also detected in the peripheral circulation (as shown by increased levels of specific biomarkers).[4,6,7,10]

Activation of these mechanisms at the early stage of HF seems to be primarily adaptive, in response to cardiac injury/dysfunction, in order to maintain an increased effort of the cardiovascular system. However, it takes a short period of time once they become maladaptive, with resultant detrimental biological effects (**Fig. 1**).

Neurohormonal activation is thought to be core of pathophysiology underlying HF and comprises numerous systems and related signaling pathways, including[4–10] the renin-angiotensin-aldosterone system (RAAS), sympathetic nervous system (with concomitant depleted activity of parasympathetic nervous system and impaired cardiopulmonary reflex control), endothelin-1 (ET-1), arginine vasopressin, and natriuretic peptides. It exerts unfavorable biological effects with further deterioration in the heart function and affects the other organs, eventually leading to a vicious circle of HF progression. The following abnormalities caused by permanent neurohormonal activation have been described: intracellular cytosolic calcium overload with impaired calcium handling, hypertrophy, apoptosis, necrosis of cardiomyocytes, myocardial fibrosis, endothelial dysfunction, oxidative stress, and sodium and water retention, with clinical consequences such as cardiac remodeling, vascular dysfunction, vasoconstriction, tachycardia, arrhythmias, prothrombotic state, volume overload.[4–10]

Identification of activated neurohormonal pathways as targets for therapy at each stage of HF natural history entirely changed patients outcomes. There is overwhelming evidence that RAAS blockade with angiotensin-converting enzyme inhibitors (ACEi) (or angiotensin receptor blockers for those who are not able to tolerate ACEi) and mineralocorticoid receptor antagonists together with a β-blocker should be always considered as a fundamental element of pharmacologic therapy for all patients with advanced HF

and reduced ejection fraction.[11] Recent introduction of a new class of drugs, angiotensin receptor-neprilysin inhibitors (ARNIs), further confirmed the view of the need for comprehensive interference with neuroendocrine activation in HF. The substrates for neprilysin include natriuretic peptides, adrenomedullin, substance P, apelin, and other vasoactive peptides.[12] PARADIGM-HF was the paramount trial that established that the combination of a neprilysin inhibitor (sacubitril) with an angiotensin receptor blocker (valsartan) was superior to an ACEi (enalapril) in reducing mortality and morbidity and also improving quality of life in patients with HF and reduced ejection fraction.[13] The results of this and subsequent studies with sacubitril-valsartan have elucidated numerous potential mechanisms of benefit and established the role of this drug as a replacement for ACEi across the whole spectrum of HF severity.[12]

Endothelial dysfunction is another dysfunctional pathway often seen in advanced HF with multiple biological consequences and impacts on the outcomes.[14] Vasoconstriction is often seen as its hallmark, being mediated by several mechanisms: activation of RAAS and sympathetic nervous systems and upregulated ET-1 secretion, which is produced and secreted by endothelial cells with pronounced vasoconstrictor effect. The endothelin system is involved in the pathophysiology of HF, and increased blood levels of ET-1 were linked to the severity of the disease and the outcomes.[14] Importantly, ET-1 also regulates renal function, and its role goes beyond controlling afferent and efferent glomerular artery tone. It directly affects the renal tubular cells, thus affecting urine production, including regulation of ion/water homeostasis.[15] Taking all these elements into account,

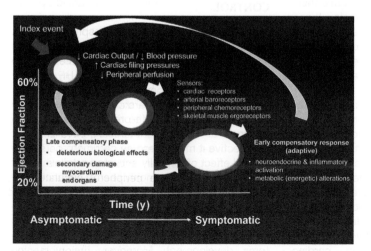

Fig. 1. Pathophysiologic mechanisms underlying progression of HF.

there were several attempts to use endothelin-receptor antagonists in the therapy for HF, but with disappointing results in clinical trials.[16,17]

Endothelial dysfunction together with proinflammatory activation and oxidative stress (described later) significantly reduce nitric oxide (NO) bioavailability in HF. NO is essential for numerous biological processes in the vascular cells and in the myocardium, because it stimulates soluble guanylate cyclase (sGC) to generate intracellular cyclic guanosine monophosphate (cGMP), which plays a fundamental role in cardiovascular function.[18,19] Disruption of the NO-sGC-cGMP signaling pathway in HF is suggested as the key pathophysiologic mechanism responsible for disease progression,[18,19] which cannot be entirely corrected by neurohormonal blockade. There were several attempts to target this mechanism with an addition of nitrates or inhibition of phosphodiesterase type-5 to slow the degradation of cGMP in patients with HF, but with disappointing results.[20] Only recently, a new class of drugs, oral sGC stimulators, has been developed that seem to act on the NO-sensitive form of sGC, stimulate the enzyme directly by mimicking NO in the absence of endogenous NO, and sensitize sGC to low levels of endogenous NO.[18,19] Riociguat was first drug in its class tested in patients with HF and showed favorable hemodynamic effects (improved cardiac index and pulmonary vascular resistance) with concomitant improvement in quality of life.[21] Vericiguat is another sGC stimulator optimized for once-daily dosage and has recently been investigated in HF studies.[18,19] VICTORIA was a randomized, double-blind, placebo-controlled trial that investigated whether vericiguat added to standard optimal guideline-based therapy would favorably affect the outcomes of patients with HF with reduced ejection fraction who had recently been hospitalized or received intravenous diuretic therapy.[22] Among these high-risk patients, those who received vericiguat showed lower incidence of death from cardiovascular causes or HF hospitalization.[22] Further studies are needed to establish the place of vericiguat in the algorithm of treatment of advanced HF.

Immune activation with proinflammatory cytokines overexpressed in the failing myocardium and present in the peripheral circulation with concurrent downregulation of antiinflammatory pathways are all considered as hallmarks of HF.[4,5,10] The levels of proinflammatory cytokines/activation correlate with the HF severity and have prognostic significance.[4,5,10] It is well established that proinflammatory cytokines unfavorably affect left ventricular function, exerting negative inotropic effects; inducing abnormalities in cardiac metabolism and energetics; possibly resulting in cardiomyocyte hypertrophy, necrosis and apoptosis, and changes in the extracellular myocardial matrix; and promoting myocardial remodeling.[4,5,10] Activation of the immune response promotes the development of endothelial dysfunction but also profound changes in the skeletal muscle with body wasting and anorexia.[4,5,10] Patients with advanced HF and particularly increased levels of circulating cytokines tend to develop cardiac cachexia, which is associated with an ominous prognosis.[23] Of note, an interaction between the neurohormonal systems and inflammatory mediators has been reported: angiotensin II stimulates the production of tumor necrosis factor alpha, aldosterone induces nuclear factor κB inflammatory signaling pathways, chronic β-adrenergic receptor stimulation results in an overexpression of proinflammatory cytokines (interleukins 1 and 6) in ventricular cardiomyocytes, and some β-blockers seem to show antiinflammatory properties in experimental models of HF.[4,10]

However, there is no clear evidence of the efficacy of specific antiinflammatory interventions in HF. Randomized clinical trials testing anti–tumor necrosis factor therapies in patients with HF (RENAISSANCE, RECOVER, ATTACH) have all shown a lack of clinical benefit.[24] The reasons for these unexpected results remain unclear, but entry criteria applied in these studies, which did not include documented overexpression of inflammatory processes, may be relevant, and a very selective approach targeting only 1 cytokine seems to be insufficient to counterbalance the detrimental and complex inflammatory pathways responsible for the progression of the disease.

IMPAIRED CARDIORESPIRATORY REFLEX CONTROL

In physiology, several cardiorespiratory reflex arches act as the guardians of adequate ventilation and hemodynamic reactivity in response to varying environmental conditions (eg, hypoxia) or intrinsic changes (eg, buildup of lactic acid in the working muscles). In the short term, this can be seen as an important life-preserving mechanism observed across different species, but in a longer perspective it might become detrimental. The untoward effect of tonically activated cardiovascular reflexes, which is commonly seen in advanced HF, is thought to be mediated mostly by the increased efferent traffic within the sympathetic nervous system.[7] Note that these reflex abnormalities contribute both to disease progression and symptoms development. Moreover, the worsening hemodynamic state further perpetuates inadequate reflex response, resulting in a vicious circle of maladaptation. The focus here is on the 3 elements of impaired reflex milieu characterizing advanced HF (blunted baroreflex response, augmented peripheral chemosensitivity, and overactive muscle ergoreceptors) because they may have potential impact on future therapies.

Low sensitivity of carotid baroreceptors can be observed in approximately 30% to 40% of patients with moderate HF, with increasing prevalence in those with advanced HF.[25] Clearly, the magnitude of baroreflex-mediated changes in blood pressure and heart rate is inversely related to the advancement of HF, with lower values seen in patients characterized by higher New York Heart Association (NYHA) class and poorer ejection fraction, peak O_2 consumption, and VE/Vco_2 slope.[25] It is thought that the unfavorable effect of low baroreflex sensitivity on the prognosis in HF is related to the autonomic imbalance with vagal withdrawal and concomitant adrenergic dominance.[26] However, recently the prognostic role (defined as influence on total mortality and appropriate implantable cardioverter-defibrillator discharges) of diminished baroreceptor sensitivity has been questioned,[25,26] most likely related to the improvements in contemporary HF therapy.

The BeAT-HF trial,[27] in which an electrical stimulation of the afferent arm of baroreflex arch was used, provided an important insight into optimization of patient selection for the modulation of the autonomic system. Based on the initial results, individuals with HF with grossly increased N-terminal pro–brain natriuretic peptide (NT-proBNP) levels might not benefit from this form of treatment. It could be speculated that in advanced HF: (1) a degree of sympathetic activation might be necessary for the maintenance of cardiac output, and (2) there is a significant irreversibility of structural and functional changes that cannot be tackled solely by manipulating the autonomic nervous system. Nonetheless, the BeAT-HF trial was underpowered for hard clinical end points, whereas such analysis was possible in the INOVATE-HF trial,[28] designed to assess the effects of direct vagus nerve stimulation. Although the quality of life, NYHA class, and 6-minute walking distance were favorably affected by the activation of the parasympathetic system, it did not reduce the rate of death and HF events.

Peripheral chemoreceptors (PChRs) are strategically located within the carotid and aortic bodies in the area of the common carotid artery bifurcation and along the aortic arch. Their stimulation by low oxygen level and/or high concentration of CO_2 leads to augmented ventilation and sympathetic surge, resulting in increases in heart rate and systemic blood pressure. High sensitivity of PChR has been described in HF and is not only related to certain clinical characteristics (low exercise tolerance, poor left ventricular ejection fraction [LVEF], high level of natriuretic peptides)[29] but is also a well-established marker of ominous long-term prognosis.[30] An augmented activity of PChR is known to contribute to exercise intolerance in the HF population. An increased ventilatory response to hypoxia/hypercapnia exacerbates the dyspnea sensation, which may directly limit exercise duration.[31] It can be hypothesized that overactive PChRs are involved in the development of poor functional capacity through 2 mechanisms: (1) by inadequately increased ventilation, as shown by reduction in VE/Vco_2 slope following hyperoxic blockade of PChR[32]; and (2) by sympathetically mediated restraint in the blood flow to working muscles.

Of note, in an animal experiment performed in HF rats carotid body denervation restored autonomic balance, prevented left ventricular remodeling, reduced propensity for arrhythmia, and improved survival.[33] In a first-in-human clinical trial performed in a small preselected group of patients with moderate-advanced congestive HF (CHF) and enhanced sensitivity of PChR, surgical carotid body resection resulted in a significant decrease in sympathetic afferent tone measured with microneurography.[34] Moreover, an improvement in the exercise tolerance (decrease in VE/Vco_2 slope) was found in all patients with CHF following bilateral resection. Nonetheless, this finding was not accompanied by improvements in LVEF and NT-proBNP. The main drawback of the interventions targeting PChR is related to the concomitant decrease (or loss in the case of bilateral denervation) in acute hypoxic sensing. This condition may lead to (1) lower minimal blood oxygen saturation (Spo_2) during mild and moderate hypoxia, and (2) markedly greater daytime short-term Spo_2 variability compared with patients with HF with intact PChR.[35]

An augmented peripheral and central chemosensitivity along with prolonged circulatory delay are the main factors determining development of periodic breathing in patients with advanced HF (including its most severe form, the Cheyne-Stokes respiration).[36] Although the prognostic role of periodic breathing in HF remains uncertain, its resolution with the novel device-based therapy using phrenic nerve stimulation was shown to improve quality of life over 12 months of follow-up.[37] Interestingly, according to recent research (BREATH study), central sleep apnea in HF may be effectively alleviated using buspirone, a $5HT_{1A}$

receptor agonist that decreases chemosensitivity to CO_2.[38]

Similarly to baroreceptors and chemoreceptors, the magnitude of ergoreflex sensitization is related to the advancement of HF (lower peak Vo_2, worse NYHA class).[39] The role of ergoreceptors in exercise intolerance was shown by selective lumbar intrathecal blockage (using fentanyl) of afferent neural traffic arising from exercising muscles of lower limbs.[40] Such experimental intervention performed in a group of patients with HF acutely led to improved peakVo_2 mediated by reduced systemic vascular resistance and improved cardiac output. Importantly, implementation of training programs in the HF population have been showed to reduce the detrimental contribution of ergoreceptors to the changes in blood pressure, ventilatory response, and peripheral vascular resistance during exercise.[41] Favorable neural resetting in response to the physical training was accompanied by improved skeletal muscle metabolism (toward aerobic changes), as shown using magnetic resonance spectroscopy.[42] Thus, normalization in ergoreflex sensitivity following regular physical activity may be attributed to a reduced production of anaerobic metabolites (eg, lactate) that directly stimulate muscle ergoreceptors.

Although the role of overactive cardiovascular reflexes in the pathophysiology of advanced HF is undisputable, the benefits of interventions targeting selected parts of the autonomic nervous system are still uncertain. Further trials focused on well-established clinical end points (such as total mortality, HF hospitalizations) are needed. Improvements observed only in the functional variables (eg, quality of life, NYHA class, 6-minute walking distance) are not entirely satisfactory, especially in the studies where sham control was not used.

FLUID RETENTION AND CONGESTION

Fluid overload with central and/or peripheral congestion characterizes the clinical picture of advanced HF and is the main reason for hospital admission in these patients. The pathophysiology underlying fluid retention, different patterns of volume overload, and association with spiral progression of HF is complex, multifactorial, and not fully understood, but the whole process starts at the early stage of HF development and seems to be associated with augmented sympathetic signaling from the diseased myocardium and neurohormonal activation.[7] At the later stage, impaired crosstalk between the heart and the kidneys tends to play a key role.[43] Numerous mechanisms are involved in the physiologic process of volume control by the kidney: intrinsic renal control related to blood pressure and hemodynamics, responses to natriuretic peptides, the arginine-vasopressin system, the activity of RAAS at the body and organ levels, just to name a few. In advanced HF, all these tuned interactions seem to be dysfunctional and/or exhausted, as in the following illustrative examples: overexpression of natriuretic peptides does not lead to increased diuresis and natriuresis, which in turn promotes fluid retention and volume overload; nonosmotic release of vasopressin further impairs water and sodium handling; low blood pressure with inadequate perfusion of the kidneys also deteriorates already dysfunctional sodium handling.[44,45]

Although traditionally an assessment of kidney function is mainly based on calculation of glomerular function (estimated glomerular filtration rate [eGFR]), it seems not to provide adequate and meaningful information about water/sodium handling. There is growing evidence of the importance of impaired water and sodium handling by the renal tubules in HF.[46,47] Recent studies have shown the need for the recognition of 2 different aspects of kidney function in HF, with an assessment of sodium/water handling using urinary biomarkers of natriuresis being at least as important as traditional assessment of renal function using creatinine/blood urea nitrogen (BUN).[48]

Although fluid accumulation starts in the intravascular compartment, with time, hydrostatic pressure increases and exceeds interstitial oncotic pressure, and fluid accumulation expands to extravascular, interstitial space. It leads to tissue congestion and is often present in advanced HF. This pattern of congestion (often referred to as cardiac congestion[11]) develops slowly, with gradual clinical deterioration and an increase in intracardiac pressures. Fluid balance at the level of the interstitium strongly depends on the lymphatic system, but the lymphatic drainage seems to be impaired in advanced HF because of increased right heart pressure caused by the decrease of the perfusion gradient at the level of the thoracic duct.[49] Recent studies show the role of the interstitial compartment in the pathophysiology of this type of congestion, with particular interest in networks of glycosaminoglycans, which may influence sodium and water homeostasis.[49] In physiology, glycosaminoglycan networks can buffer a large amount of sodium and maintain tissue water content in stable conditions. Nijst and colleagues[50] showed that patients with HF have higher interstitial glycosaminoglycan density and degree of sulfation compared with healthy controls, and the magnitude of these changes is related to the clinical presence of peripheral edema and correlated with total water content. Interestingly, because patients not receiving ACEi/angiotensin receptor blockers tended to have higher levels of interstitial glycosaminoglycans, the investigators hypothesized that the neurohormonal system may be involved in the structure and function of this interstitial network.[50] More studies are needed to clarify the role of the interstitial compartment in order to improve management of volume overload in advanced HF.

IMPAIRED CARDIAC CONTRACTILITY

Impaired myocardial contractility is at the core of HF development and progression. As discussed earlier, reduced contractility is associated with increased wall stress, underlies cardiac remodeling, and triggers unfavorable compensatory mechanisms, including neurohormonal activation and dysfunctional reflex responses within the cardiorespiratory system. This framework has led to numerous attempts to directly improve cardiac contractility with inotropic agents, all of which have consistently failed to meet expectations.[51,52] Virtually all of these studies reported adverse events related to use of inotropic agents in patients with HF, such as ventricular arrhythmias, atrial fibrillation, hypotensive events, increased myocardial oxygen consumption with subsequent ischemia, or direct toxic effects at the level of myocardium.[51,52] It seems that these drugs have a common mechanism because they increase intracellular calcium levels to increase myocardial force production and improve cardiac function, and are therefore classified as calcitropes.[52] In chronic stable HF settings, they are contraindicated because they are related to increased risk of poor outcome. In acute HF in the short term, intravenous infusion of inotropic agents (dobutamine, dopamine, levosimendan, phosphodiesterase III inhibitors) may be considered in patients with hypotension (systolic blood pressure <90 mm Hg) and/or signs/symptoms of hypoperfusion despite adequate filling status, to increase cardiac output, increase blood pressure, improve peripheral perfusion, and maintain end-organ function.[11]

Recently, a new class of drugs that improve cardiac contractility has been developed, called cardiac myotropes, which target the myosin, actin, the associated regulatory proteins, or other structural elements of the sarcomere through calcium-independent mechanisms.[52,53] One of these therapeutics, omecamtiv mecarbil, is now being investigated in clinical trials in patients with HF.[52,53] Omecamtiv mecarbil is a selective cardiac myosin activator that increases cardiac contractility by specifically binding to myosin at an allosteric site. Omecamtiv mecarbil stabilizes the pre–power stroke state of myosin, enabling more myosin heads to undergo a power stroke during systole.[52,53] This effect of increased contraction is independent of changes in the intracellular calcium.

The GALACTIC trial investigated the effects of omecamtiv mecarbil on the cardiovascular outcomes in HF.[54] Patients with symptomatic, chronic HF and reduced LVEF (≤35%) (of whom 25% were included as inpatients) received omecamtiv mecarbil (using pharmacokinetic-guided dosing), in addition to standard HF therapy. Those treated with omecamtiv mecarbil had a lower incidence of a composite of an HF event (HF hospitalization or urgent visit for HF) or cardiovascular death.[54] Interestingly, a preplanned subgroup analysis showed an interaction of the effect with LVEF, and patients with LVEF less than the median (<28%) tended to benefit more. The results of all these studies seem to show that omecamtiv mecarbil may be of particular applicability for patients with advanced HF and severely impaired LVEF.

ADVANCED HEART FAILURE: A MULTIMORBID CLINICAL SYNDROME

In everyday practice, patients with an isolated diagnosis of advanced HF are virtually never seen, in contrast with those with multiple chronic diseases and/or coexisting conditions (both cardiovascular and noncardiovascular). Intriguing common pathophysiologic pathways and risk factors underlying such prevalent coexistence, adverse influences on the natural course of HF and patients' outcomes, and important therapeutic consequences of these interrelationships all explain the growing interest in the topic.[55,56]

HF evolution has been characterized as 4 consecutive stages: the pre-HF category (stage A), when only cardiovascular risk factors are present, followed by a latent period of structural heart disease without HF symptoms (stage B), eventually leading to development of symptomatic HF (stages C and D).[2] This model can be applied to explain the multimorbid nature of HF. At early disease stages, there is an interaction between risk factors/comorbidities and multiple adverse effects on the cardiovascular system leading to HF development. For example, arterial hypertension, obesity, and diabetes are increasingly coexisting worldwide and are risk factors for HF and almost all major HF-related comorbidities.[57] It is evident in patients with HF with preserved ejection fraction, where systemic proinflammatory activation, with overproduction of reactive oxygen species, limits nitric oxide bioavailability for cardiomyocytes, with resultant hypertrophy, stiffening, and increased collagen deposition by myofibroblasts causing myocardial remodeling and diastolic dysfunction.[58] Many of these patients now tend to reach advanced stages of the disease because of a lack of effective therapies. At later stages, once HF is already present, it may give rise to conditions that adversely affect the cardiovascular system, with further disease progression and adverse outcomes. As discussed earlier, HF is no longer seen in isolation as cardiac/hemodynamic disease, and numerous pathophysiologic pathways have been identified in this syndrome that may be shared with other chronic cardiovascular and noncardiovascular conditions.

Comorbidities complicating natural course of HF represent a mixture of different categories (**Box 2**). The evidence that targeting a certain non-HF comorbidity would favorably affect HF outcomes is still fairly limited, particularly at the late, advanced stage of the disease. However, in this context, recent studies tend to indicate that at least 3 comorbidities may become specific therapeutic targets for interventions in HF: atrial fibrillation, diabetes mellitus, and iron deficiency. The last 2 are briefly discussed here.

Box 2
Categories of comorbidities complicating advanced heart failure

Traditional cardiovascular risk factors for HF development (eg, arterial hypertension, diabetes mellitus, obesity, dyslipidemia)

Causal factors leading to HF (eg, coronary artery disease, arterial hypertension, diabetes mellitus, valvular heart disease)

Cardiovascular conditions often coexisting with HF (eg, atrial fibrillation, peripheral artery disease, stroke)

Chronic noncardiovascular diseases associated with higher HF prevalence (eg, chronic kidney disease, chronic obstructive pulmonary disease, depression, osteoarthritis)

Conditions characterizing chronic diseases including HF syndrome (eg, anemia, iron deficiency, sleep-disordered breathing, cachexia/sarcopenia)

Malignant diseases (often reflecting cardiotoxic effects of certain chemotherapeutic agents with subsequent development of HF)

Age-related disorders typically characterizing elderly populations, not necessarily specific for HF syndrome (eg, frailty, dementia)

Type 2 diabetes mellitus is a common comorbidity in HF, occurring in 25% to 45% of these patients.[59] These diseases are closely related in terms of common pathophysiologic pathways, including neurohormonal activation and insulin resistance, as well as common risk factors. They tend to worsen each other's courses; the occurrence of HF is one of the most serious complications of diabetes in terms of prognosis, and patients with HF and coexisting diabetes have an increased risk of death and hospitalization for HF compared with patients with nondiabetic HF.[60] Data from large clinical trials with drugs tested in the treatment of HF indicate that the coexistence of diabetes may increase the risk of all-cause and cardiovascular mortality by nearly 2-fold, and the risk of hospitalization caused by exacerbation of HF by 1.2-fold to 1.9-fold.[59]

Among the mechanisms underlying the adverse effect of diabetes on the course of HF, in addition to the long-known harmful effects of hyperglycemia, insulin resistance, and advanced glycation end products on metabolism, function, and structural remodeling of myocardium, in recent years much attention has been paid to excessive activation of the sodium-hydrogen exchanger (NHE).[61,62] The NHE is present in at least a few isoforms in cell membranes, the NHE1 isoform being predominant in cardiomyocytes and blood vessels and the NHE3 isoform being found in the renal tubular epithelial cells. The activity of both of these isoforms in patients with HF is initially increased as a result of stimulation of the RAAS and sympathetic activation, but in the presence of diabetes mellitus, as a result of the stimulating effect of hyperglycemia, insulin resistance, and adipokines, it further increases significantly.[61,62] At the level of the myocardium, this leads to an overload of cardiomyocytes with calcium ions (exchange for sodium ions by the sodium-calcium exchanger) and their subsequent injury and apoptosis, and, as a result, fibrosis and unfavorable remodeling of the heart and, at the level of the proximal renal tubules, to a significant increase in sodium ion reabsorption, resulting in fluid overload and the development of resistance to diuretics.[61,62]

Inhibition of overactive NHE1 and NHE3 seems to be a therapeutic target and most likely is one of the mechanisms determining favorable action of the new drug class, sodium-glucose cotransporter (SGLT) 2 inhibitors. In clinical trials assessing cardiovascular safety in diabetic patients, SGLT2 inhibitors proved not only to be safe in terms of the impact on cardiovascular mortality and ischemic events but also to significantly reduce the risk of hospitalization because of HF.[63,64] Moreover, 2 SGLT2 inhibitors, dapagliflozin and empagliflozin, significantly reduced the risk of the composite end point of cardiovascular death and the worsening of HF not only in patients with HF and diabetes but also in patients without coexisting diabetes.[65,66] These effects cannot be fully explained by a hypoglycemic effect alone. SGLT2 inhibitors are likely to have several other favorable cardiovascular and cardioprotective effects, including promoting ketone bodies as the main energy substrate used by the myocardium, which allows the optimization of ATP production with limited oxygen supply; induction of osmotic diuresis, which promotes proportionally greater fluid loss from the extravascular space compared with the intravascular space; and the aforementioned inhibition of the NHE.[67]

Iron deficiency (ID) is one of the most common comorbidities in HF, present in approximately 50% to 70% of patients with HF, with increasing prevalence in those with advanced disease.[68,69] Among the mechanisms underlying ID in HF, the following tend play leading roles: (1) reduced dietary intake (because of malnutrition, poor absorption caused by impaired duodenal iron transport, interaction with certain drugs or food reducing iron absorption); (2) increased iron loses (caused by edema of the gut, impaired integrity of intestinal mucosa, occult gastrointestinal/genitourinary bleeding caused by use of antithrombotics); (3) functional impairment of iron availability/use caused by proinflammatory activation, seen in HF with increased levels of hepcidin and impaired duodenal iron absorption and iron retention in the reticuloendothelial system (which may coincide with normal iron stores in the body).[68,70]

Iron is a micronutrient essential for numerous biological processes, thus ID is associated with deleterious consequences far more extensive and independent than those related to low hemoglobin level. ID alone results in decreased oxygen storage, abnormal oxidative metabolism and cellular energy handling, and impaired reactive oxygen species defense, all of which contribute to mitochondrial dysfunction. Tissues with high energetic demand (such as cardiomyocytes) are particularly susceptible to the deleterious pathologic effects of ID. Because ID deteriorates energy homoeostasis, already impaired in the HF syndrome,[71,72] it may further accelerate progression of HF and lead to increased risk of poor outcomes. There is clear evidence that ID in HF predicts increased long-term all-cause mortality independently of the presence of anemia and is associated with impaired functional capacity and decreased health-related quality of life.[68,70] All these findings form a strong background to expect beneficial effects of correcting ID in patients with HF, which has been confirmed by several studies. They used intravenous iron (ferric carboxymaltose [FCM]) to correct ID in HF and showed an improvement of functional status, exercise capacity, and health-related quality of life.[73,74] Recently, it was also shown that correction of ID with FCM in patients admitted to hospital with decompensated HF significantly reduces the risk of HF hospital admissions and improves quality of life.[75]

Patients with advanced HF often have impaired renal function, which accelerates spiral progression of the disease but also significantly limits therapeutic options. The importance of cardiorenal interactions led to the introduction of 5 types of cardiorenal syndromes.[76] The mechanisms of their development have already been extensively characterized and include neurohormonal and sympathetic activation; toxicity of some HF drugs and contrast media; decreased kidney perfusion; increased intravascular volume; and proinflammatory cytokine secretion with subclinical inflammation, vasoconstriction, and anemia.[76] Clinically, 2 main manifestations of renal dysfunction in advanced HF can be distinguished: gradual progression of eGFR decline and an inability to restore/keep volume balance.[77] From a clinical perspective, it is important to understand that those 2 could be disconnected and do not always overlap.[48] There is a robust evidence that renal function (defined by eGFR/creatinine/BUN) has critical prognostic significance in HF. The lower the eGFR, the higher the risk of HF complications and poor outcome. The failure in the control of body volume homeostasis (leading to congestion, as mentioned earlier) is the most frequent cause of advanced HF hospitalizations. The increasing sodium avidity with advanced HF leads to early fluid overload and attenuates diuretic responsiveness.[78] To overcome the phenomenon, higher doses of diuretics need to be used to maintain the fluid balance. In extreme situations, diuretic resistance develops, in which kidneys fail to increase fluid and sodium excretion sufficiently to relieve congestion, despite high doses of diuretic.[78] Importantly, the total diuretic dose is also an important clinical marker of disease severity and poor outcome. Recently, the net interactions between failing heart, liver, and kidney (described by Model for End-stage Liver Disease [MELD] XI score) have been also studied, showing the clinical relevance and prognostic significance in HF.[79–83] Importantly, the causative interaction between HF progression and peripheral organ dysfunction (kidney, liver) has been shown because organ function can improve after heart transplant or left ventricular assist device implantation.

As already mentioned, the problem of growing coexistence of advanced HF and malignant diseases also needs to be acknowledged. For many years, this relation has been mainly seen through the prism of drug cardiotoxicity; however, it now becomes clear that it goes far beyond these boundaries. The general population, especially of industrialized countries, is progressively aging, resulting in significant increase in patients with both HF and malignant diseases.[84] The incidence of malignancy in previously diagnosed HF has been estimated in the range of 19 to 34 per 1000 person-years.[85] The combination of these 2 diseases with the need for simultaneous treatments is becoming serious challenge in clinical practice. Interestingly, there is growing evidence of the overlap of risk factors for HF and cancer. Some epidemiologic studies suggest that cancer may be more common among patients with preexisting HF.[86,87] An intriguing explanation considers systemic pathophysiologic processes, such as neurohormonal activation, inflammation, and oxidative stress, superimposed by genetic predisposition to promote development of both conditions, HF and cancer.[86] However, the results are still equivocal,[88] and more studies are needed to confirm the potential pathophysiologic and epidemiologic link between HF and cancer. From a clinical perspective, the similarity of symptoms should also be noted, because many patients with malignancies report HF-like symptoms, such as dyspnea, fatigue, weakness, muscle wasting, edema, and anorexia.[84–86] Of note, cachexia, defined as a generalized process that affects most body compartments (skeletal muscle, fat, and bone tissue), associated with progressive loss of body weight may complicate both advanced HF and malignant diseases.[89,90] Regardless of other coexisting factors, the occurrence of cachexia significantly worsens a patient's prognosis. Treatment options for patients who develop cachexia are very limited and include nutritional counseling support (with polyunsaturated fatty acids; high-calory, protein-rich nutritional supplements; and essential amino acids), various forms of exercise, optimized HF therapy (with β-blockers and ACEi to prevent skeletal muscle wasting/cachexia), anabolic steroids, other anabolic therapies such as antimyostatin antibodies and ghrelin-receptor agonists, antiinflammatory substances, appetite stimulants, and proteasome inhibitors.[89,90] Taking into account the growing number of patients with coexistent advanced HF and malignancies who may develop wasting conditions, there is a clinical need to identify novel safe and effective strategies to prevent and treat cachexia.

CLINICS CARE POINTS

For the pathophysiologic mechanisms in advanced HF, remember:

- To target activation of the neurohormonal system and sympathetic nervous system
- To assess congestion and, if present, to identify different patterns of congestions with subsequent therapeutic decisions.
- To evaluate and manage coexisting comorbidities, because their underlying pathophysiologies may interfere with the progression of the disease.
- That novel pathophysiologic pathways have become therapeutic targets with the following therapies: vericiguat, a soluble guanylate cyclase stimulator; omecamtiv mecarbil, a selective cardiac myosin activator; sodium-glucose cotransporter 2 inhibitors; and FCM for patients with concomitant ID

DISCLOSURE

Prof. P. Ponikowski declares consultancy fees and speaker's honoraria from AstraZeneca, Boehringer Ingelheim, Vifor Pharma, Amgen, Servier, Novartis, Bayer, Pfizer, and Impulse Dynamics, and a research grant from Vifor Pharma. Other authors have nothing to disclose.

REFERENCES

1. Crespo-Leiro MG, Metra M, Lund LH, et al. Advanced heart failure: a position statement of the Heart Failure Association of the European Society of Cardiology. Eur J Heart Fail 2018;20(11):1505–35.
2. Bozkurt B, Coats AJS, Tsutsui H, et al. Universal definition and classification of heart failure: a report of the Heart Failure Society of America, Heart Failure Association of the European Society of Cardiology, Japanese Heart Failure Society and Writing Committee of the Universal Definition of Heart Failure: Endorsed by the Canadian Heart Failure Society, Heart Failure Association of India, Cardiac Society of Australia and New Zealand, and Chinese Heart Failure Association. Eur J Heart Fail 2021;23(3): 352–80.
3. Wilcox JE, Fang JC, Margulies KB, et al. Heart Failure With Recovered Left Ventricular Ejection Fraction: JACC Scientific Expert Panel. J Am Coll Cardiol 2020;76(6):719–34.
4. Jankowska EA, Ponikowski P, Piepoli MF, et al. Autonomic imbalance and immune activation in chronic heart failure —Pathophysiological links. Cardiovasc Res 2006;70:434–45.

5. Epelman S, Liu PP, Mann DL. Role of innate and adaptive immune mechanisms in cardiac injury and repair. Nat Rev Immunol 2015;15(2):117–29.

6. Hartupee J, Mann DL. Neurohormonal activation in heart failure with reduced ejection fraction. Nat Rev Cardiol 2017;14(1):30–8. https://doi.org/10.1038/nrcardio.2016.163.

7. Floras JS, Ponikowski P. The sympathetic/parasympathetic imbalance in heart failure with reduced ejection fraction. Eur Heart J 2015;36:1974–82.

8. McMurray JJ, Ray SG, Abdullah I, et al. Plasma endothelin in chronic heart failure. Circulation 1992;85:1374–9.

9. Goldsmith SR. Arginine vasopressin antagonism in heart failure: Current status and possible new directions. J Cardiol 2019;74(1):49–52.

10. Adamo L, Rocha-Resende C, Prabhu SD, et al. Reappraising the role of inflammation in heart failure. Nat Rev Cardiol 2020;17(5):269–85.

11. Ponikowski P, Voors AA, Anker SD, et al, ESC Scientific Document Group. 2016 ESC guidelines for the diagnosis and treatment of acute and chronic heart failure: The Task Force for the diagnosis and treatment of acute and chronic heart failure of the European Society of Cardiology (ESC)Developed with the special contribution of the Heart Failure Association (HFA) of the ESC. Eur Heart J 2016;37(27):2129–200.

12. Docherty KF, Vaduganathan M, Solomon SD, et al. Sacubitril/Valsartan: Neprilysin Inhibition 5 Years After PARADIGM-HF. JACC Heart Fail 2020;8(10):800–10.

13. McMurray JJV, Packer M, Desai AS, et al. Angiotensin-neprilysin inhibition versus enalapril in heart failure. N Engl J Med 2014;371:993–1004.

14. Alem MM. Endothelial Dysfunction in Chronic Heart Failure: Assessment, Findings, Significance, and Potential Therapeutic Targets. Int J Mol Sci 2019;20(13):3198.

15. Ramseyer VD, Cabral PD, Garvin JL. Role of endothelin in thick ascending limb sodium chloride transport, . Endothelin in renal physiology and disease. p. 76–83.

16. Packer M, McMurray JJV, Krum H, et al. Long-Term Effect of Endothelin Receptor Antagonism With Bosentan on the Morbidity and Mortality of Patients With Severe Chronic Heart Failure: Primary Results of the ENABLE Trials. JACC: Heart Fail 2017;5:317–26.

17. McMurray JJV, Teerlink JR, Cotter G, et al. Effects of tezosentan on symptoms and clinical outcomes in patients with acute heart failure: The VERITAS randomized controlled trials. JAMA 2007;298:2009–19.

18. Gheorghiade M, Marti CN, Sabbah HN, et al. Soluble guanylate cyclase: a potential therapeutic target for heart failure. Heart Fail Rev 2013;18:123–34.

19. Emdin M, Aimo A, Castiglione V, et al. Targeting Cyclic Guanosine Monophosphate to Treat Heart Failure: JACC Review Topic of the Week. J Am Coll Cardiol 2020;76(15):1795–807.

20. Singh P, Vijayakumar S, Kalogeroupoulos A, et al. Multiple avenues of modulating the nitric oxide pathway in heart failure clinical trials. Curr Heart Fail Rep 2018;15:44–52.

21. Bonderman D, Ghio S, Felix SB, et al. Riociguat for patients with pulmonary hypertension caused by systolic left ventricular dysfunction: a phase IIb double-blind, randomized, placebo-controlled, dose-ranging hemodynamic study. Circulation 2013;128:502–11.

22. Armstrong PW, Pieske B, Anstrom KJ, et al. Vericiguat in patients with heart failure and reduced ejection fraction. N Engl J Med 2020;382:1883–93.

23. Anker SD, Ponikowski PP, Clark AL, et al. Cytokines and neurohormones relating to body composition alterations in the wasting syndrome of chronic heart failure. Eur Heart J 1999;20(9):683–93.

24. Anker SD, Coats AJ. How to RECOVER from RENAISSANCE? The significance of the results of RECOVER, RENAISSANCE, RENEWAL and ATTACH. Int J Cardiol 2002;86(2–3):123–30.

25. Paleczny B, Olesińska-Mader M, Siennicka A, et al. Assessment of baroreflex sensitivity has no prognostic value in contemporary, optimally managed patients with mild-to-moderate heart failure with reduced ejection fraction: a retrospective analysis of 5-year survival. Eur J Heart Fail 2019;21(1):50–8.

26. La Rovere MT, Pinna GD, Maestri R, et al. Prognostic implications of baroreflex sensitivity in heart failure patients in the beta-blocking era. J Am Coll Cardiol 2009;53(2):193–9.

27. Zile MR, Lindenfeld JA, Weaver FA, et al. Baroreflex Activation Therapy in Patients With Heart Failure With Reduced Ejection Fraction. J Am Coll Cardiol 2020;76(1):1–13.

28. Gold MR, Van Veldhuisen DJ, Hauptman PJ, et al. Vagus Nerve Stimulation for the Treatment of Heart Failure: The INOVATE-HF Trial. J Am Coll Cardiol 2016;68(2):149–58.

29. Niewinski P, Engelman ZJ, Fudim M, et al. Clinical predictors and hemodynamic consequences of elevated peripheral chemosensitivity in optimally treated men with chronic systolic heart failure. J Card Fail 2013;19(6):408–15.

30. Ponikowski P, Chua TP, Anker SD, et al. Peripheral chemoreceptor hypersensitivity: an ominous sign in patients with chronic heart failure. Circulation 2001;104(5):544–9.

31. Buchanan GF, Richerson GB. Role of chemoreceptors in mediating dyspnea. Respir Physiol Neurobiol 2009;167(1):9–19.

32. Chua TP, Ponikowski PP, Harrington D, et al. Contribution of peripheral chemoreceptors to ventilation and the effects of their suppression on exercise tolerance in chronic heart failure. Heart 1996;76(6):483–9.

33. Del Rio R, Marcus NJ, Schultz HD. Carotid chemore-ceptor ablation improves survival in heart failure: rescuing autonomic control of cardiorespiratory function. J Am Coll Cardiol 2013;62(25):2422–30.

34. Niewinski P, Janczak D, Rucinski A, et al. Carotid body resection for sympathetic modulation in sys-tolic heart failure: results from first-in-man study. Eur J Heart Fail 2017;19(3):391–400.

35. Niewinski P, Tubek S, Paton JFR, et al. Oxygenation pattern and compensatory responses to hypoxia and hypercapnia following bilateral carotid body resection in humans. J Physiol 2021;JP281319. https://doi.org/10.1113/JP281319.

36. Dempsey JA, Smith CA, Blain GM, et al. Role of cen-tral/peripheral chemoreceptors and their interde-pendence in the pathophysiology of sleep apnea. Adv Exp Med Biol 2012;758:343–9.

37. Costanzo MR, Ponikowski P, Coats A, et al. Phrenic nerve stimulation to treat patients with central sleep apnoea and heart failure. Eur J Heart Fail 2018; 20(12):1746–54.

38. Giannoni A, Borrelli C, Mirizzi G, et al. Benefit of bus-pirone on chemoreflex and central apnoeas in heart failure: a randomized controlled crossover trial. Eur J Heart Fail 2020. https://doi.org/10.1002/ejhf.1854.

39. Ponikowski PP, Chua TP, Francis DP, et al. Muscle er-goreceptor overactivity reflects deterioration in clin-ical status and cardiorespiratory reflex control in chronic heart failure. Circulation 2001;104(19): 2324–30.

40. Smith JR, Joyner MJ, Curry TB, et al. Locomotor muscle group III/IV afferents constrain stroke volume and contribute to exercise intolerance in human heart failure. J Physiol 2020;598(23):5379–90.

41. Piepoli M, Clark AL, Volterrani M, et al. Contribution of muscle afferents to the hemodynamic, autonomic, and ventilatory responses to exercise in patients with chronic heart failure: Effects of physical training. Circulation 1996;93(5):940–52.

42. Stratton JR, Dunn JF, Adamopoulos S, et al. Training partially reverses skeletal muscle metabolic abnor-malities during exercise in heart failure. J Appl Phys-iol 1994;76(4):1575–82.

43. Schrier RW, Abraham WT. Hormones and hemody-namics in heart failure. N Engl J Med 1999;341: 577–85.

44. Miller WL. Fluid Volume Overload and Congestion in Heart Failure: Time to Reconsider Pathophysiology and How Volume Is Assessed. Circ Heart Fail 2016;9(8):e002922.

45. Mullens W, Verbrugge FH, Nijst P, et al. Renal so-dium avidity in heart failure: from pathophysiology to treatment strategies. Eur Heart J 2017;38: 1872–82.

46. Damman K, Maaten JM Ter, Coster JE, et al. Clinical importance of urinary sodium excretion in acute heart failure. Eur J Heart Fail 2020. ejhf.1753.

47. Biegus J, Zymliński R, Sokolski M, et al. Serial assessment of spot urine sodium predicts effective-ness of decongestion and outcome in patients with acute heart failure. Eur J Heart Fail 2019;21:624–33.

48. Biegus J, Zymliński R, Testani J, et al. Renal profiling based on estimated glomerular filtration rate and spot urine sodium identifies high-risk acute heart failure patients. Eur J Heart Fail 2020. https://doi.org/10.1002/ejhf.2053.

49. Boorsma EM, Ter Maaten JM, Damman K, et al. Congestion in heart failure: a contemporary look at physiology, diagnosis and treatment. Nat Rev Car-diol 2020;17(10):641–55.

50. Nijst P, Olinevich M, Hilkens P, et al. Dermal Interstitial Alterations in Patients With Heart Failure and Reduced Ejection Fraction: A Potential Contributor to Fluid Accu-mulation? Circ Heart Fail 2018;11(7):e004763.

51. Maack C, Eschenhagen T, Hamdani N, et al. Treat-ments targeting inotropy. Eur Heart J 2019;40(44): 3626–44.

52. Psotka MA, Gottlieb SS, Francis GS, et al. Cardiac Calcitropes, Myotropes, and Mitotropes: JACC Re-view Topic of the Week. J Am Coll Cardiol 2019; 73(18):2345–53.

53. Teerlink JR, Diaz R, Felker GM, et al. Omecamtiv Me-carbil in Chronic Heart Failure With Reduced Ejection Fraction: Rationale and Design of GALACTIC-HF. JACC Heart Fail 2020;8(4):329–40.

54. Teerlink JR, Diaz R, Felker GM, et al. Cardiac Myosin Activation with Omecamtiv Mecarbil in Systolic Heart Failure. N Engl J Med 2021;384(2):105–16.

55. Luo N, Mentz RJ. A Gordian knot: disentangling co-morbidities in heart failure. Eur J Heart Fail 2016; 18(7):759–61.

56. Mentz RJ, Kelly JP, von Lueder TG, et al. Noncardiac comorbidities in heart failure with reduced versus preserved ejection fraction. J Am Coll Cardiol 2014;64(21):2281–93.

57. Triposkiadis F, Giamouzis G, Parissis J, et al. Refram-ing the association and significance of co-morbidities in heart failure. Eur J Heart Fail 2016;18(7):744–58.

58. Paulus WJ, Tschöpe C. A novel paradigm for heart failure with preserved ejection fraction: comorbidi-ties drive myocardial dysfunction and remodeling through coronary microvascular endothelial inflam-mation. J Am Coll Cardiol 2013;62(4):263–71.

59. Ofstad AP, Atar D, Gullestad L, et al. The heart fail-ure burden of type 2 diabetes mellitus – a review of pathophysiology and interventions. Heart Fail Rev 2018;23:303–23.

60. McMurray JJ, Gerstein HC, Holman RR, et al. Heart failure: a cardiovascular outcome in diabetes that can no longer be ignored. Lancet Diabetes Endocri-nol 2014;2:843–51.

61. Lee BL, Sykes BD, Fliegel L. Structural and func-tional insights into the cardiac Na/H exchanger. J Moll Cell Cardiol 2013;61:60–7.

62. Packer M. Activation and inhibition of sodium-hydrogen exchanger is a mechanism that links the pathophysiology and treatment of diabetes mellitus with that of heart failure. Circulation 2013;136: 1548–59.

63. Zinman B, Wanner C, Lachin IM, et al. Empagliflozin, cardiovascular outcomes, and mortality in type 2 diabetes. N Engl J Med 2015;373:2117–28.

64. Neal B, Perkovic V, Mahaffey KW, et al. Canagliflozin and cardiovascular and renal events in type 2 diabetes. N Engl J Med 2017;373:644–57.

65. McMurray JJV, Solomo SD, Inzucchi SE, et al. Dapagliflozin in patients with heart failure and reduced ejection fraction. N Engl J Med 2019;381: 1995–2008.

66. Packer M, Anker SD, Butler J, et al. EMPEROR-Reduced Trial Investigators. Cardiovascular and Renal Outcomes with Empagliflozin in Heart Failure. N Engl J Med 2020;383(15):1413–24.

67. Zelniker TA, Braunwald E. Mechanisms of cardiorenal effects of sodium-glucose cotransporter 2 inhibitors. JACC state-of-the-art. Review. J Am Coll Cardiol 2020;75:422–34.

68. Ghafourian K, Shapiro JS, Goodman L, et al. Iron and Heart Failure: Diagnosis, Therapies, and Future Directions. JACC Basic Transl Sci 2020;5(3):300–13.

69. Jankowska EA, Kasztura M, Sokolski M, et al. Iron deficiency defined as depleted iron stores accompanied by unmet cellular iron requirements identifies patients at the highest risk of death after an episode of acute heart failure. Eur Heart J 2014;35:2468–76.

70. Jankowska EA, von Haehling S, Anker SD, et al. Iron deficiency and heart failure: diagnostic dilemmas and therapeutic perspectives. Eur Heart J 2013;34: 816–29.

71. Neubauer S. The failing heart – an engine out of fuel. N Engl J Med 2007;356:1140–51.

72. Biegus J, Zymliński R, Sokolski M, et al. Elevated lactate in acute heart failure patients with intracellular iron deficiency as identifier of poor outcome. Kard Pol 2019;77:347–54.

73. Anker SD, Comin CJ, Filippatos G, et al. Ferric carboxymaltose in patients with heart failure and iron deficiency. N Engl J Med 2009;361:2436–48.

74. Ponikowski P, van Veldhuisen DJ, Comin-Colet J, et al. Beneficial effects of long-term intravenous iron therapy with ferric carboxymaltose in patients with symptomatic heart failure and iron deficiency. Eur Heart J 2015;36:657–68.

75. Ponikowski P, Kirwan BA, Anker SD, et al. Ferric carboxymaltose for iron deficiency at discharge after acute heart failure: a multicentre, double-blind, randomised, controlled trial. Lancet 2020; 396(10266):1895–904.

76. Ronco C, McCullough P, Anker SD, et al. Acute Dialysis Quality Initiative (ADQI) consensus group. Cardio-renal syndromes: report from the consensus conference of the acute dialysis quality initiative. Eur Heart J 2010;31(6):703–11.

77. Mullens W, Damman K, Testani JM, et al. Evaluation of kidney function throughout the heart failure trajectory – a position statement from the Heart Failure Association of the European Society of Cardiology. Eur J Heart Fail Eur J Heart Fail 2020;22(4):584–603.

78. Mullens W, Damman K, Harjola VP, et al. The use of diuretics in heart failure with congestion - a position statement from the Heart Failure Association of the European Society of Cardiology. Eur J Heart Fail 2019;21(2):137–55.

79. Zymliński R, Sokolski M, Biegus J, et al. Multi-organ dysfunction/injury on admission identifies acute heart failure patients at high risk of poor outcome. Eur J Heart Fail 2019;21(6):744–50.

80. Biegus J, Demissei B, Postmus D, et al. Hepatorenal dysfunction identifies high-risk patients with acute heart failure: insights from the RELAX-AHF trial. ESC Heart Fail 2019;6(6):1188–98.

81. Biegus J, Zymliński R, Sokolski M, et al. Impaired hepato-renal function defined by the MELD XI score as prognosticator in acute heart failure. Eur J Heart Fail 2016;18:1518–21.

82. Biegus J, Hillege HL, Postmus D, et al. Abnormal liver function tests in acute heart failure: relationship with clinical characteristics and outcome in the PROTECT study. Eur J Heart Fail 2016;18:830–9.

83. Biegus J, Zymliński R, Sokolski M, et al. Liver function tests in patients with acute heart failure. Pol Arch Intern Med 2012;122:471–9.

84. Meijers WC, de Boer RA. Common risk factors for heart failure and cancer. Cardiovasc Res 2019; 115(5):844–53.

85. Ameri P, Canepa M, Anker MS, et al. Heart Failure Association Cardio-Oncology Study Group of the European Society of Cardiology. Cancer diagnosis in patients with heart failure: epidemiology, clinical implications and gaps in knowledge. Eur J Heart Fail 2018;20(5):879–87.

86. Bertero E, Canepa M, Maack C, et al. Linking Heart Failure to Cancer: Background Evidence and Research Perspectives. Circulation 2018;138(7): 735–42.

87. Hasin T, Gerber Y, McNallan SM, et al. Patients with heart failure have an increased risk of incident cancer. J Am Coll Cardiol 2013;62(10):881–6.

88. Selvaraj S, Bhatt DL, Claggett B, et al. Lack of association between heart failure and incident cancer. J Am Coll Cardiol 2018;71:1501–10.

89. von Haehling S, Ebner N, Dos Santos MR, et al. Muscle wasting and cachexia in heart failure: mechanisms and therapies. Nat Rev Cardiol 2017;14(6): 323–41.

90. Bauer J, Morley JE, Schols AMWJ, et al. Sarcopenia: A Time for Action. An SCWD Position Paper. J Cachexia Sarcopenia Muscle 2019;10(5):956–61.

Advanced Heart Failure
Definition, Epidemiology, and Clinical Course

Maria Generosa Crespo-Leiro, MD, PhD[a,b,c,d],*,
Eduardo Barge-Caballero, MD, PhD[a,b,c]

KEYWORDS

- Advanced heart failure • Definition • Prognosis • Referral criteria • Selection criteria
- Heart transplantation • Mechanical circulatory support • Coordination and networking

KEY POINTS

- Advanced heart failure is characterized by a progressive worsening of symptoms that are disabling for daily life, refractory to all therapies, and with high mortality.
- Patients with advanced heart failure may be candidates for life-prolonging therapies, such as heart transplantation or long-term mechanical circulatory support, or just require palliative therapies.
- The 2018 Heart Failure Association definition of advanced heart failure requires 4 criteria that must be present despite optimal guideline-directed treatment.
- Timely referral of patients to advanced heart failure centers and careful selection for heart transplantation or long-term mechanical circulatory support are key to good clinical outcomes.

DEFINITION OF ADVANCED HEART FAILURE

Although medical, surgical, and device therapies, according to scientific evidence, have progressively improved the quality of life and survival of patients with heart failure (HF), some patients evolve unfavorably with a progressive worsening of symptoms that are disabling for daily life, refractory to all therapies, and with high mortality. This stage is recognized as advanced HF, also known as American College of Cardiology (ACC)/American Heart Association (AHA) "Stage D" HF, meaning refractory HF requiring specialized interventions or end-stage HF.[1–3]

Patients at this stage may be candidates for life-prolonging therapies, such as heart transplantation (HT) or long-term mechanical circulatory support (MCS) devices, or may just require palliative therapies (eg, intermittent ionotropic infusions,

ultrafiltration, or peritoneal dialysis to control congestion or end-of-life comfort care). The 1-year survival after HT and left ventricular assist devices (LVAD) for bridge to transplant or destination therapy is approaching 80% to 90%,[4,5] being patient selection and timing critical for optimal outcomes. Each patient should be individually assessed for their specific needs, and in case of being noneligible for advanced therapies, treatment goals should be aimed at reducing symptomatic burden and improving quality of life.

The search for a definition of advanced HF has been of a great interest for clinicians, because the proper identification of patients in need of a particular treatment, especially those potentially benefiting from advanced therapies (such as HT or MCS), who are to be referred to advanced therapy centers, needs to be done at an appropriate time. Not too early, but not too late.[6]

[a] Heart Failure and Heart Transplant Unit, Cardiology Department, Complexo Hospitalario Universitario A Coruña (CHUAC), Xubias 84, 15006 A Coruña, Spain; [b] Instituto Investigación Biomedica A Coruña (INIBIC); [c] Centro de Investigación Biomedica en Red Cardiovascular (CIBERCV); [d] Universidade da Coruña (UDC)
* Corresponding author. Heart Failure and Heart Transplant Unit, Cardiology Department, Complexo Hospitalario Universitario A Coruña (CHUAC), Xubias 84, 15006 A Coruña, Spain.
E-mail address: marisacrespo@gmail.com
Twitter: @marisa1109 (M.G.C.-L.); @eduardo_barge (E.B.-C.)

Heart Failure Clin 17 (2021) 533–545
https://doi.org/10.1016/j.hfc.2021.06.002

There is no single symptom, sign, or test that can identify these patients, and this advance stage cannot be compared with patients with an acute HF hospitalization in whom, in most cases, the cause can be treated, the symptoms controlled, and the treatment implemented with improved clinical outcomes. The clinical course of patients with HF is highly unpredictable and a challenge even for experts in HF, as there are many influencing factors such as different responses to treatment or sudden instability due to pathologies and/or intercurrent circumstances, both of cardiac or extracardiac origin. Therefore, over time different scientific societies have suggested criteria to identify patients in advanced HF, which are shown in **Boxes 1–3**.

There are some overlaps and complementarities between them, but as a whole they gather the main clinical features that accompany patients with advanced HF and allow us to identify them with information that is easily accessible in daily clinical practice. Most of the proposed criteria are based on severity of symptoms, end-stage heart disease, absence of other treatments, recurrent hospitalizations, inability to tolerate neurohormonal activation blocking treatments such as renin-angiotensin-aldosterone system inhibitors (RAASi), beta-blockers (BB), or angiotensin receptor-neprilysin inhibitor (ARNI), recurrent hospitalizations, implantable cardioverter-defibrillator shocks, refractory congestion, poor functional capacity, cardiac cachexia and progressive multiorgan impairment, especially kidney or liver dysfunction, and pulmonary hypertension.[1,3]

The Interagency Registry for Mechanically Assisted Circulatory Support (INTERMACS) profiles[7] were developed to classify patients who were to be considered for long-term MCS device implantation, based on the symptoms, hemodynamic compromise, and characteristics consistent with a need for advanced therapies. The classification includes 7 profiles from highest to lowest clinical severity and shorter to longer recommended maximum time frame for intervention. Profiles 1 to 3 refer to inpatients and profiles 4 to 7 to outpatients. INTERMACS profiles comprise profile 1 "Critical cardiogenic shock" in which the patient requires definitive intervention within hours, profile 2 "Progressive decline" in which definitive intervention is needed within few days, profile 3 "Stable but inotrope-dependent" in which definitive intervention elective over a period of weeks to few months, followed by profiles 4 to 6 in which the urgency for intervention is variable to profile 7 "advanced NYHA Class III" in which neither cardiac transplantation nor an MCS is yet indicated. Specific descriptions of each profile and the

Box 1
Previous definitions or advanced heart failure: Heart Failure Association-ESC (2007)

1. Severe symptoms of HF with dyspnea and/or fatigue at rest or with minimal exertion (NYHA functional class III or IV)

2. Episodes of fluid retention (pulmonary and/or systemic congestion, peripheral edema) and/or of reduced cardiac output at rest (peripheral hypoperfusion)

3. Objective evidence of severe cardiac dysfunction, shown by at least one of the following:
   a. A low LVEF (<30%)
   b. A severe abnormality of cardiac function on Doppler-echocardiography with a pseudonormal or restrictive mitral inflow pattern
   c. High LV filing pressures (mean PCWP >16 mm Hg, and/or mean RAP >12 mm Hg by pulmonary artery catheterization)
   d. High BNP or NT-proBNP plasma levels, in the absence of noncardiac causes

4. Severe impairment of functional capacity shown by one of the following:
   a. Inability to exercise
   b. 6-MWT distance less than 300 m or less in women and/or patients older than 75 years
   c. pVO$_2$ less than 12 to 14 mL/kg/min

5. History of more than or equal to 1 heart failure hospitalization in the past 6 months

Presence of all the previous features despite "attempts to optimize" therapy, including diuretics, inhibitors of the renin-angiotensin-aldosterone system, and beta-blockers, unless these are poorly tolerated or contraindicated, and CRT, when indicated

Abbreviations: 6-MWT, 6-minute walk test; BNP, B-type natriuretic peptide; CRT, cardiac resynchronization therapy; LV, left ventricular; LVEF, left ventricular ejection fraction; NT-proBNP, N-terminal pro-B-type natriuretic peptide; NYHA, New York Heart Association; PCWP, pulmonary capillary wedge pressure; RAP, right atrial pressure.
From Crespo-Leiro MG, Metra M, Lund LH, Milicic D, Costanzo MR, Filippatos G, Gustafsson F, Tsui S, Barge-Caballero E, De Jonge N, Frigerio M, Hamdan R, Hasin T, Hülsmann M, Nalbantgil S, Potena L, Bauersachs J, Gkouziouta A, Ruhparwar A, Ristic AD, Straburzynska-Migaj E, McDonagh T, Seferovic P, Ruschitzka F. Advanced heart failure: a position statement of the Heart Failure Association of the European Society of Cardiology. Eur J Heart Fail. 2018 Nov;20(11):1505-1535.

Box 2
Previous definitions or advanced heart failure: American College of Cardiology/American Heart Association

1. Repeated ($\geq$2) hospitalizations or ED visits for HF in the past year

2. Progressive deterioration in renal function (eg, increase in BUN and creatinine)

3. Weight loss without other cause (eg, cardiac cachexia)

4. Intolerance to ACE inhibitors due to hypotension and/or worsening renal function

5. Intolerance to beta-blockers due to worsening HF or hypotension

6. Frequent systolic blood pressure less than 90 mm Hg

7. Persistent dyspnea with dressing or bathing requiring rest

8. Inability to walk 1 block on the level ground due to dyspnea or fatigue

9. Recent need to escalate diuretics to maintain volume status, often reaching daily furosemide equivalent dose greater than 160 mg/d and/or use of supplemental metolazone therapy

10. Progressive decline in serum sodium, usually to less than 133 mEq/L.

11. Frequent ICD shocks

Abbreviations: ACE, angiotensin-converting enzyme; BUN, blood urea nitrogen; ED, emergency department; ICD, implantable cardioverter-defibrillator.
From Crespo-Leiro MG, Metra M, Lund LH, Milicic D, Costanzo MR, Filippatos G, Gustafsson F, Tsui S, Barge-Caballero E, De Jonge N, Frigerio M, Hamdan R, Hasin T, Hülsmann M, Nalbantgil S, Potena L, Bauersachs J, Gkouziouta A, Ruhparwar A, Ristic AD, Straburzynska-Migaj E, McDonagh T, Seferovic P, Ruschitzka F. Advanced heart failure: a position statement of the Heart Failure Association of the European Society of Cardiology. Eur J Heart Fail. 2018 Nov;20(11):1505-1535.

recommended timing of different interventions are shown in **Table 1**. The INTERMACS classification includes 3 modifiers for profiles: temporary circulatory support (TCS), arrhythmia (A), and frequent flyer (FF). This classification has been useful to predict outcomes after durable MCS devices implantation[8] and also for patients undergoing urgent HT.[9] It has also been found useful for risk stratifying ambulatory patients with advanced HF (profiles 4, 5, 6, and 7) and for identifying and triaging candidates for advanced therapies.[10–12]

For patients in cardiogenic shock or at risk of developing it, the Society for Cardiovascular Angiography and Interventions developed a classification in 5 stages from "A" to "E" based on physical examination, laboratory values, and hemodynamics (**Fig. 1**). Stage A is "at risk" for cardiogenic shock, stage B is "beginning" shock, stage C is "classic" cardiogenic shock, stage D is "deteriorating", and E is "extremis." The difference between stages B and C is the presence of hypoperfusion, which is present in stages C and higher. Stage D defines the patient in whom the initial set of interventions chosen have not restored stability and adequate perfusion despite at least 30 minutes of observation, and stage E is the patient in extremis, highly unstable, often with cardiovascular collapse. This classification is simple, with clinical criteria readily available to both critical care and referral center health care professionals and provides a common language for physicians and surgeons,[13] and it facilitates a paradigm shift in the care of patients in cardiogenic shock, with a focus on early identification and aggressive treatment and with important logistical implications because not all the necessary resources, in particular temporary MCS devices, are available at each center and patients need to be referred in a timely manner. The Society of Cardiovascular Angiography and Interventions classification has proved its prognostic usefulness in contemporary, real-world cohorts of patients with cardiogenic shock.[14]

For patients with less severe HF who are being followed by nonadvanced HF specialists, a useful mnemonic "I NEED HELP" has been proposed to aid in the identification of patients with advanced HF and timely referral for consideration of advanced therapies.[15] This mnemonic integrates typical features such as a decline in functional status; severe reduction in LVEF; the need for inotropes; refractory congestion; hypotension; inability to uptitrate or maintain previously well-tolerated drugs such as RAASi, BB, or ARNI; hospitalizations, and electric instability or persistently high natriuretic peptide levels. **Table 2**.

The 2018 position statement of the Heart Failure Association of the European Society of Cardiology (HFA-ESC) on advanced HF[16] updated the 2007 criteria taking into account the availability of new therapies and emphasizing both the need for patients to be optimized on such therapies before being considered for advanced HF therapies and to refer the patient timely to advanced HF units. The updated HFA-ESC criteria are outlined in **Box 4**.

Compared with the former HFA-ESC definition[1] the main 2 changes in 2018 were in criterion 2 and 3. Criterion 2, which refers to severe cardiac dysfunction, was based on the 2016 ESC HF

Box 3
Previous definitions or advanced heart failure:
Heart Failure Society of America

The presence of progressive and/or persistent severe signs and symptoms of HF despite optimized medical, surgical, and device therapy. It is generally accompanied by frequent hospitalization, severely limited exertional tolerance, and poor quality of life and is associated with high morbidity and mortality. Importantly, the progressive decline should be primarily driven by the HF syndrome.

Indicators of advanced HF in the setting of optimal medical and electrical therapies that should trigger consideration of referral for evaluation of advanced therapies include

- Need for intravenous inotropic therapy for symptomatic relief or to maintain end-organ function
- Peak V_{O_2} less than 14 mL/kg/min or less than 50% of predicted
- 6MWT distance less than 300 m more than or equal to 2 HF admissions in the last 12 months
- More than 2 unscheduled visits (eg, ED or clinic) in the last 12 months
- Worsening right HF and secondary pulmonary hypertension
- Diuretic refractoriness associated with worsening renal function
- Circulatory–renal limitation to RAAS inhibition or beta-blocker therapy
- Progressive/persistent NYHA functional class III–IV symptoms
- Increased 1-year mortality (eg, 20%–25%) predicted by HF survival models (eg, SHFS, HFSS, and so forth)
- Progressive renal or hepatic end-organ dysfunction
- Persistent hyponatremia (serum sodium <134 mEq/L)
- Recurrent refractory ventricular tachyarrhythmias; frequent ICD shocks
- Cardiac cachexia
- Inability to perform ADL

Abbreviations: 6MWT, 6-minute walk test; ADL, activities of daily living; ED, emergency department; HFSS, Heart Failure Survival Score; ICD, implantable cardioverter-defibrillator; NYHA, New York Heart Association; RAAS, renin-angiotensin-aldosterone system; SHFS, Seattle Heart Failure Score.
From Crespo-Leiro MG, Metra M, Lund LH, Milicic D, Costanzo MR, Filippatos G, Gustafsson F, Tsui S, Barge-Caballero E, De Jonge N, Frigerio M, Hamdan R, Hasin T, Hülsmann M, Nalbantgil S, Potena L, Bauersachs J, Gkouziouta A, Ruhparwar A, Ristic AD,

Straburzynska-Migaj E, McDonagh T, Seferovic P, Ruschitzka F. Advanced heart failure: a position statement of the Heart Failure Association of the European Society of Cardiology. Eur J Heart Fail. 2018 Nov;20(11):1505-1535.

guidelines.[17] The ESC criteria were considered sufficient to define cardiac dysfunction, and they can be used for the definition of advanced HF when accompanied by other criteria that characterize patient severity. Using the ESC criteria for cardiac dysfunction gives the same importance to all patients with HF, independent of left ventricular ejection fraction (LVEF). Indeed, with a few exceptions, such as patients with hypertrophic cardiomyopathy or restrictive cardiomyopathy, most of the patients with an indication for HT or MCS have a reduced LVEF. However, at least 50% of patients hospitalized for acute HF have a preserved LVEF, and these patients can also be considered advanced, provided the other criteria outlined in the definition are present. Criterion 3 refers to HF hospitalization. In this sense, unplanned visits for HF were added and given the same value as hospital admissions. Malignant arrhythmias were added as major causes of acute events. This criterion acknowledge that acute events leading to one or more unplanned visits or hospitalizations within 12 months were the hallmark of advanced HF, independent of treatment, with emphasis placed on the instability of the clinical course and resource utilization.

This position statement on advanced HF includes proposals on triage of patients and appropriate timing of referral to advanced HF (**Fig. 2**).

EPIDEMIOLOGY

The prevalence of advanced HF is not well known and quite difficult to estimate. Epidemiologic studies of HF usually categorize patients according to functional status (eg, New York Heart Association [NYHA] class) and LVEF but do not according to advanced HF versus other less progressed stages.[18–20] Most of the information we have come from LVAD clinical trials and/or referral population to advanced HF centers, sometimes excluding the rest of the patients with advanced HF from the health care area, not referred to these centers, and who are, in fact, most of the patients. But even in centers with availability of advanced HF therapies, an unrecognized need for these therapies has been observed.[6]

A study conducted more than 2 decades ago, in Olmstead County, Minnesota (USA), population-based, cross-sectional design, in a random

Table 1
Interagency Registry for Mechanically Assisted Circulatory Support profile descriptions in patients with advanced heart failure

Profile	Time Frame for Intervention
Profile 1: Critical cardiogenic shock Patient with life-threatening hypotension despite rapidly escalating inotropic support, critical organ hypoperfusion, often confirmed by worsening acidosis and/or lactate levels. "Crash and burn."	Definitive intervention needed within hours.
Profile 2: progressive decline Patient with declining function despite intravenous inotropic support may be manifested by worsening renal function, nutritional depletion, or inability to restore volume balance. "Sliding on inotropes." Also describes declining status in patients unable to tolerate inotropic therapy.	Definitive intervention needed within few days.
Profile 3: stable but inotrope dependent Patient with stable blood pressure, organ function, nutrition, and symptoms on continuous intravenous inotropic support (or a temporary circulatory support device or both) but demonstrating repeated failure to wean from support due to recurrent symptomatic hypotension or renal dysfunction. "Dependent stability."	Definitive intervention elective over a period of weeks to few months.
Profile 4: resting symptoms Patient can be stabilized close to normal volume status but experiences daily symptoms of congestion at rest or during ADL. Doses of diuretics generally fluctuate at very high levels. More intensive management and surveillance strategies should be considered, which may in some cases reveal poor compliance that would compromise outcomes with any therapy. Some patients may shuttle between 4 and 5.	Definitive intervention elective over a period of weeks to few months.
Profile 5: exertion intolerant Comfortable at rest and with ADL but unable to engage in any other activity, living predominantly within the house. Patients are comfortable at rest without congestive symptoms, but may have underlying refractory elevated volume status, often with renal dysfunction. If underlying nutritional status and organ function are marginal, patients may be more at risk than INTERMACS 4 and require definitive intervention.	Variable urgency, depends on maintenance of nutrition, organ function, and activity.
Profile 6: exertion limited Patient without evidence of fluid overload is comfortable at rest and with ADL and minor activities outside the home but fatigues after the first few minutes of any meaningful activity. Attribution to cardiac limitation requires careful measurement of peak oxygen consumption, in some cases with hemodynamic monitoring to confirm severity of cardiac impairment "walking wounded."	Variable, depends on maintenance of nutrition, organ function, and activity level.
Profile 7: advanced NYHA class III A placeholder for more precise specification in future; this level includes patients who are without current or recent episodes of unstable fluid balance, living comfortably with meaningful activity limited to mild physical exertion.	Transplantation or circulatory support may not currently be indicated.

Modifiers for Profiles	Possible Profiles to Modify
TCS: temporary circulatory support can modify only patients in hospital (other devices would be INTERMACS devices). This includes IABP, ECMO. TandemHeart, Levitronix, BVS 5000 or AB5000, Impella.	1, 2, 3 in hospital.
A: arrhythmia can modify any profile. Recurrent ventricular tachyarrhythmias that have recently contributed substantially to clinical compromise. This includes frequent ICD shocks or requirement for external defibrillator, usually more than twice weekly.	Any profile.
FF: frequent flyer can modify only outpatients, designating a patient requiring frequent emergency visits or hospitalizations for diuretics, ultrafiltration, or temporary intravenous vasoactive therapy.	3 if at home, 4, 5, 6. A Frequent Flyer would rarely be profile 7.

Abbreviations: ADL, activities of daily living; ECMO, extracorporeal membrane oxygenation; IABP, intraaortic balloon pump; ICD, implantable cardioverter-defibrillator; NYHA, New York Heart Association.

From Stevenson LW, Pagani FD, Young JB, Jessup M, Miller L, Kormos RL, et al. INTERMACS profiles of advanced heart failure: the current picture. J Heart Lung Transplant. 2009;28:535-41; with permission.

sample of 2029 residents 45 years and older, found that advanced HF (stage D) affected 0.2% of the population assessed and 2% of those with HF. However, in this study stage D was operationally defined as history of HF and functional class IV according to a self-administered questionnaire, in which the participant was able to perform activity—less than 2 metabolic equivalents (METS).[21] Criteria for defining advanced HF have changed over time,[22] and the difficulty in making estimates is well illustrated in a systematic review by Bjork and colleagues (2016) (#7721 of criteria used in clinical trials, including 134 publications). In this study, in addition to the 2 most commonly

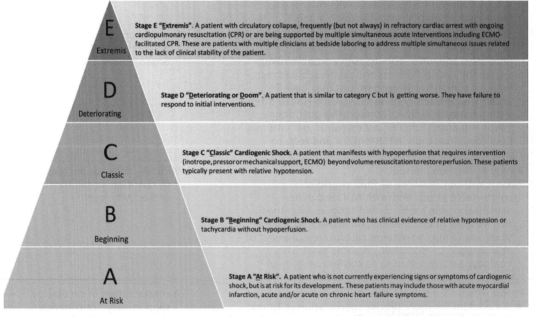

Fig. 1. Society for the cardiovascular angiography and intervention classification of cardiogenic shock. (*From* Baran DA, Grines CL, Bailey S, Burkhoff D, Hall SA, Henry TD, et al. SCAI clinical expert consensus statement on the classification of cardiogenic shock: This document was endorsed by the American College of Cardiology (ACC), the American Heart Association (AHA), the Society of Critical Care Medicine (SCCM), and the Society of Thoracic Surgeons (STS) in April 2019. Catheter Cardiovasc Interv. 2019;94(1):29-37.)

Table 2
I NEED HELP. Markers of advanced heart failure

_I_	Inotropes	Previous or ongoing requirement for dobutamine, milrinone, dopamine, or levosimendan
_N_	NYHA class/ natriuretic peptides	Persisting NYHA class III or IV and/or persistently high BNP or NT-proBNP
_E_	End-organ dysfunction	Worsening renal or liver dysfunction in the setting of heart failure
_E_	Ejection fraction	Very low ejection fraction <20%
_D_	Defibrillator shocks	Recurrent appropriate defibrillator shocks
_H_	Hospitalizations	More than 1 hospitalization with heart failure in the last 12 mo
_E_	Edema/escalating diuretics	Persisting fluid overload and/or increasing diuretic requirement
_L_	Low-blood pressure	Consistently low BP with systolic <90–100 mm Hg
_P_	Prognostic medication	Inability to uptitrate (or need to decrease/cease) ACEI, beta-blockers, ARNIs, or MRAs

Abbreviation: ACEI, angiotensin-converting enzyme inhibitor.
From Baumwol J. "I Need Help"-A mnemonic to aid timely referral in advanced heart failure. J Heart Lung Transplant. 2017;36(5):593-4; with permission.

Box 4
Heart Failure Association of the European Society of Cardiology 2018 criteria for defining advanced heart failure

All the following criteria must be present despite optimal guideline-directed treatment:

1. Severe and persistent symptoms of heart failure (NYHA class III [advanced] or IV).

2. Severe cardiac dysfunction defined by a reduced LVEF less than or equal to 30%, isolated RV failure (eg, ARVC) or nonoperable severe valve abnormalities or congenital abnormalities or persistently high (or increasing) BNP or NT-proBNP values and data of severe diastolic dysfunction or LV structural abnormalities according to the ESC definition of HFpEF and HFmrEF.[9]

3. Episodes of pulmonary or systemic congestion requiring high-dose intravenous diuretics (or diuretic combinations) or episodes of low output requiring inotropes or vasoactive drugs or malignant arrhythmias causing more than 1 unplanned visit or hospitalization in the last 12 months.

4. Severe impairment of exercise capacity with inability to exercise or low 6MWTD (<300 m) or pVO$_2$ (<12–14 mL/kg/min), estimated to be of cardiac origin.

In addition to the aforementioned criteria, extracardiac organ dysfunction due to heart failure (eg, cardiac cachexia, liver, or kidney dysfunction) or type 2 pulmonary hypertension may be present but are not required.

Criteria 1 and 4 can be met in patients who have cardiac dysfunction (as described in criterion #2) but who also have substantial limitation due to other conditions (eg, severe pulmonary disease, noncardiac cirrhosis, or most commonly by renal disease with mixed etiology). These patients still have limited quality of life and survival due to advanced disease and warrant the same intensity of evaluation as someone in whom the only disease is cardiac, but the therapeutic options for these patients are usually more limited.

Abbreviations: 6MWTD, 6-minute walk test distance; ARVC, arrhythmogenic right ventricular cardiomyopathy; BNP, B-type natriuretic peptide; ESC, European society of cardiology; HFA, heart failure association; HFmrEF, heart failure with mid-range ejection fraction; HFpEF, heart failure with preserved ejection fraction; LV, left ventricular; LVEF, left ventricular ejection fraction; NT-proBNP, N-terminal pro-B-type natriuretic peptide; NYHA, New York Heart Association; pVO$_2$, peak exercise oxygen consumption; RV, right ventricular.
From Crespo-Leiro MG, Metra M, Lund LH, Milicic D, Costanzo MR, Filippatos G, Gustafsson F, Tsui S, Barge-Caballero E, De Jonge N, Frigerio M, Hamdan R, Hasin T, Hülsmann M, Nalbantgil S, Potena L, Bauersachs J, Gkouziouta A, Ruhparwar A, Ristic AD, Straburzynska-Migaj E, McDonagh T, Seferovic P, Ruschitzka F. Advanced heart failure: a position statement of the Heart Failure Association of the European Society of Cardiology. Eur J Heart Fail. 2018 Nov;20(11):1505-1535.

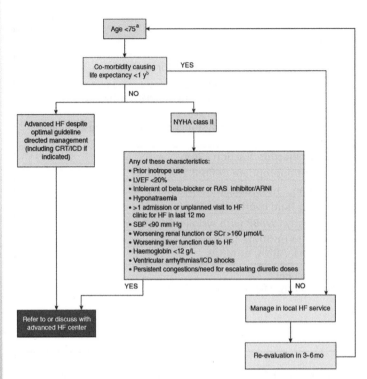

Fig. 2. Triage of patients with advanced HF and appropriate timing of referral.[a] >75 years if good functional status apart from HF (mono-organ disease). [b]e.g. untreatable cancer, dementia, severe COPD (*From* Crespo-Leiro MG, Metra M, Lund LH, Milicic D, Costanzo MR, Filippatos G, Gustafsson F, Tsui S, Barge-Caballero E, De Jonge N, Frigerio M, Hamdan R, Hasin T, Hülsmann M, Nalbantgil S, Potena L, Bauersachs J, Gkouziouta A, Ruhparwar A, Ristic AD, Straburzynska-Migaj E, McDonagh T, Seferovic P, Ruschitzka F. Advanced heart failure: a position statement of the Heart Failure Association of the European Society of Cardiology. Eur J Heart Fail. 2018 Nov;20(11):1505-1535.)

used criteria (NYHA and LVEF), there were a wide array of criteria used such as inotrope-dependent status in 12.7%, peak oxygen consumption in 10.4%, previous hospitalizations in 10.4%, cardiac index in 10.4%, or transplant listing status in 5.2%, and it was found there is little consistency both in criteria selection and quantitative cut-off points.[20] The sequential development of more disease-modifying therapies over the past several decades has dramatically changed the prognosis of patients with HF and explain that the prevalence of advanced disease is increasing, due to growing number of patients with HF and their better treatment and survival.[23–25] Until now, none of the available therapies can cure HF. Current treatments can maintain clinical stability for a certain period of time, even with quite good quality of life, but the risk of disease progression persists over time. More recent studies estimate that patients with advanced HF account for 1% to 10% of the overall HF population[3,26] and from patients who receive care in a referral center, 4.5% progressed to advanced HF every year.[27]

In the absence of life-prolonging therapies such as HT or LVADs the prognosis of patients with advanced HF is poor. In the landmark trial REMATCH[28] in which patients ineligible for HT were randomized to first-generation LVAD implantation or optimal medical management, the 1- and 2-year survival of patients in the medical therapy

group was 25% and 8%, respectively. However, since this study different criteria for defining the patient population may have modified these estimates. In addition to the poor survival and quality of life of these patients, the medical therapy is associated with significant costs and resource consumption, which increase as death approaches, as it was shown in one study that 50% of costs was spent in the last 6 months.[29]

CLINICAL COURSE

In patients with NYHA functional class III or ACC/AHA stage C, the clinical course is mainly determined by congestion due to volume overload from LV dysfunction with elevated LV end-diastolic pressure but still normal systemic blood pressure and stroke volume. When patients progress to advanced HF a progressive reduction in stroke volume determinates the clinical picture with consequent multiorgan damage, declining renal function, liver congestion, pulmonary hypertension, and cardiac cachexia. In patients with HF with reduced ejection fraction the reduction on stroke volume is often accompanied by LV dilation and varying degrees of secondary mitral regurgitation, which further reduces the stroke volume. In addition, the progression of HF is followed by greater electrical instability.[18,30]

The typical signs and symptoms of advanced HF include a progressive decline in functional status, with symptoms at rest or with minimal effort, refractory congestion needing escalating doses of diuretics or the use of combinations of diuretics, hypotension, inability to maintain disease-modifying therapies, the need for inotropes, and symptomatic ventricular arrhythmias. These characteristics are well reflected in the definitions and criteria discussed earlier.

However, the clinical course of patients with advanced HF can be highly unpredictable even for experienced clinicians for many reasons, including persistent activation of disease pathways that are not fully blocked by neurohormonal antagonists, new episodes of myocardial damage or valvular dysfunction, development of pulmonary hypertension, right ventricular failure and

cardiorenal syndrome, as well as the cumulative effect of multiorgan damage, environmental factors, and comorbidities.[31] Moreover, some comorbidities (renal dysfunction, pulmonary hypertension) can be consequences, as well as causes of advanced HF, and sometimes a proper treatment of the cardiac disease can lead to improvement in the comorbid condition.

Patients who are considered as potential candidates for advanced therapies should be referred in a timely manner to an Advanced HF Center, and parameters have been established to refer the patient before it is too late. The concept is that patients are not necessarily referred to receive these advanced HF therapies immediately, but they can be evaluated for a potential candidacy for HT and/or LVAD—that is, a thorough evaluation aimed to confirm indications rule out

Table 3
Suggested clinical, laboratory, and echocardiographic criteria to trigger referral

Clinical[a]	Laboratory	Imaging	Risk Score Data
• >1 HF hospitalization in last year • NYHA class III–IV • Intolerant of optimal dose of any GDMT HF drug • Increasing diuretic requirement • SBP ≤90 mm Hg • Inability to perform CPET • 6MWT • CRT nonresponder clinically • Cachexia, unintentional weight loss • KCCQ • MLHFQ	• eGFR <45 mL/min • SCr ≥160 mmol/L • K >5.2 or <3.5 mmol/L • Hyponatraemia • Hb ≤120 g/L • NT-proBNP ≥1000 pg/mL • Abnormal liver function test • Low albumin	• LVEF ≤30% • Large area of akinesis/dyskinesis or aneurysm • Moderate[b]–severe mitral regurgitation • RV dysfunction • PA pressure ≥50 mm Hg • Moderate-severe tricuspid regurgitation • Difficult to grade aortic stenosis • IVC dilated or without respiratory variation	• MAGGIC predicted survival ≤80% at 1 y • SHFM predicted survival ≤80% at 1 y

Abbreviations: 6MWT, 6-minute walk test; CPET, cardiopulmonary exercise test; CRT, cardiac resynchronization therapy; eGFR, estimated glomerular filtration rate; GDMT, guideline-directed medical therapy; Hb, hemoglobin; HF, heart failure; IVC, inferior vena cava; K, potassium; KCCQ, Kansas City Cardiomyopathy Questionnaire; LVEF, left ventricular ejection fraction; MAGGIC, Meta-Analysis Global Group in Chronic Heart Failure; MLHFQ, Minnesota Living with Heart Failure Questionnaire; Na, sodium; NT-proBNP, N-terminal pro-B-type natriuretic peptide; NYHA, New York Heart Association; PA, pulmonary artery; RV, right ventricular; SCr, serum creatinine; SBP, systolic blood pressure; SHFM, Seattle Heart Failure Model.

[a] Note that this table reflects many clinically relevant but sometimes subjective and nonspecific criteria. With these criteria, sensitivity has been prioritized over specificity, that is, many criteria may be present in patients who do not need referral, but by considering these criteria in a comprehensive assessment, there is a lower risk that high-risk patients may be missed or referred too late. Although cut-offs exist for transplantation listing or LVAD implantation, there are no data to support specific cut-offs for referral to an HF center.

[b] Moderate MR alone is not sufficient, but moderate MR is one factor suggesting risk of progression and should be considered together with other variables.

From Crespo-Leiro MG, Metra M, Lund LH, Milicic D, Costanzo MR, Filippatos G, Gustafsson F, Tsui S, Barge-Caballero E, De Jonge N, Frigerio M, Hamdan R, Hasin T, Hülsmann M, Nalbantgil S, Potena L, Bauersachs J, Gkouziouta A, Ruhparwar A, Ristic AD, Straburzynska-Migaj E, McDonagh T, Seferovic P, Ruschitzka F. Advanced heart failure: a position statement of the Heart Failure Association of the European Society of Cardiology. Eur J Heart Fail. 2018 Nov;20(11):1505-1535.

Table 4
Prognostic scores in heart failure

Score	Components	Comments
HFSS	• Presence/absence coronary artery disease • Resting heart rate • Left ventricular ejection fraction • Mean arterial blood pressure • Presence/absence of intraventricular conduction delay • Serum sodium • Peak oxygen uptake HFSS = [(0.0216 * resting HR) + (−0.0255 * mean BP) + (−0.0464 * LVEF) + (−0.047 * serum sodium) + (−0.0546 * peak V_{O_2}) + (0.608 * presence or absence of IVCD) + (0.6931 * presence or absence of ischemic heart disease)]	Score is based on a sum of these variables multiplied by defined coefficients Low risk: ≥8.1 Medium-risk: HFSS 7.20–8.09 High-risk: HFSS ≤7.1
SHFM	• Demographics • Clinical characteristics • Medications • Laboratory data • Devices www.seattleheartfailuremodel.org/	Incorporates impact of interventions (medical and device) and provides estimates of 1, 2, and 5-y survival
MECKI	• Percent predicted peak V_{O_2} • VE/VCO$_2$ slope • Hemoglobin • Serum sodium • LVEF • eGFR by MDRD	Incorporates data from the CPET as well as kidney function
MAGGIC	• Age • Gender • Left ventricular ejection fraction • Systolic blood pressure • Body mass index • Serum creatinine • NYHA class • Smoking history • Comorbidities (eg, diabetes, COPD) • Length of heart failure diagnosis • Medications www.heartfailurerisk.org/	Risk model converted into integer score Generalizable to broad spectrum of patients

Abbreviations: BP, blood pressure; COPD, chronic obstructive pulmonary disease; CPET, cardiopulmonary exercise test; eGFR, estimated glomerular filtration rate; HFSS, Heart Failure Survival Score; HR, heart rate; IVCD, intraventricular conduction defect; LVEF, left ventricular ejection fraction; MAGGIC, Meta-Analysis Global Group in Chronic Heart Failure; MDRD, modification of diet in renal disease; NYHA, New York Heart Association; SHFM, Seattle Heart Failure Model, VE/VCO2, minute ventilation carbon dioxide production relationship; V_{O_2}, oxygen consumption.

From Crespo-Leiro MG, Metra M, Lund LH, Milicic D, Costanzo MR, Filippatos G, Gustafsson F, Tsui S, Barge-Caballero E, De Jonge N, Frigerio M, Hamdan R, Hasin T, Hülsmann M, Nalbantgil S, Potena L, Bauersachs J, Gkouziouta A, Ruhparwar A, Ristic AD, Straburzynska-Migaj E, McDonagh T, Seferovic P, Ruschitzka F. Advanced heart failure: a position statement of the Heart Failure Association of the European Society of Cardiology. Eur J Heart Fail. 2018 Nov;20(11):1505-1535.

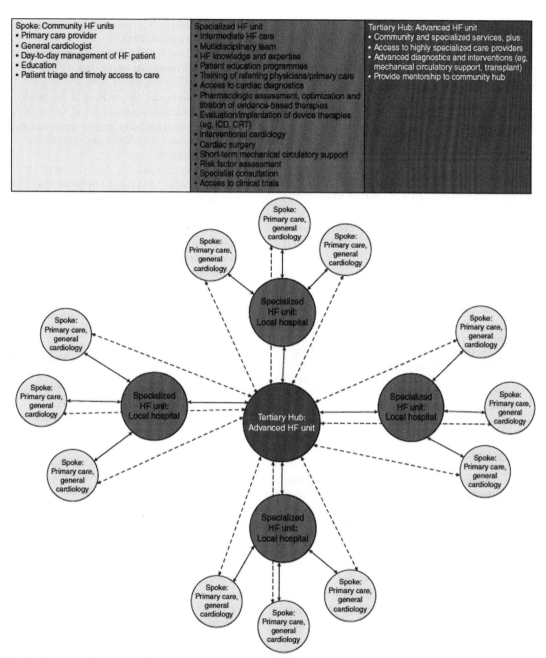

Spoke: Community HF units
- Primary care provider
- General cardiologist
- Day-to-day management of HF patient
- Education
- Patient triage and timely access to care

Specialized HF unit
- Intermediate HF care
- Multidisciplinary team
- HF knowledge and expertise
- Patient education programmes
- Training of referring physicians/primary care
- Access to cardiac diagnostics
- Pharmacologic assessment, optimization and titration of evidence-based therapies
- Evaluation/implantation of device therapies (eg, ICD, CRT)
- Interventional cardiology
- Cardiac surgery
- Short-term mechanical circulatory support
- Risk factor assessment
- Specialist consultation
- Access to clinical trials

Tertiary Hub: Advanced HF unit
- Community and specialized services, plus:
- Access to highly specialized care providers
- Advanced diagnostics and interventions (eg, mechanical circulatory support, transplant)
- Provide mentorship to community hub

Fig. 3. Conceptual structure of a hub and spoke model of care for patients with advanced HF. (*From* Crespo-Leiro MG, Metra M, Lund LH, Milicic D, Costanzo MR, Filippatos G, Gustafsson F, Tsui S, Barge-Caballero E, De Jonge N, Frigerio M, Hamdan R, Hasin T, Hülsmann M, Nalbantgil S, Potena L, Bauersachs J, Gkouziouta A, Ruhparwar A, Ristic AD, Straburzynska-Migaj E, McDonagh T, Seferovic P, Ruschitzka F. Advanced heart failure: a position statement of the Heart Failure Association of the European Society of Cardiology. Eur J Heart Fail. 2018 Nov;20(11):1505-1535.)

contraindications and establish the proper time of intervention—if required. **Table 3** shows the suggested clinical, laboratory, and echocardiographic criteria to trigger referral, with specific comments on the prognostic scores more used in HF (**Table 4**), established in the 2018 HFA-ESC position statement. This document was intended primarily for professionals unfamiliar with advanced therapies who are caring for patients with HF, to correctly identify which patients are at an advanced stage and may be candidates for specific therapies that require timely referral to centers that can offer them and suggest an operational interactional "Hub and Spoke" networking, facilitating both communication and transitional care of patients between centers with different HF resources[18] (Fig. 3).

CLINICS CARE POINTS

Evidence-based pearls:

- The 1-year survival after HT and/or long-term MCS is approaching 80% to 90%.
- Timely referral to advanced HF centers and careful patient selection are critical for optimal outcomes.

Pitfalls

- The prevalence of advanced HF is not well known.
- The clinical course of patients with HF is highly unpredictable and a challenge even for experts in HF, as there are many influencing factors such as different responses to treatment or sudden instability due to pathologies and/or intercurrent circumstances, both of cardiac or extracardiac origin.

DISCLOSURE

Maria Generosa Crespo-Leiro and Eduardo Barge-Caballero, are members of the "CIBERCV" network of the Instituto de Salud Carlos III, which provides research funds to their institution.

REFERENCES

1. Metra M, Ponikowski P, Dickstein K, et al. Advanced chronic heart failure: a position statement from the study group on advanced heart failure of the Heart Failure Association of the European Society of Cardiology. Eur J Heart Fail 2007;9(6–7):684–94.
2. Yancy CW, Jessup M, Bozkurt B, et al. 2013 ACCF/AHA guideline for the management of heart failure: executive summary: a report of the American College of Cardiology Foundation/American Heart Association Task Force on practice guidelines. Circulation 2013;128(16):1810–52.
3. Fang JC, Ewald GA, Allen LA, et al. Advanced (stage D) heart failure: a statement from the Heart Failure Society of America Guidelines Committee. J Card Fail 2015;21(6):519–34.
4. Khush KK, Potena L, Cherikh WS, et al. The international thoracic organ transplant registry of the international society for heart and lung transplantation: 37th adult heart transplantation report-2020; focus on deceased donor characteristics. J Heart Lung Transpl 2020;39(10):1003–15.
5. Mehra MR, Uriel N, Naka Y, et al. A fully magnetically levitated left ventricular assist device - final report. N Engl J Med 2019;380(17):1618–27.
6. Lund LH, Trochu JN, Meyns B, et al. Screening for heart transplantation and left ventricular assist system: results from the ScrEEning for advanced Heart Failure treatment (SEE-HF) study. Eur J Heart Fail 2018;20(1):152–60.
7. Stevenson LW, Pagani FD, Young JB, et al. INTERMACS profiles of advanced heart failure: the current picture. J Heart Lung Transpl 2009;28:535–41.
8. Kirklin JK, Naftel DC, Kormos RL, et al. Fifth INTERMACS annual report: risk factor analysis from more than 6,000 mechanical circulatory support patients. J Heart Lung Transpl 2013;32:141–56.
9. Barge-Caballero E, Segovia-Cubero J, Almenar-Bonet L, et al. Preoperative INTERMACS profiles determine postoperative outcomes in critically ill patients undergoing emergency heart transplantation: analysis of the Spanish National Heart Transplant Registry. Circ Heart Fail 2013;6(4):763–72.
10. Kittleson MM, Shah P, Lala A, et al. INTERMACS profiles and outcomes of ambulatory advanced heart failure patients: a report from the REVIVAL Registry. J Heart Lung Transpl 2020;39(1):16–26.
11. Hedley JS, Samman-Tahhan A, McCue AA, et al. Definitions of Stage D heart failure and outcomes among outpatients with heart failure and reduced ejection fraction. Int J Cardiol 2018;272:250–4.
12. Ambardekar AV, Kittleson MM, Palardy M, et al. Outcomes with ambulatory advanced heart failure from the Medical Arm of Mechanically Assisted Circulatory Support (MedaMACS) registry. J Heart Lung Transpl 2019;38(4):408–17.
13. Baran DA, Grines CL, Bailey S, et al. SCAI clinical expert consensus statement on the classification of cardiogenic shock: This document was endorsed by the American College of Cardiology (ACC), the American Heart Association (AHA), the Society of Critical Care Medicine (SCCM), and the Society of Thoracic Surgeons (STS) in April 2019. Catheter Cardiovasc Interv 2019;94(1):29–37.
14. Baran DA, Long A, Badiye AP, et al. Prospective validation of the SCAI shock classification: single center analysis. Catheter Cardiovasc Interv 2020;96(7):1339–47.
15. Baumwol J. "I Need Help"-A mnemonic to aid timely referral in advanced heart failure. J Heart Lung Transpl 2017;36(5):593–4.
16. Crespo-Leiro MG, Metra M, Lund LH, et al. Advanced heart failure: a position statement of the Heart Failure Association of the European Society of Cardiology. Eur J Heart Fail 2018;20(11):1505–35.
17. Ponikowski P, Voors AA, Anker SD, et al. 2016 ESC guidelines for the diagnosis and treatment of acute

and chronic heart failure: the task force for the diagnosis and treatment of acute and chronic heart failure of the European Society of Cardiology (ESC). Developed with the special contribution of the Heart Failure Association (HFA) of the ESC. Eur J Heart Fail 2016;18(8):891–975.

18. Crespo-Leiro MG, Anker SD, Maggioni AP, et al. European Society of Cardiology Heart Failure Long-Term Registry (ESC-HF-LT): 1-year follow-up outcomes and differences across regions. Eur J Heart Fail 2016;18(6):613–25.

19. Virani SS, Alonso A, Benjamin EJ, et al. Heart disease and stroke statistics-2020 update: a report from the American Heart Association. Circulation 2020;141(9):e139–596.

20. Bjork JB, Alton KK, Georgiopoulou VV, et al. Defining advanced heart failure: a systematic review of criteria used in clinical trials. J Card Fail 2016; 22(7):569–77.

21. Ammar KA, Jacobsen SJ, Mahoney DW, et al. Prevalence and prognostic significance of heart failure stages: application of the American College of Cardiology/American Heart Association heart failure staging criteria in the community. Circulation 2007; 115(12):1563–70.

22. Abouezzeddine OF, Redfield MM. Who has advanced heart failure?: definition and epidemiology. Congest Heart Fail 2011;17(4):160–8.

23. Bhatt AS, Abraham WT, Lindenfeld J, et al. Treatment of HF in an era of multiple therapies: statement from the HF Collaboratory. JACC Heart Fail 2021; 9(1):1–12.

24. Truby LK, Rogers JG. Advanced heart failure: epidemiology, diagnosis, and therapeutic approaches. JACC Heart Fail 2020;8(7):523–36.

25. Gidding SS, Lloyd-Jones D, Lima J, et al. Prevalence of American Heart Association Heart Failure Stages in black and white young and middle-aged adults: the CARDIA study. Circ Heart Fail 2019; 12(9):e005730.

26. Xanthakis V, Enserro DM, Larson MG, et al. Prevalence, neurohormonal correlates, and prognosis of heart failure stages in the community. JACC Heart Fail 2016;4(10):808–15.

27. Kalogeropoulos AP, Samman-Tahhan A, Hedley JS, et al. Progression to Stage D heart failure among outpatients with stage c heart failure and reduced ejection fraction. JACC Heart Fail 2017;5(7):528–37.

28. Rose EA, Gelijns AC, Moskowitz AJ, et al. Long-term use of a left ventricular assist device for end-stage heart failure. N Engl J Med 2001;345(20):1435–43.

29. Russo MJ, Gelijns AC, Stevenson LW, et al. The cost of medical management in advanced heart failure during the final two years of life. J Card Fail 2008; 14(8):651–8.

30. Guglin M, Zucker MJ, Borlaug BA, et al. Evaluation for heart transplantation and LVAD implantation: JACC council perspectives. J Am Coll Cardiol 2020;75(12):1471–87.

31. Greenberg B, Fang J, Mehra M, et al. Advanced heart failure: trans-atlantic perspectives on the Heart Failure Association of the European Society of Cardiology position statement. Eur J Heart Fail 2018; 20(11):1536–9.

Echocardiography in Advanced Heart Failure for Diagnosis, Management, and Prognosis

Enrico Melillo, MD[a],*, Daniele Masarone, MD, PhD[a], Jae K. Oh, MD[b],
Marina Verrengia, MD[a], Fabio Valente, MD[a], Rossella Vastarella, MD[a],
Ernesto Ammendola, MD[a], Roberta Pacileo, MD[a], Giuseppe Pacileo, MD[a]

KEYWORDS

- Advanced heart failure • Advanced imaging • Echocardiography • Prognosis
- Therapeutic management

KEY POINTS

- Echocardiography plays a key role in diagnosis, risk stratification, and decision-making in advanced heart failure.
- A multiparametric approach, including anatomic and functional diagnostic tools, is highly advised for complete evaluation of patients with advanced heart failure.
- The primary focus is to identify an exhaustive imaging framework of right ventricle systolic performance, which is crucial for prognosis and therapy.
- Novel advanced echocardiographic imaging has been widely studied in the last few years and is being progressively integrated into daily practice.

INTRODUCTION

Advanced heart failure (AHF) represents an end-stage disease in which patients present a severe impairment of functional capacity despite optimized guideline-directed medical therapy (GDMT) and frequent episodes of congestive or low-output decompensated phases causing repetitive hospitalizations and requiring consideration of more aggressive therapeutic options like mechanical circulatory support or heart transplant (HTx).[1] Proper and early recognition of the transition to such end-stage phase is crucial to timely selection of tailored therapeutic options and improving survival and prognosis. Despite a recent transition to a multimodality imaging approach in the cardiovascular field, echocardiography remains the gold standard and first-line approach for evaluation of patients with heart failure (HF),

providing fundamental diagnostic tools and defining the prognostic and therapeutic landscapes in AHF. Moreover, recent technological advances have improved the daily clinical practice diagnostic armamentarium for evaluating patients with HF. In the present chapter, we provide an overview of the role of echocardiography in the management of patients with AHF, underscoring its pivotal role for diagnostic and prognostic assessment and guiding the therapeutic decision-making process.

Echocardiographic Evaluation of Heart Failure Severity and Prognosis

Echocardiography remains the mainstay for diagnostic assessment of AHF, thanks to its noninvasive nature, which enables accurate depictions of cardiac anatomy and physiology with high

[a] Heart Failure Unit, AORN dei Colli, Monaldi Hospital, Naples, Italy; [b] Department of Cardiovascular Medicine, Mayo Clinic, Rochester, MN, USA
* Corresponding author.
E-mail address: doc.emelillo88@gmail.com

Heart Failure Clin 17 (2021) 547–560
https://doi.org/10.1016/j.hfc.2021.05.001
1551-7136/21/© 2021 Elsevier Inc. All rights reserved.

sensitivity and specificity.[2] The presence of resting symptoms, severe impairment of functional capacity, and identification of irreversible causes of HF are key elements for defining AHF. In this setting, raw bidimensional echocardiography can identify the HF anatomic phenotype, such as the dilated or hypertrophic remodeling of the left ventricle (LV) with eventual primary involvement of the right ventricle (RV) and functional classification according to the prevalence of systolic (HF with reduced ejection; HFrEF; HF with midrange ejection fraction; HFmEF) or diastolic impairment (eg, HF with preserved ejection fraction; HFpEF).[2,3] Ischemic heart disease, suggested by the presence of scarred/akinetic wall motion anomalies, dilated cardiomyopathy resulting in globally hypokinetic LV, congenital heart disease, primary RV enlargement and impairment, pericardial effusion/constriction or severe valvular heart disease with potentially reversible as well as irreversible causes of AHF, can be assessed by echocardiographic study along with clinical (NYHA class, 6-minute walking distance, Vo_2 max of cardiopulmonary exercise test) and biochemical (NT-proBNP) assessment.[4] Alongside diagnostic phenotyping, echocardiography can preliminary provide prognostic elements. In the Beta-Blocker Evaluation in Survival trial, independent echocardiographic predictors of adverse outcome among patients with HF and LVEF less than 35% were index left ventricle end-diastolic volume (cutoff 120 mL/m^2), mitral deceleration time (cutoff 150 ms), and degree of mitral regurgitation (MR).[5] The severe impairment of LV systolic function,[6] the coexistence of RV impairment, and pulmonary hypertension (PH)[7–9] are further risk markers emphasizing a worse outcome and an early referral to an AHF specialist center.[1]

Assessment of Left Ventricle Systolic Function and Geometry: Beyond Ejection Fraction

Systolic contraction of the LV is a dynamic process that involves coordinated contraction of subendocardial, midwall, and subepicardial muscle fibers. Midwall fibers have a circumferential disposition, and their contractions are responsible for a shortening of the minor axis of the LV with a major contribution to the generation of stroke volume (SV). Subepicardial and subendocardial muscle fibers have a longitudinal disposition and generate a shortening of the long axis of the LV. Furthermore, the apex of the LV rotates counterclockwise in systole and the base clockwise in diastole in a twisting motion. The main variables influencing LV systolic performance are preload, afterload, myocardial contractility, and heart rate.

The most recommended echocardiographic parameter for evaluating LV systolic function is LVEF, calculated as (end-diastolic volume − end-systolic volume)/end-diastolic volume and should be calculated using the biplane disk's summation method on apical 4-chamber and 2-chamber views[10] (Fig. 1, Panel A). LVEF is a universally recognized prognostic marker and classifier of different HF profiles and phenotypes.[11] Main advantages are easy bedside and visual assessment. However, acute changes in loading conditions can significantly influence LVEF; moreover, calculation of LV volumes can be operator-dependent and require experienced hands because foreshortened acquisitions of apical views (resulting in lack of visualization of the apex) and incorrect definition of endocardial borders can result in significant underestimation.

LV, SV, and cardiac output (CO) are integrative echocardiographic measures of pump function. These indexes are evaluated using the PW Doppler sample of LV outflow tract (LVOT) velocity at the aortic annulus height in apical 5-chamber view and measuring LVOT diameter in mid-systole from parasternal long axis view[10] (see Fig. 1, panel B), and several studies have shown a good agreement between noninvasive measures and right heart catheterization assessment in patients with HF.[12,13] LVEF should be integrated with the SV measure when evaluating patients with AHF because SV provides an effective hemodynamic measure of anterograde pump function, and in presence of a severely enlarged LV, a frequent mismatch between reduced LVEF and preserved SV can be observed in chronic compensated AHF in patients, probably explained by the adaptive remodeling of the failing LV and physically by means of Laplace's law. In this regard, an extensive echocardiographic study in HF patients with different ranges of LVEF showed that SV was preserved until a reduction in LVEF less than 20% was observed, suggesting that this threshold could be used as a red flag for transition to AHF.[14] An SV index (SVi) < 30 mL/m^2 is a powerful predictor of all-cause mortality in hospitalized HF patients, with a stronger risk stratification than a per-minute approach (cardiac index) and the traditional cutoff of low flow state defined as an SVi less than 35 mL/m^2.[15] Furthermore, uptitration of GDMT through an echo-guided approach based on the evaluation of LV filling pressures and SV resulted in significantly lower mortality and HF hospitalization rates than a non-echo-guided strategy.[16] This evidence suggests that SV is a clinically meaningful tool for therapeutic decision-making and driving prognosis in patients with AHF,

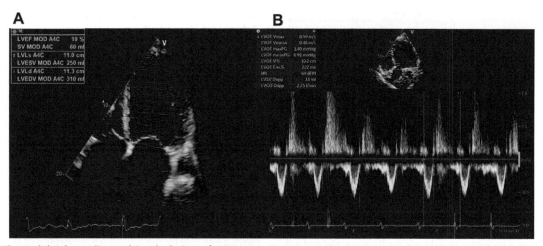

Fig. 1. (A) Echocardiographic calculation of LVEF using Simpson method, tracing endocardial border of the LV in apical 4-chamber view with estimation of left ventricle end-diastolic and end-systolic volumes. (B) PW Doppler sampling of the left ventricle outflow tract in apical 5-chamber view with measurement of SV and CO by tracing LVOT trace and measuring heart rate.

promoting its routine assessment in daily clinical practice.

Even though LVEF and SV are reference indexes for diagnosis and risk stratification, LV analysis of myocardial deformation through 2-D speckle tracking echocardiography (STE) can provide further depiction of LV contractile function beyond ejection fraction. STE measures local myocardial deformation during cardiac cycle through the longitudinal, circumferential, and radial planes, also enabling assessment of LV twist and rotation. Strain is a dimensionless parameter depicting change in length at 2 different time points. The speckles are created by interaction between ultrasound beams and myocardium on a 2-D echocardiographic grayscale, and their motions serve as markers to display regional shortening or lengthening using dedicated automated software. During systole, the LV undergoes longitudinal and circumferential shortening, expressed as negative values, and radial thickening, displayed as a positive value.[17] Global longitudinal strain (GLS) is the most representative parameter and reflects the global myocardial deformation measured from 3 apical LV views (**Fig. 2**). In HF, strain analysis can provide further diagnostic and prognostic refinements. A well-established inverse relationship between reduction in LVEF and mortality is described in HF patients, which plateaus between LVEF values of 40% to 45%,[18] and patients falling in the range of HFmEF and HFpEF have similar 1-year mortality irrespective of LVEF.[19] In contrast, GLS has shown an additive and independent prognostic value regardless of LVEF in HFrEF patients, with a further risk prediction also in patients

with LVEF less than 35%.[20–22] The prognostic impact of reduced GLS has also been demonstrated in acute HF, across the broad spectrum of LVEF,[23] and in stable outpatients with ischemic HF for prediction of HF hospitalization.[24] In HF with recovered LVEF, an abnormal GLS (<-16%) has been shown to be a quite accurate predictor for future deterioration of LVEF.[25] Furthermore, the main established role of GLS is to provide further information on the extent of LV impairment in initial stages of HF and to provide possible future evolutions of HF phenotype. A recent observational study performed in 2104 patients admitted for acute HF confirmed that HF patients with improved LVEF in follow-up had lower cardiovascular mortality.[26] Interestingly, in multivariable analysis, a 1% increase in GLS, suggesting better contractility, was associated with a 10% increased odds for HF with improved ejection fraction among patients with HFrEF at baseline and 7% reduced odds for HF with declined ejection fraction among patients with HFpEF at baseline, suggesting a close relationship between strain deformation in initial stages of HF and longitudinal changes in LVEF in HF patients. Patients with AHF requiring HTx often present a severe reduction in global myocardial longitudinal deformation (GLS < 8%), reflecting extended myocardial damage and fibrosis.[27] In end-stage disease, a reduction in circumferential strain and twisting can also be observed, suggesting an impairment of compensatory mechanisms of myocardial contractility and dynamics.[28]

Three-dimensional echocardiography has provided a further technological advancement in the

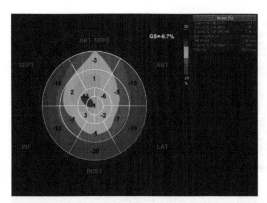

Fig. 2. Standard GLS assessment expressed as bull's eye plot derived from 2-D STE gives an overview of global and local myocardial deformation. In this case, a patient with ischemic cardiomyopathy and apical aneurysm present positive values of myocardial strain, suggesting regional lengthening.

quantification of the degree of LV enlargement and impairment. Thanks to high spatial and temporal resolution and a multimodality display imaging (surface rendering, volume rendering, cropping, real-time single-beat and multibeat imaging), 3-D echocardiography allows some limitations of 2-D examination, like potential image foreshortening and geometric assumptions on cardiac chambers shape, to be overcome, thus providing a more accurate representation of the LV endocardial surface, which is crucial for a precise definition of LV geometry and systolic function. Full-volume multibeat acquisitions currently offer the best resolution for evaluation of LV volumes (**Fig. 3**) In order to overcome "time-consuming" image acquisition and offline analysis, the development of automated instantaneous software has allowed accurate definition of LV volumes and ejection fraction without a need for cavity geometry.[29] When comparing with cardiac magnetic resonance (CMR), 3-D echo shows closer agreement for LV volume quantification than 2-D echo. In a meta-analysis comparing 3-D echocardiography with CMR, 3-D echo underestimated the LV end-diastolic volume by -14 ± 5 mL and the LV end-systolic volume by -7 ± 3 mL, while 2-D-derived volumes showed a larger difference.[30] The derivation of SV and LVEF are accurate also in HF patients with a good prognostic impact.[31,32] Furthermore, while traditional 2-D parameters like LV mass, relative wall thickness and sphericity index (LV short/long axis ratio) provide a global and generic estimate of LV geometry, 3-D echo can most accurately define anatomy and function in cases of distorted ventricles (eg, LV aneurysm) and in the presence of local shape abnormalities.[33]

Evaluation of Diastolic Dysfunction in Advanced Heart Failure

The diastolic phase of the cardiac cycle can be divided into 4 phases: isovolumic relaxation, rapid filling, diastasis, and atrial systole occurring in end-diastole. The main factors influencing diastolic function are myocardial relaxation, LV compliance, left atrium (LA) function, heart rate, and pericardium. In HF, adequate organ perfusion occurs at the expense of increased LV filling pressures, and therefore, evaluation of markers of diastolic dysfunction like LV end-diastolic pressure, LA pressure and pulmonary capillary wedge pressure (PCWP) is crucial for prognostic stratification and therapeutic management.[2] Echocardiography plays a key role for noninvasive assessment of diastolic function in HF. Echocardiographic evaluation of LV filling patterns mainly relies on PW Doppler sampling of transmitral flow, identifying E wave (early diastolic flow velocity), A wave (end-diastole atrial contraction phase) and deceleration time (DT).[34] These variables are affected by age, heart rhythm and loading condition and integration with tissue Doppler imaging (TDI) interrogation of early diastolic septal and lateral mitral annulus velocity (e' velocity), which reflects the status of LV myocardial relaxation, is mandatory for a correct assessment of LV filling pressure in HF patients.[34] In the majority of patients with reduced LVEF, 3 stages of diastolic dysfunction can be observed, ranging from predominant abnormal relaxation pattern with normal filling pressure (stage I; E/A ratio < 0.8), pseudonormal pattern (stage II, E/A ratio >0.8 < 2), restrictive pattern (stage III; E/A ratio >2, DT < 150 ms), which are associated with progressive increase in LA pressure.[34] Measure of TDI derived early mitral annulus velocities (e') is mandatory for assessment of LA pressure in stage II, together with LA volume index and tricuspid regurgitation jet velocity.[34] Moreover, because e' is less dependent from acute load changes, the ratio E/e' provides an accurate noninvasive measure of PCWP.[35] In significant MR, widened QRS, and cardiac resynchronization device, the E/è ratio may not always be well correlated with PCWP.[36] Patients with AHF, regardless of preserved or reduced EF, frequently present a restrictive inflow physiology characterized by a prominent E wave, with markedly reduced A wave and an E/e' greater than 15, suggesting high LV filling pressures, a shortened isovolumic relaxation time (<80 ms) due to early mitral valve opening related to high LV pressures, a DT < 150 ms, with significant reduction in e' velocities (<5 cm/s) indicating extended derangement of myocardial disease[34]

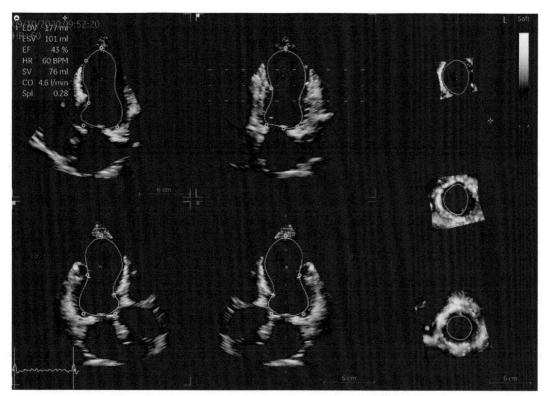

Fig. 3. Three-dimensional assessment of LVEF in a patient with ischemic cardiomyopathy and apical aneurysm, obtained tracing endocardial border in a simultaneous triplanar view.

(Fig. 4). Despite the well-established prognostic weight of echocardiographic diastolic variables in HF,[5,37] an E/è ratio greater than 14 and particularly greater than 20 indicates high risk and increased short-term and long-term mortality in HFrEF under medical treatment[38] and should be used to guide follow-up timing and uptitration of GDMT. Therefore, in cardiac imaging of patients with AHF, diastolic measures are not simple markers of cardiac hemodynamics but are key complements to LVEF measurement and should be routinely implemented in daily clinical practice.

The Left Atrium: A Watershed Between the Left Ventricle and Pulmonary Circulation

In the pathophysiology of HF, the LA plays a key role in keeping optimal CO despite increased LV filling pressure.[39] The LA is directly exposed to pressure and volume overload deriving from decreased LV compliance and MR. The pathophysiological result is progressive LA dilatation and remodeling, with an increase in LA pressure to maintain adequate LV filling. The most widely accepted echocardiographic measure of LA volumetry is maximal left atrium volume index for body surface area (LAVI), with normal values < 34 mL/m².[40] LAVI is an established independent prognostic factor among HF patients.[41] LA enlargement in HF patients suggests underlying diastolic dysfunction and is the primary driver in the development of postcapillary PH due to retrograde transmission of increased LA pressure to the pulmonary venous system.[42] Evaluation of LA function is a key and complementary measure to the simple LA dimension because while LA dilatation can occur early during HF process, LA function may be both increased or decreased depending on the stage of disease, with different physiopathological consequences. Ideally, during the HF timeline, a dilated but stiff and functionally impaired LA cannot tolerate high LV filling pressures, causing an early increase in pulmonary pressure and worsening of RV function, while a dilated but active and functioning LA can better preserve the RV-pulmonary artery unit.[43] Therefore, considering the role of LA as a "watershed" between impaired LV and pulmonary circulation, it derives that assessment of LA function is fundamental for monitoring potential transition to AHF.[44] LA function modulates LV filling during the 3 main phases in the cardiac cycle, acting as a *reservoir* for pulmonary venous blood during systole, as a *conduit* for passive pulmonary venous return

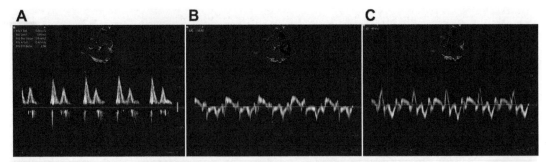

Fig. 4. Features of diastolic dysfunction frequently observed in patients with AHF: restrictive-like physiology with reduced deceleration time (*A*), estimated high LV filling pressures assessed with the E/è ratio (*B*) and shortened isovolumic relaxation time (*C*).

during early diastole, and as a *booster pump* in end-diastole through active LA contraction.[45] Echocardiographic assessment of LA function can be performed using a volumetric method, based on 2-D measure of LA maximal volume, LA minimal volume and LA volume before atrial contraction at P-wave onset. Combining this phasic parameters, we can describe the LA expansion index as a surrogate of reservoir function, LA passive emptying fraction as an expression of conduit function, and LA active emptying fraction as a surrogate of the booster pump phase[45] (**Fig. 5** panel A). Two-dimensional STE allows a more sensitive analysis of LA deformation despite being more time consuming and influenced by LA anatomy (LA appendage, pulmonary veins).[45] Using dedicated softwares and offline analysis, it is possible to derive the peak atrial longitudinal strain (PALS), an expression of reservoir function, and measure the pump function just before P-wave onset. Consequently, conduit function can be estimated as the difference between PALS and pump function (see **Fig. 5** panel B). Evaluation of LA reservoir function assessed with 2-D STE can provide additive and independent

prognostic value of LA volume, E/è ratio, and GLS in HFrEF patients.[46] Furthermore, LA reservoir function is highly correlated with degree of diastolic dysfunction and elevated PCWP.[47,48] Therefore, despite being limited by time-consumption, high frame rate imaging and the need for offline analysis, the addition of echocardiographic assessment of LA strain to volume measurement can provide further diagnostic and prognostic stratification in HF patients.

The Right Ventricle: Gatekeeper of Advanced Heart Failure Therapeutic Options

With increasing LV filling pressures and backward transmission to the pulmonary venous system, the ultimate development of pulmonary hypertension (PH) and RV dysfunction marks a dismal prognosis in patients with AHF.[49] The RV forms the majority of the anterior and inferior bord of the heart, is heavily trabeculated, and has a complex geometry with a crescent shape in short axis view due to shifting of interventricular toward RV cavity. RV contraction initially involves the inflow portion followed by contraction of the conus region, and a

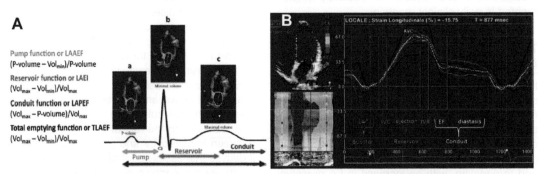

Fig. 5. (*A*): Evaluation of LA function with phasic-volumetric method, based on the calculation of LA volume maximum (Vol Max), minimum (Vol Min) and before atrial contraction (P-volume). (*B*): Assessment of LA function using 2-D STE. The result is a time-dependent curve where three different phases are depicted: reservoir, which corresponds to the peak of longitudinal strain curve, pump function, measured before P-wave onset, and conduit phase.

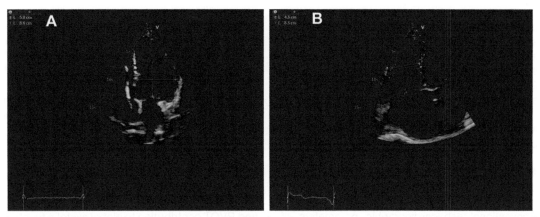

Fig. 6. Left ventricular (*A*) and right ventricular (*B*) sphericity index, measured as the ratio between the end-diastolic mid-basal-apical and transverse diameters.

main contributor of systolic function is longitudinal shortening, which closely correlates with RVEF and global RV stroke work.[50,51] RV responds to chronic volume/pressure overload with a compensatory remodeling process leading to hypertrophy and progressive dilatation with transition to a spherelike shape mainly due to enlargement of the basal and middle portions. When adequate SV can no longer be sustained, and with persistent pressure/volume overload, compensatory mechanisms fail, and RV failure ensues. In the presence of advanced RV failure and enlargment, there is a leftward shifting of the interventricular septum (IVS) with a bigger RV basal diameter than the

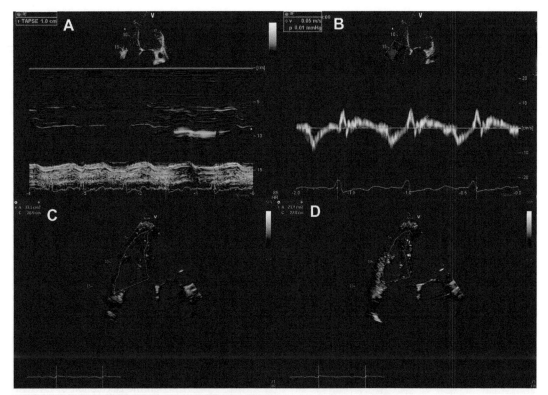

Fig. 7. Echocardiographic assessment of right ventricular systolic function: (*A*) measurement of tricuspid annular systolic excursion in apical 4-chamber view. (*B*): measurement of TDI derived systolic wave velocity of the basal inflow region. (*C*) calculation of end-diastole and (*D*) end-systole right ventricular area, used to determine fractional area change as percentage in area change.

LV. The LV eccentricity index, the ratio between LV anteroposterior and septolateral diameters in short axis view, and the sphericity index, expressed as the ratio between RV midventricular and longitudinal diameters in 4-chamber view, are 2 echocardiographic markers of RV remodeling and shape and predictors of worse outcome in HF patients with PH.[52,53] (**Fig. 6**). The RV sphericity index also showed a good correlation with outcome in AHF referred for HTx.[54]

The complex geometry of the RV makes global and objective evaluation of its systolic function difficult and challenging, and a multiparametric echocardiographic approach is highly advised. Conventional echocardiographic parameters of RV systolic function are tricuspid annular plane systolic excursion (TAPSE), TDI-derived S' wave velocity, and fractional area change (FAC).[10]

TAPSE expresses RV longitudinal function as the amount of apical displacement of tricuspid annulus in 4-chamber view with normal values > 16 mm (**Fig. 7** panel A). Easy reproducibility and measurement are its main advantages; however, TAPSE is highly load-dependent and angle-dependent and can be misleading after cardiac surgery and in presence of pericardial effusion.[10] Importantly, TAPSE does not account for the contribution of RVOT and IVS to the global RV systolic function process, and this is an important issue in the evaluation of patients with AHF. Despite a renowned prognostic impact in HF,[55] TAPSE must be integrated with other echo indexes of RV performance, especially when considering potential eligibility for a left ventricle assist device (LVAD).[56,57]

Peak systolic TDI velocity of the tricuspid annulus (S' wave) is another index of RV longitudinal function with normal values > 9.5 cm/s[10] (see **Fig. 7** Panel B). Like TAPSE, it is a measure of regional RV function and disregards the septal and RVOT contribution to global systolic function. Furthermore, it can be affected by the tethering effect of adjacent myocardial segments, considering that a velocity gradient between basal and apical regions has been described in healthy subjects.[58] Indeed, being a Doppler-derived measure, it is angle-dependent, and correct alignment with the region of interest is necessary to avoid misleading values.[10] S' wave is a further index for risk stratification in HF patients[59]; however, it must be integrated in a multiparametric approach.

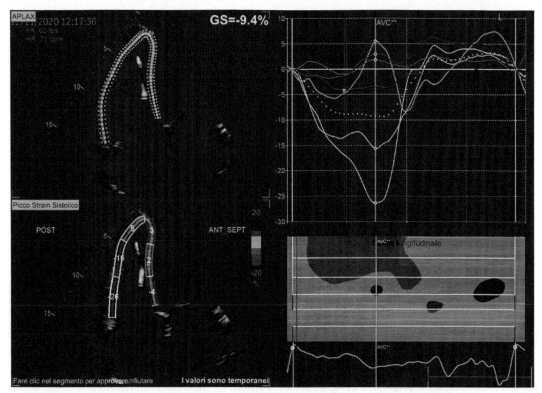

Fig. 8. Measurement of right ventricle global longitudinal strain and free wall longitudinal strain in a patient with AHF. Note that apical segments present positive deformation values, suggestion lengthening rather than shortening, and due to pacemaker-related dyssynchrony.

FAC is a quantitative index of global RV function measured as the percentage of change in RV area at end-diastole and end-systole obtained by carefully tracing RV endocardial borders including trabeculations and tricuspid leaflets, with normal values > 35%[10] (see **Fig. 7**, Panel C-D). The main disadvantage is the low interobserver reproducibility due to difficult precise remarking of endocardial border and an overall limited bidimensional analysis of RV function. FAC has a good agreement with CMR assessment of RV function[60] and is a predictor of worse outcome in patients with AHF.[61]

Advanced echocardiographic imaging, including 3-D evaluation of RVEF and RV strain, are key complementary measures of RV systolic function in patients with AHF.

Three-dimensional echocardiographic evaluation of RVEF has an incremental value compared with standard methods because it provides an overall measure of systolic function including inflow, infundibular, and apical RV regions, has high correlation with CMR assessment and less

underestimation of RV volumes than 2-D methods,[62] and normal reported values are greater than 45%.[10] It requires high experience, a semiautomated dedicated software for image analysis, and is influenced by septal motion and load conditions, with women reporting higher values because of smaller RV volumes.[10] Preliminary evidence shows that 3-D RVEF (cutoff 24.8%) is associated with RV failure and long-term outcome after LVAD surgery,[63] although larger studies are needed in this setting.

The application of STE to analyze RV longitudinal deformation provides second-level additive parameters of RV systolic function, allowing quantification of RVGLS, measured in apical 4-chamber view including IVS and lateral RV wall, and of RV free wall lateral strain (normal reported values > - 20%[10]), which measures longitudinal deformation of RV lateral wall only, excluding IVS contribution that can be influenced by paradoxic motion and LV dyssynergy (**Fig. 8**). RVFWS has showed an additive and incremental prognostic stratification in patients with HFrEF and preserved TAPSE values[64]

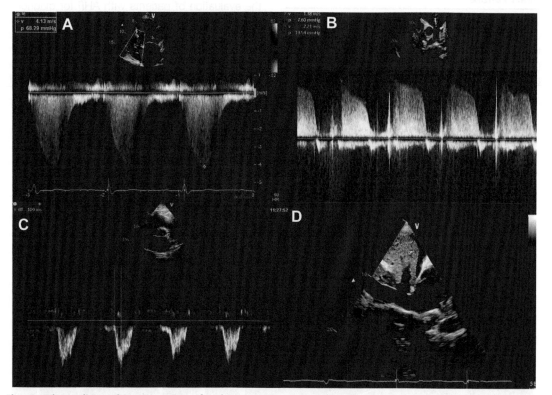

Fig. 9. Echocardiographic estimation of pulmonary pressure with different measures: (*A*) estimate of right ventricular systolic pressure with application of modified Bernoulli equation ($P = 4 \times v^2$) from peak tricuspid regurgitation velocity. (*B*) The diastolic pulmonary artery pressure can be estimated from the velocity of the end-diastolic pulmonary regurgitant velocity using the modified Bernoulli equation. The mean pulmonary artery pressure (mPAP) can be estimated from the following equation: mPAP = 4V (early peak pulmonary regurgitation velocity)2 + right atrial pressure. (*C*) measurement of acceleration time from PW sampling of the right ventricle outflow tract. (*D*) the size and collapsibility of inferior vena cava are used to estimate right atrial pressure.

and in patients with AHF referred for HTx.[54] Further-more, there is growing evidence addressing the po-tential predictive value of RV strain for early RV failure after LVAD. Two retrospective studies showed that RVFWS (cutoff peak > -9.6%) and RVGLS (cutoff > -10%) may be associated with an increased risk of RV failure in patients with AHF undergoing LVAD placement.[56,65] Ongoing larger study data are needed to standardize and confirm these findings. Current recommendations highly advise a multiparametric approach, including echocardiographic measures of RV remodeling (sphericity index could be employed in this setting) and systolic function including advanced indexes like RV strain for selection of LVAD candidates.[66] Overall, echocardiographic evaluation of RV sys-tolic function and geometry definitively has a major role for therapeutic decision-making in patients with AHF, representing an effective tool in the selection of LVAD candidates and a prognostic element for patients awaiting HTx.

Type II Pulmonary Hypertension in Advanced Heart Failure

Type II PH portends a dismal prognosis in patients with AHF, influencing therapeutic strategy and timing.[67] Elevated pulmonary vascular resistance (PVR > 3 wood unit) is a risk factor for mortality and RV failure after HTx, and such patients should

receive vasodilator therapy or LVAD as a bridge to eligibility in order to reduce PVR.[68] Echocardio-graphic estimation of systolic pulmonary pressure requires adding estimates of right ventricular sys-tolic pressure (calculated by applying the Bernoulli equation to the peak tricuspid regurgitation veloc-ity) and estimates of right atrial pressure (based on size and collapse of inferior vena cava size). Mean and diastolic pulmonary pressure can be esti-mated by tracing the tricuspid regurgitation jet curve and adding right atrial pressure or with end-diastolic pulmonary regurgitation velocity, respectively.[69] Indeed, echo can provide determi-nants of precapillary versus postcapillary PH like the apex-forming chamber, RV/LV ratio, and E/è ratio.[70] The noninvasive measure of PVR is also reliable with PW trace of RVOT,[69] and overall Doppler echocardiography has a good agreement with gold standard invasive assessment of pulmo-nary hemodynamics[12] (**Fig. 9**)

Hepatic Vein Doppler Velocities

Hepatic vein Doppler velocity pattern is essential in the evaluation of patients with AHF for diagnosis. Right atrial pressure can be estimated by the timing of predominant forward flow velocity in sinus rhythm. As RA pressure increases, systolic forward flow velocity decreases while diastolic forward flow velocity increases. When RA pressure is severely

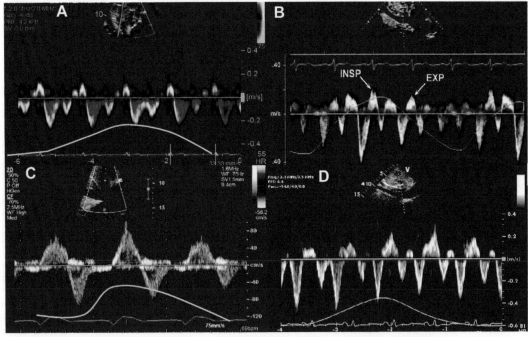

Fig. 10. Pulsed wave hepatic vein velocity recording by Doppler echocardiography, simultaneously with respirom-eter recording at the bottom demonstrating inspiration by upward deflection and expiration by downward deflection. (A). Normal, (B). Restrictive Cardiomyopathy, (C). Severe Tricuspid Regurgitation, (D). Constrictive Pericarditis.

increased or tricuspid regurgitation is severe, prominent systolic flow reversal occurs. Marked diastolic flow reversal in hepatic vein indicates a clinically significant elevation in RV end-diastolic and right atrial pressure. The timing of hepatic vein diastolic flow reversal in reference to the respiratory cycle can separate constrictive pericardial from restrictive myocardial hemodynamics that occur with expiration and inspiration, respectively (**Fig. 10**).

Role of Echocardiography in Management and Prognosis in Advanced Heart Failure

Finally, echocardiography plays a key role in therapeutic management and prognostic stratification of patients with AHF. The echo estimate of central venous pressure and fluid overload through inferior cava vein size and collapsibility and assessment of LV filling pressures and LV SV are meaningful tools complementary to clinical examination for uptitration of disease-modifying drugs and regulating diuretic therapy.[16] Indeed, echocardiography provides several markers of dismal prognosis in AHF, such as extreme impairment of LVEF, degree of diastolic dysfunction and MR, and the presence of RV impairment with PH.[5–9] Moreover, STE-derived parameters, such as GLS and LA strain, are prognostic factors with an additive effect beyond "traditional" measures such as LV dimensions, systolic function, and LA volume.[20,46]

SUMMARY

Echocardiography is a pivotal imaging tool for assessing patients with AHF, providing elements for diagnostic and hemodynamic assessment and to address the prognostic stratification and therapeutic decision-making of end-stage HF. In the last few years, there has been a growing application of second-level advanced imaging techniques, including 3-D echocardiography and 2-D and 3-D STE, and the future should lead to progressive integration of these "new" techniques in daily practice to allow more accurate definition and classification of AHF profiles with consequent choice of tailored therapeutic options.

CLINICS CARE POINTS

- AHF is characterized by high mortality and frequent hospitalization, and thus, aggressive therapeutic options and timely recognition of the evolution to such end-stage disease are crucial to improve patient outcomes.

- Echocardiography is the first-line imaging technique for providing the diagnostic markers necessary for early identification of the transition to AHF and allows risk stratification and a therapeutic decision-making process.

- Assessment of LV dimension and LVEF, degree of diastolic dysfunction and MR, and LV filling pressure provide clinical and hemodynamic insights to guide uptitration of disease modification and optimization of decongestive therapies.

- Evaluation of RV systolic function and size as well as pulmonary pressures is a key element when considering eligibility for advanced therapeutic options like HTx and long-term mechanical circulatory support.

- Progressive integration of novel echocardiographic indexes in daily clinical practice, like STE analysis and three-dimensional assessment of LV and LA, will provide a deeper and more comprehensive assessment of AHF physiology and prognosis.

DISCLOSURE STATEMENT

The authors have nothing to disclose.

REFERENCES

1. Crespo-Leiro MG, Metra M, Lund LH, et al. Advanced heart failure: a position statement of the Heart Failure Association of the European Society of Cardiology. Eur J Heart Fail 2018;20(11):1505–35.
2. Ponikowski P, Voors AA, Anker SD, et al. ESC Scientific Document Group 2016 ESC guidelines for the diagnosis and treatment of acute and chronic heart failure. Eur Heart J 2016;37:2129–200.
3. Kirkpatrick JN, Vannan MA, Narula J, et al. Echocardiography in heart failure: applications, utility, and new horizons. J Am Coll Cardiol 2007;50(5):381–96.
4. Garbi M, Edvardsen T, Bax J, et al. EACVI appropriateness criteria for the use of cardiovascular imaging in heart failure derived from European National Imaging Societies voting. Eur Heart J Cardiovasc Imaging 2016;17(7):711–21.
5. Grayburn P, Appleton C, DeMaria A, et al. Echocardiographic predictors of morbidity and mortality in patients with advanced heart failure. The Beta-blocker Evaluation of Survival Trial (BEST). J Am Coll Cardiol 2005;45:1064.e71.
6. Solomon SD, Anavekar N, Skali H. Influence of ejection fraction on cardiovascular outcomes in a broad spectrum of heart failure patients. Circulation 2005;112:3738–44.

7. Ghio S, Gavazzi A, Campana C, et al. Independent and additive prognostic value of right ventricular systolic function and pulmonary artery pressure in patients with chronic heart failure. J Am Coll Cardiol 2001;37:183–8.

8. Juilliere Y, Barbier G, Feldmann L, et al. Additional predictive value of both left and right ventricular ejection fractions on long-term survival in idiopathic dilated cardiomyopathy. Eur Heart J 1997;18:276–80.

9. Palazzini M, Dardi F, Manes A, et al. Pulmonary hypertension due to left heart disease: analysis of survival according to the haemodynamic classification of the 2015 ESC/ERS guidelines and insights for future changes. Eur J Heart Fail 2018;20:248–55.

10. Lang MR, Badano PL, Mor-Avi V, et al. Recommendations for Cardiac Chamber Quantification by Echocardiography in Adults: An Update from the American Society of Echocardiography and the European Association of Cardiovascular Imaging. Eur Heart J Cardiovasc Imaging 2015;16:233–71.

11. Mele D, Nardozza M, Ferrari R. Left ventricular ejection fraction and heart failure: an indissoluble marriage? Eur J Heart Fail 2018;20(3):427–30.

12. Temporelli PL, Scapellato F, Eleuteri E, et al. Doppler echocardiography in advanced systolic heart failure. A noninvasive alternative to Swan-Ganz catheter. Circ Heart Fail 2010;3:387–94.

13. Nagueh SF, Bhatt R, Vivo RP, et al. Echocardiographic evaluation of hemodynamics in patients with decompensated systolic heart failure. Circ Cardiovasc Imaging 2011;4:220–7.

14. Ky B, Plappert T, Kirkpatrick J, et al. Left ventricular remodeling in human heart failure: quantitative echocardiographic assessment of 1,794 patients. Echocardiography 2012;29(7):758–65.

15. Mele D, Pestelli G, Dal Molin D, et al. Echocardiographic Evaluation of Left Ventricular Output in Patients with Heart Failure: A Per-Beat or Per-Minute Approach? J Am Soc Echocardiogr 2020;33(2):135–47.

16. Hsiao SH, Lin SK, Chiou YR, et al. Utility of Left Atrial Expansion Index and Stroke Volume in Management of Chronic Systolic Heart Failure. J Am Soc Echocardiogr 2018;31(6):650–9.e1.

17. Potter E, Marwick TH. Assessment of Left Ventricular Function by Echocardiography: The Case for Routinely Adding Global Longitudinal Strain to Ejection Fraction. JACC Cardiovasc Imaging 2018;11:260–74.

18. Curtis JP, Sokol SI, Wang Y, et al. The association of left ventricular ejection fraction, mortality, and cause of death in stable outpatients with heart failure. J Am Coll Cardiol 2003;42:736–42.

19. Bhatia RS, Tu JV, Lee DS, et al. Outcome of heart failure with preserved ejection fraction in a population-based study. N Engl J Med 2006;355:260–9.

20. Zhang KW, French B, May Khan A, et al. Strain improves risk prediction beyond ejection fraction in chronic systolic heart failure. J Am Heart Assoc 2013;3:e000550.

21. Sengelov M, Jorgensen PG, Jensen JS, et al. Global longitudinal strain is a superior predictor of all-cause mortality in heart failure with reduced ejection fraction. J Am Coll Cardiol Img 2015;8:1351–9.

22. Stanton T, Leano R, Marwick TH. Prediction of all-cause mortality from global longitudinal speckle strain: comparison with ejection fraction and wall motion scoring. Circ Cardiovasc Imaging 2009;2:356–64.

23. Park JJ, Park JB, Park JH, et al. Global longitudinal strain to predict mortality in patients with acute heart failure. J Am Coll Cardiol 2018;71:1947–57.

24. Kaufmann D, Szwock M, Kwiatkowska J, et al. Global longitudinal strain can predict heart failure exacerbation in stable outpatients with ischemic left ventricular systolic dysfunction. PLoS One 2019;14(12):e0225829.

25. Adamo L, Perry A, Novak E, et al. Abnormal Global Longitudinal Strain Predicts Future Deterioration of Left Ventricular Function in Heart Failure Patients With a Recovered Left Ventricular Ejection Fraction. Circ Heart Fail 2017;10(6):e003788.

26. Park JJ, Mebaza A, Hwang CI, et al. Phenotyping Heart Failure According to the Longitudinal Ejection Fraction Change: Myocardial Strain, Predictors, and Outcomes. J Am Heart Assoc 2020;9(12):e015009.

27. Cameli M, Mondillo S, Righini MR, et al. Left Ventricular Deformation and Myocardial Fibrosis in Patients With Advanced Heart Failure Requiring Transplantation. J Card Fail 2016;22:901–7.

28. Wang J, Khoury DS, Yue Y, et al. Preserved left ventricular twist and circumferential deformation, but depressed longitudinal and radial deformation in patients with diastolic heart failure. Eur Heart J 2008;29:1283–9.

29. Zhang J, Gajjala S, Agrawal P, et al. Fully automated echocardiogram interpretation in clinical practice. Feasibility and diagnostic accuracy. Circulation 2018;138:1623–35.

30. Rigolli M, Anandabaskaran S, Christiansen JP, et al. Bias associated with left ventricular quantification by multimodality imaging: a systematic review and metaanalysis. Open Heart 2016;3:e000388.

31. Fleming SM, Cumberledge B, Kiesewetter C, et al. Usefulness of real-time three-dimensional echocardiography for reliable measurement of cardiac output in patients with ischemic or idiopathic dilated cardiomyopathy. Am J Cardial 2005;95:308–10.

32. Mancuso FJN, Moises VA, Almeida DR, et al. Prognostic value of real-time three-dimensional

echocardiography compared to two-dimensional echocardiography in patients with systolic heart failure. Int J Cardiovasc Imaging 2018;34:553–60.

33. Monaghan MJ. Role of real time 3D echocardiography in evaluating the left ventricle. Heart 2006;92: 131–6.

34. Nagueh SF, Smiseth OA, Appleton CP, et al. Recommendations for the evaluation of left ventricular diastolic function by echocardiography: an update from the American Society of Echocardiography and the European Association of Cardiovascular Imaging. J Am Soc Echocardiogr 2016;29:277–314.

35. Nagueh SF, Middleton KJ, Kopelen HA, et al. Doppler tissue imaging: a noninvasive technique for evaluation of left ventricular relaxation and estimation of filling pressures. J Am Coll Cardiol 1997; 30:1527–33.

36. Nagueh SF. Letter by Nagueh et al regarding article, "Tissue Doppler imaging in the estimation of intracardiac filling pressure in decompensated patients with advanced systolic heart failure". Circulation 2009;120(7):e44.

37. Rigolli M, Rossi A, Quintana M, et al. The prognostic impact of diastolic dysfunction in patients with chronic heart failure and post-acute myocardial infarction: Can age-stratified E/A ratio alone predict survival? Int J Cardiol 2015;181:362–8.

38. Benfari G, Miller LW, Antoine C, et al. Diastolic Determinants of Excess Mortality in Heart Failure With Reduced Ejection Fraction. JACC Heart Fail 2019; 7:808–17.

39. Rosca M, Lancellotti P, Popescu BA, et al. Left atrial function: pathophysiology, echocardiographic assessment, and clinical applications. Heart 2011; 97:1982–9.

40. Galderisi M, Cosyns B, Edvardsen T, et al. Standardization of adult transthoracic echocardiography reporting in agreement with recent chamber quantification, diastolic function, and heart valve disease recommendations: an expert consensus document of the European Association of Cardiovascular Imaging. Eur Heart J Cardiovasc Imaging 2017;18: 1301–10.

41. Tamura H, Watanabe T, Nishiyama S, et al. Increased left atrial volume index predicts a poor prognosis in patients with heart failure. J Card Fail 2011;17(3):210–6.

42. Guazzi M. Pulmonary hypertension and heart failure: a dangerous liaison. Heart Failure Clin 2018;14: 297–309.

43. Palmiero G, Melillo E, Ferro A, et al. Significant functional mitral regurgitation affects left atrial function in heart failure patients: haemodynamic correlations and prognostic implications. Eur Heart J Cardiovasc Imaging 2019;20:1012–9.

44. Melenovsky V, Hwang SJ, Redfield MM, et al. Left atrial remodeling and function in advanced heart failure with preserved or reduced ejection fraction. Circ Heart Fail 2015;8:295–303.

45. Hoit BD. Left atrial size and function. J Am Coll Cardiol 2014;63:493–505.

46. Carluccio E, Biagioli P, Mengoni A, et al. Left Atrial Reservoir Function and Outcome in Heart Failure With Reduced Ejection Fraction. Circ Cardiovasc Imaging 2018;11(11):e007696.

47. Frydas A, Morris DA, Belyavskiy E, et al. Left atrial strain as sensitive marker of left ventricular diastolic dysfunction in heart failure. ESC Heart Fail 2020;7: 1956–65.

48. CameliM, Mandoli GE, Loiacono F, et al. Left atrial strain: a new parameter for assessment of left ventricular filling pressure. Heart Fail Rev 2016;21: 65–76.

49. Ghio S, Temporelli PL, Klersy C, et al. Prognostic relevance of a non-invasive evaluation of right ventricular function and pulmonary artery pressure in patients with chronic heart failure. Eur J Heart Fail 2013;15:408–14.

50. Rushmer RF, Crystal DK, Wagner C. The functional anatomy of ventricular contraction. Circ Res 1953; 1:162–70.

51. Kaul S, Tei C, Hopkins JM, et al. Assessment of right ventricular function using two-dimensional echocardiography. Am Heart J 1984;107:526–31.

52. Raymond RJ, Hinderliter LA, Willis PK, et al. Echocardiographic predictors of adverse outcomes in primary pulmonary hypertension. J Am Coll Cardiol 2002;39:1214–9.

53. Grapsa J, Gibbs JS, Cabrita IZ, et al. The association of clinical outcome with right atrial and ventricular remodelling in patients with pulmonary arterial hypertension: study with real-time three-dimensional echocardiography. Eur Heart J Cardiovasc Imaging 2012;13:666–72.

54. Cameli M, Righini FM, Lisi M, et al. Comparison of right versus left ventricular strain analysis as a predictor of outcome in patients with systolic heart failure referred for heart transplantation. Am J Cardiol 2013;112:1778–84.

55. Ghio S, Recusani F, Klersy C, et al. Prognostic usefulness of the tricuspid annular plane systolic excursion in patients with congestive heart failure secondary to idiopathic or ischemic dilated cardiomyopathy. Am J Cardiol 2000;85(7):837–42.

56. Grant ADM, Smedira NG, Starling RC, et al. Independent and incremental role of quantitative right ventricular evaluation for the prediction of right ventricular failure after left ventricular assist device implantation. J Am Coll Cardiol 2012;60:521–8.

57. Patil NP, Mohite PN, Sabashnikov A, et al. Preoperative predictors and outcomes of right ventricular assist device implantation after continuous-flow left ventricular assist device implantation. J Thorac Cardiovasc Surg 2015;150:1651–8.

58. Kukulski T, Hübbert L, Arnold M, et al. Normal regional right ventricular function and its change with age: a Doppler myocardial imaging study. J Am Soc Echocardiogr 2000;13:194–204.

59. Donal E, Coquerel N, Bodi S, et al. Importance of ventricular longitudinal function in chronic heart failure. Eur J Echocardiogr 2011;12:619–27.

60. Anavekar NS, Gerson D, Skali H, et al. Two-dimensional assessment of right ventricular function: an echocardiographic-MRI correlative study. Echocardiography 2007;24:452–6.

61. Cameli M, Pastore MC, Mandoli GE, et al. Prognosis and Risk Stratification of Patients With Advanced Heart Failure (from PROBE). Am J Cardiol 2019; 124:55–62.

62. Sugeng L, Mor-AviV, Weinert L, et al. Multimodality comparison of quantitative volumetric analysis of the right ventricle. JACC Cardiovasc Imaging 2010;3:10–8.

63. Magunia H, Dietrich C, Langer HF, et al. 3D echocardiography derived right ventricular function is associated with right ventricular failure and mid-term survival after left ventricular assist device implantation. Int J Cardiol 2018;272:348–55.

64. Carluccio E, Biagioli P, Alunni G, et al. Prognostic Value of Right Ventricular Dysfunction in Heart Failure With Reduced Ejection Fraction: Superiority of Longitudinal Strain Over Tricuspid Annular Plane Systolic Excursion. Circ Cardiovasc Imaging 2018; 11(1):e006894.

65. Liang LW, Birati EY, Justice C, et al. Right Ventricular Strain as a Predictor of Post-LVAD Early Right Ventricular Failure. J Heart Lung Transplant 2019;38: s18.

66. Stainback RF, Estep JD, Agler AD, et al. Echocardiography in the management of patients with left ventricle assist devices: recommendations from the American Society of Echocardiography. J Am Soc Echocardiogr 2015;28:853–909.

67. Guazzi M, Galiè N. Pulmonary hypertension in left heart disease. Europ Resp Rev 2012;21:338–46.

68. Beyersdorf F, Schlensak C, Berchtold-Herz M, et al. Regression of "fixed" pulmonary vascular resistance in heart transplant candidates after unloading with ventricular assist devices. J Thorac Cardiovasc Surg 2010;140:747–9.

69. Parasuraman S, Walker S, Loudon BL, et al. Assessment of pulmonary artery pressure by echocardiography—A comprehensive review. Int J Cardiol Heart Vasc 2016;12:45–51.

70. D'Alto M, Romeo E, Argiento P, et al. Echocardiographic prediction of pre- versus postcapillary pulmonary hypertension. J Am Soc Echocardiogr 2015;28:108–15.

Disease-modifier Drugs in Patients with Advanced Heart Failure
How to Optimize Their Use?

Massimo Iacoviello, MD, PhD*, Enrica Vitale, MD, Maria Delia Corbo, MD,
Michele Correale, MD, PhD, Natale Daniele Brunetti, MD, PhD, FESC

KEYWORDS

• Advanced heart failure • Therapy • Prognosis

KEY POINTS

- The presence of an optimal medical therapy based on disease-modifier drugs is one of the criteria to diagnose advanced heart failure.
- However, several conditions such as hospitalization, hypotension, renal dysfunction, and electrolyte disorders, but also medical inertia and poor patients' adherence, may limit the continuation or introduction of the disease-modifier drugs.
- A disease management program in advanced heart failure should consider these conditions and should try to overcome them.
- A close clinical follow-up, a tailored therapy based on the monitoring of blood pressure, renal function, and electrolyte levels, as well as the promotion of patients' self-management, could represent successful strategies.

INTRODUCTION

Over recent decades, several therapeutic approaches have been shown to improve the prognosis of patients affected by heart failure (HF) with reduced ejection fraction (HFrEF)[1–11] because of their effects on the pathophysiologic mechanisms underlying the onset and progression of the syndrome.[12,13] The optimal use of the disease-modifier drugs currently recommended[1,14] is one of the main criteria to diagnose advanced HF (AdvHF).[15]

However, some of the clinical conditions characterizing AdvHF, such as hospitalization because of acute decompensated heart failure (ADHF), hypotension, renal dysfunction, or electrolyte abnormalities,[15–17] could make the therapeutic optimization challenging. Beside these factors, medical inertia and inadequate patients'

adherence[18,19] could also lead to an underuse of the recommended therapy. Finally, the new classes of disease-modifier drugs[20–23] are still not widely adopted among patients with HFrEF.[24,25]

This article focuses on the issues influencing the optimal use of disease-modifier drugs as well as on the possible usefulness of new therapeutic opportunities in AdvHF patients.

THE PATHOPHYSIOLOGIC MECHANISMS OF DISEASE-MODIFIER DRUGS IN HFrEF

The cornerstone of HFrEF treatment is the modulation of the neurohormonal systems responsible for HF progression.[12,13] Initially, in HFrEF, the activation of renin-angiotensin-aldosterone system (RAAS) and the increased of sympathetic nervous activity (SNA) play a compensatory role in the presence of a systolic dysfunction, by increasing

Cardiology Unit, Department of Medical and Surgical Sciences, University of Foggia, Viale Luigi Pinto 1, Foggia, Italy
* Corresponding author.
E-mail address: massimo.iacoviello@unifg.it

Heart Failure Clin 17 (2021) 561–573
https://doi.org/10.1016/j.hfc.2021.05.002
1551-7136/21/© 2021 Elsevier Inc. All rights reserved.

inotropism and peripheral vascular resistances, and promoting fluid and salt retention.[12,13] However, in the long term, they have negative effects by leading to further left ventricular remodeling through alterations in myocyte biology, myocardial structure, and in left ventricular chamber geometry.[12] From this pathophysiologic background, angiotensin-converting enzyme (ACE) inhibitors (ACEi),[26–28] β-blockers,[4–9] mineralocorticoid receptor (MR) antagonists (MRAs),[10,11] and, with less evidence, angiotensin (AT) II receptor blockers (ARBs)[1,29] have been shown to improve HFrEF prognosis.

Recently, the neurohormonal approach has been further improved by the introduction of sacubitril/valsartan,[20] which is a new class of drugs able to block both the ATII receptor and a neutral endopeptidase, the neprilysin, which is involved in degradation of natriuretic peptides (NPs).[30] The NP system (NPS) counteracts RAAS and SNA[30] by promoting natriuresis and diuresis, exerting an antifibrotic effect at cardiac level as well as vasodilation and inhibition of RAAS. Although NPs (ie, atrial NP [ANP] and brain NP [BNP]) serum levels increase with worsening of HF, their effectiveness is progressively reduced because of several factors: an altered target organ responsiveness, overactivation of RAAS and SNA, and decreased availability of biologically active NPs.[31] This last condition could be related to the neprilysin overactivity.[32,33] Consequently, neprilysin inhibition by sacubitril, combined with ATII receptor antagonism of valsartan, exerts a reduced NP degradation[34] and a more effective neurohormonal modulation by the enhancement of the NPS. In HFrEF, compared with enalapril, sacubitril/valsartan has been shown to be associated with an improved prognosis[20,21] as well as with a greater reverse remodeling and improvement of left ventricular ejection fraction (LVEF).[35,36] Although the earlier the use of the neurohormonal approach the greater is the observed efficacy,[37–39] in patients with more severe HF, neurohormonal modulation also exerts favorable effects.[7,10,21,26]

In addition to neurohormonal modulation, another therapeutic approach that has been found to modify the natural history of HFrEF is that based on the type 2 sodium-glucose cotransporter (SGLT2) inhibitors (SGLT2i). SGLT2i were initially tested for their hypoglycemic effects in patients with type 2 diabetes mellitus (T2DM), but they have since shown the extraordinary ability of reducing hospitalizations related to HF.[40–43] More recently, it has been published the Study to Evaluate the Effect of Dapagliflozin on the Incidence of Worsening Heart Failure or Cardiovascular Death in Patients With Chronic Heart Failure

(DAPA-HF). In a population of patients with HFrEF, dapagliflozin, compared with placebo, reduced HF hospitalization and cardiovascular (CV) and all-cause mortality both in diabetic and nondiabetic patients.[22] Similarly, in EMPagliflozin outcomE tRial in Patients With chrOnic heaRt Failure With Reduced Ejection Fraction (EMPEROR-Reduced), empagliflozin reduced the first and the recurrent HF hospitalizations, although not CV and all-cause mortality.[23]

The mechanisms by which the SGLT2i are able to reduce the risk of HF-related events have not been fully clarified.[44,45] SGLT2i could exert, by glycosuria, a diuretic osmotic effect,[44,46–48] thus potentiating the loop diuretics and favoring hemodynamic stability without inducing electrolyte abnormalities and RAAS activation. In contrast, the increased delivery of sodium at the level of the macula densa is associated with the inhibition of tubule-glomerular feedback and the consequent vasoconstriction of the glomerular afferent arteriole and the reduction of renin activity.[49] This mechanism is considered the main driver of the nephroprotection observed in HF[23] as well as in patients with chronic kidney disease (CKD).[50] The metabolic,[51,52] inflammatory,[53] and cardiac effects[44] represent the other mechanisms by which SGLT2i improve prognosis. In particular, the myocardial energetics could be improved by the increase in hematocrit[51] and oxygen delivery as well as the changes of energetic substrates.[52]

The global picture of the disease-modifier drugs (**Fig. 1**) is that of different therapeutic approaches which potentiate each other by interfering with different pathophysiologic backgrounds, thus exerting their favorable effects. For this reason, their combined use maximizes the improvement of HFrEF prognosis[54] and should represent the current approach to preventing HF progression in HFrEF.

THE CLINICAL CONDITIONS INFLUENCING DISEASE-MODIFIER DRUGS IN ADVANCED HEART FAILURE

Several clinical features of AdvHF are able to influence the possibility of starting, continuing, or uptitrating disease-modifier drug therapy (**Fig. 2**).

Acute Decompensated Heart Failure Hospitalization

Because of its prognostic relevance, ADHF is one of the criteria to diagnose AdvHF.[15] Compared with outpatients with chronic HF, patients admitted for ADHF have a 1-year mortality about 4 times higher, and in a high percentage of patients hospitalized for HF a new HF hospitalization occurs within 1 year.[55]

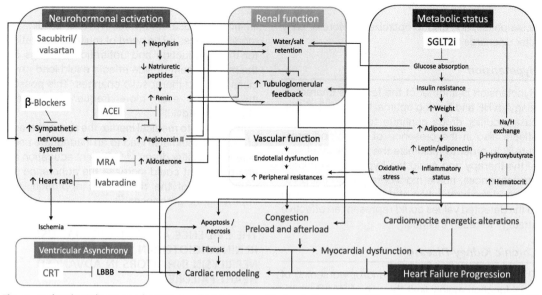

Fig. 1. Pathophysiologic mechanisms underlying the effects of disease-modifier therapeutic approach in HFrEF. CRT, cardiac resynchronization therapy; LBBB, left bundle branch bock.

Despite this epidemiologic relevance, there are few randomized controlled trials (RCTs) which evaluated the effects of the initiation, continuation, switching, and withdrawal of disease-modifier drugs in ADHF patients.[56] Available data suggest that their in-hospital discontinuation as well as their missed introduction is associated with a worse prognosis.[56,57] In patients with AdvHF, every effort should be made to eventually restore the disease-modifier drug therapy that was modified during the

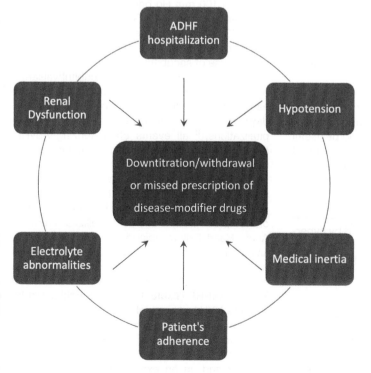

Fig. 2. The principal factors influencing the underuse of disease-modifier drugs in AdvHF.

acute phase, and also to optimize it before or early after discharge.

Hypotension

Hypotension is another of the features characterizing AdvHF and limiting optimal therapy.[15–17] Disease-modifier drugs continue to exert favorable effects also in the presence of low blood pressure.[58] In order to maximize the beneficial effects of the therapy and avoid the hypotension-related consequences, home monitoring of arterial pressure and the modulation of drug doses according to the detected values could represent an effective strategy to reach this goal.

Chronic Kidney Disease

The presence of severe CKD and/or worsening of renal function mainly limit the use of RAAS inhibitors (RAASi). ACEi and ARBs,[59–61] and especially angiotensin receptor neprilysin inhibitors (ARNi)[62] and SGLT2i,[23,51] exert a protective effect toward the progression of renal dysfunction.

Nevertheless, the introduction of these nephroprotective drugs could be associated with an initial decrease of glomerular filtration rate (GFR) caused by their interference with the mechanisms underlying the autoregulation of renal perfusion.[63–65] Moreover, RAAS blockade could favor an acute worsening of renal function in patients experiencing hypovolemia,[66,67] although this is generally transient and without prognostic implications.[68,69] In patients with AdvHF, because of their hemodynamic instability and the risk of hypotension, which could favor acute renal failure, a careful monitoring of renal function is useful for the optimal use of RAASi as well as of ARNi.

Renal dysfunction, as with hepatic dysfunction, should also be considered for its pharmacokinetic consequences. In general, the different pharmacokinetic characteristics of the drugs could be useful for a tailored pharmaceutical approach, designed to obtain the maximal efficacy and to minimize the risk of drug intolerance (supplement Table).

Electrolyte Disorders

An effective RAASi could be also limited by hyperkalemia, particularly in patients with MRAs.[70] An adequate management of hyperkalemia could allow optimization of therapy in AdvHF, thus allowing a better prognosis.[71]

Medical Inertia and Patient Adherence

The missed or inadequate use of disease-modifier drugs is not only related to clinical conditions. Medical inertia could be one of the main factors limiting the use and effectiveness of disease-modifier drugs.[72] The need of multiple evaluations for the introduction and uptitration of drugs and the management of side effects could lead physicians to avoid therapeutic changes. This possibility could be even more frequent in patients affected by AdvHF.

In addition to medical inertia, the non-adherence of patients could also lead to an inadequate use of disease-modifier drugs.[73,74] Patient education and empowerment could increase the adherence and optimization of the therapeutic approach, thus improving the prognoses.[75]

THE EVIDENCE AND THE OPTIMAL USE OF RENIN ANGIOTENSIN SYSTEM AND NEPRILYSIN INHIBITORS IN ADVANCED HEART FAILURE

Despite evidence of its greater favorable effect on prognosis compared with ACEi,[20,21] sacubitril/valsartan is still underused in real-world practice.[24,56] The larger trial that evaluated sacubitril/valsartan, PARADIGM-HF (Efficacy and Safety of LCZ696 Compared to Enalapril on Morbidity and Mortality of Patients With Chronic Heart Failure),[20] enrolled outpatients with HFrEF mainly without clinical features of AdvHF. In fact, they were all in stable clinical conditions, most of them in New York Heart Association (NYHA) class II, without symptomatic hypotension or systolic blood pressure (SBP) less than 100 mm Hg before or less than 95 mm Hg after run-in and with GFR greater than 30 mL/min/1.73 m^2. In contrast, some of the available evidence coming from the PARADIGM-HF suggests that the use of sacubitril/valsartan in AdvHF could still exert a favorable effect. Sacubitril/valsartan was able to reduce the HF hospitalization very early during the follow-up,[76] as well as the 30-day readmission[77] and the total number of HF hospitalizations,[76] all events characterizing AdvHF. Moreover, the benefit was also present in patients with prior decompensation.[78]

The possible efficacy in AdvHF has been also supported by the PIONEER-HF trial (Comparison of Sacubitril/Valsartan Versus Enalapril on Effect on NT-proBNP in Patients Stabilized From an Acute Heart Failure Episode),[21] which compared sacubitril/valsartan and enalapril among patients with HFrEF admitted for ADHF. The patients enrolled in PIONEER-HF, compared with those of PARADIGM-HF (**Table 1**), were characterized by a worse NYHA class, higher amino-terminal brain natriuretic peptide (NT-proBNP) levels, and lower LVEF. In these patients, sacubitril/valsartan was more effective than enalapril in reducing NT-proBNP and, in an exploratory analysis, it was

Table 1
Clinical characteristics and adverse events of the main trials evaluating sacubitril/valsartan

	PARADIGM-HF[20]		Transition[82]		PIONEER-HF[21]	
	Sacubitril/ Valsartan	Enalapril	Pre-discharge	Post-discharge	Sacubitril/ Valsartan	Enalapril
Number of patients	4187	4212	495	496	440	441
Age (years)	63.8 ± 11.5	63.8 ± 11.3	66.7	66.9	61	63
Male (%)	79.0	77.4	74.9	75.2	74.3	69.8
NYHA class, (%)						
I	4.3	5.0	0.0	0.6	0.9	1.1
II	71.6	69.3	64.6	63.5	22.7	27.7
III	23.1	24.9	33.5	34.9	64.3	61.0
IV	0.8	0.6	1.4	0.8	8.9	8.2
LVEF (%)	29.6 ± 6.1	29.4 ± 6.3	28.6 ± 7.5	29.0 ± 7.6	24	25
GFR (ml/min *1.73 m2)	-	-	61.6 ± 20.5	62.5 ± 19.4	58.4	58.9
Serum creatinine (mg/dL)	1.13 ± 0.3	1.12 ± 0.3	-	-	-	-
Median NT-proBNP (pg/mL)	1631	1594	1902	1669	2883	2536
Therapy (%)						
ACEi/ARBs	-	-	24.6	24.0	47.3	48.5
ACEi	78.0	77.5	50.5	51.0	-	-
ARBs	22.2	22.9	24.8	25.0	-	-
Beta-blockers	93.1	92.9	59.5	59.6	59.5	59.6
MRA	54.2	57.0	34.1	36.5	10.9	9.1
Follow-up duration	27 mo (median)		10 wk		8 wk	
Adverse events (%)						
Hypotension	14.0	9.2	12.7	9.5	15.0	12.7
Elevated serum potassium.	16.1	17.3	11.3	11.3	11.6	9.3
Worsening renal function (%)	2.2[a]	2.6 [a]	5.1 [b]	3.2 [b]	13.6 [b]	14.7 [b]
Discontinuation	17.8	19.8	7.1	5.6	11.5	10.1

Abbreviation: ACEi, ACE inhibitors; ARBs: Angiotensin II receptor blockers; GFR, glomerular filtration rate; LVEF, left ventricular ejection fraction; MRA, mineralcorticoid receptor antagonists; NT-proBNP, amino-terminal brain natriuretic peptide; PARADIGM-HF, Efficacy and Safety of LCZ696 Compared to Enalapril on Morbidity and Mortality of Patients With Chronic Heart Failure; PIONEERHF, Comparison of Sacubitril/Valsartan Versus Enalapril on Effect on NT-proBNP in Patients Stabilized From an Acute Heart Failure Episode; TRANSITION-HF, Initiation of sacubitril/valsartan in haemodynamically stabilised heart failure patients in hospital or early after discharge.

[a] Decline in renal function was defined as end-stage renal disease or a decrease greater than or equal to 50% from the value at randomization or a decrease in the estimated GFR (eGFR) of more than 30 mL/min/1.73 m², to less than 60 mL/min/1.73 m².

[b] Worsening renal function defined by an increase in the serum creatinine concentration greater than or equal to 0.5 mg/dL and a decrease in eGFR greater than or equal to 25%.

associated with lower incidence of HF-related events.[21,79] In addition, in observational studies enrolling patients with AdvHF, sacubitril/valsartan was associated with the improvement of filling pressures,[80] 6-minute walking test distance, and depressive symptoms.[81]

From this evidence, in patients with features of AdvHF and low LVEF, who are still not taking sacubitril/valsartan, an attempt to introduce this therapy should be made. Its prescription could be considered in the setting of an outpatients clinic or after in-hospital admission for ADHF. In this last case, according with the design of PIONEER-HF[21] or TRANSITION (Initiation of sacubitril/valsartan in haemodynamically stabilised heart failure patients in hospital or early after discharge),[82] sacubitril/valsartan could be started early during hospitalization or just before/after discharge. In the first case, patients should be in stable hemodynamic condition, without infusion of inotropes or vasodilatory drugs and with a stable dose of diuretics.[21] In the second case, sacubitril/valsartan could be started before or after discharge, when patients are not receiving intravenous drugs.[82]

In all these cases, the sacubitril/vaslartan starting dose should be carefully considered in order to avoid hypotension.[20,21,82] The dose of 24/26 mg twice a day should be preferred and the uptitration should be slow in order to achieve a better drug tolerance.[83] In patients with SBP less than 100 mm Hg, the successful introduction of sacubitril/valsartan is even more challenging, whereas, in those with SBP less than 90 mm Hg, it could be harmful. Although not tested in any trial, in patients with SBP between 90 and 100 mm Hg, it could be useful to evaluate the initial response to the drug with a starting dose even lower (24/26 mg once a day before increasing to 24/26 mg twice a day).

In order to better reduce the risk of hypotension, vasodilators and alpha-antagonists should be stopped and the loop diuretic dose should be also reconsidered. Sacubitril/valsartan could exert a diuretic response resulting in a reduction of pulmonary arterial pressure[80] and in reduced loop diuretic use in outpatients.[84] This response seems to be initially related to the increased availability of NPs, but it is then sustained by the reverse remodeling and reduced filling pressures.[85] As a consequence, when sacubitril/valsartan is introduced, the loop diuretic dose could be reduced, in the case of hypotension. In addition, education of patients in the self-management of sacubitril/valsartan dose according to arterial pressure home monitoring could be useful to maximize the efficacy of the drug and to minimize intolerance.

After sacubitril/valsartan introduction in AdvHF, a routine evaluation of renal function should also be recommended. Sacubitril/valsartan has been found to be associated with a greater nephroprotective effect,[86] particularly in patients with T2DM.[62] However, in the case of a reduction of low cardiac output and mean arterial pressure, analogously to ACEi and ARBs, its use could expose patients to an acute worsening of renal function,[63] Moreover, in the presence of renal dysfunction, the patients could be exposed to greater serum levels of sacubitrilat,[87] the active metabolite of sacubitril, thus further supporting the use of a low starting dose and a slow titration of sacubitril/valsartan. In addition, all the RCTs but one[88] that have tested sacubitril/valsartan considered a minimum GFR of 30 mL/min, which represents the lower limit to introduce the drugs.

As far as hyperkalemia is concerned, during PARADIGM-HF, sacubitril/valsartan treatment, compared with enalapril, was associated with its lower occurrence,[89] thus further strengthening its safety in patients with CKD.

In the case of ARNi intolerance in AdvHF patients, therapy with ACEi or ARBs should be adopted, if tolerated. The choice of ACEi can also be related to the pharmacokinetic properties. A very low dosage of ACEi/ARBs and/or the choice of a drug with a short half-life, such as captopril (see supplement Table), could be preferable in patients at higher risk of hypotension. Patients' education and self-management of drug doses according to blood pressure monitoring could also be useful in the management of ACEi/ARBs dose.

MINERALOCORTICOID RECEPTOR ANTAGONISTS AND HYPERKALEMIA IN ADVANCED HEART FAILURE

The most effective strategy for RAASi is based on the combination of ARNi/ACEi/ARBs with MRAs.[1,90] The MRs are present in the human body not only at the level of renal tubule but also in the myocardium, vascular wall, endothelium, macrophages, intestines, and eye.[90] At the renal level, MR activation promotes sodium retention, potassium loss, and fibrosis, leading to the progression of renal dysfunction. At the myocardium level, there is hypertrophy, fibrosis, and cell death.[90] At the vascular level, there is endothelial dysfunction, perivascular fibrosis, and increased vascular stiffness.[91] MR activation also leads to an overexpression of angiotensin I and ACE and to a vicious circle responsible for RAAS overactivation in HF. In addition, the simple blocking of ACE or ARBs is not able to effectively reduce the aldosterone overactivity that can be stimulated by other conditions, responsible for the so-called aldosterone escape.[92] According to this pathophysiologic background, MRA should be used in all patients with HFrEF, and this need is even more relevant in AdvHF patients. In the RALES (The Effect of Spironolactone on Morbidity and Mortality in Patients with Severe Heart Failure) trial,[10] among patients with severe functional limitation, spironolactone significantly reduced mortality and hospitalization compared with placebo.

Interestingly, the beneficial effects were still present in patients with renal dysfunction and/or worsening of renal function[93] as well as in those with mild hyperkalemia.[94] In addition, the withdrawal of MRA or its missed use because of renal dysfunction and hyperkalemia is associated with an increased risk of death.[95,96]

In the presence of mild hyperkalemia, current guidelines recommend the continuation of MRA.[1,71] In order to avoid the worsening of hyperkalemia, the presence of possible favorable factors, such as nonsteroidal antiinflammatory drugs, should be excluded and recommendations about the potassium intake in the diet should be provided to the patients.[71] In the case of moderate to severe hyperkalemia, MRA should be downtitrated or stopped according to the serum potassium levels. Note that, in the RALES trial, the dose of spironolactone in hyperkalemic patients could have been reduced to 25 mg every other day and the mean dose during the trial was 26 mg daily.[10] In the near future, in hyperkalemia, the new potassium binders could play an important role optimizing RAASi and improving patients' prognoses.[71] In addition, spironolactone is not the only MRA available. As shown in supplement Table, the molecules derived from spironolactone could have less influence on sex hormones and gynecomastia.

β-BLOCKERS AND HEART RATE IN ADVANCED HEART FAILURE

In the COPERNICUS (The Carvedilol Prospective Randomized Cumulative Survival) study,[4] β-blockers were tested in severely symptomatic HFrEF (dyspnea or fatigue at rest or on minimal exertion for at least 2 months and an LVEF≤25%). The administration of carvedilol, initially at very low dose (3.125 mg twice a day) and then uptitrated (mean final dose 37 mg daily), was associated with a significant reduction of mortality.[4] In patients treated with AdvHF, the beneficial effects of β-blockers were also observed in a subanalysis of the FIRST study.[97] The greater withdrawal rates at 1 year of carvedilol were observed among patients with recent or recurrent cardiac decompensation or severely depressed cardiac function (17.5%).[4]

In patients in whom β-blockers cannot be continued and/or are not uptitrated, or who are not able to reach a sinus rhythm heart rate lower than 70 beats per minute, the introduction or uptitration of ivabradine should be considered.[1] Ivabradine is a selective inhibitor of If current at the level of sinus node and it is able to slow heart rate in patients in sinus rhythm.[98] In the SHIFT (Ivabradine and outcomes in chronic heart failure)

trial, its administration in addition to the optimal therapy with β-blockers was associated with a reduced incidence of hospitalization because of ADHF and of death caused by HF worsening.[99] In patients with features of AdvHF, ivabradine could be safe and beneficial because the reduction of heart rate could be associated with an increased stroke volume and a preserved cardiac output.[100]

TYPE 2 SODIUM-GLUCOSE COTRANSPORTER INHIBITION IN ADVANCED HEART FAILURE

The evidence coming from DAPA-HF and EMPEROR-reduced trials has focused on the usefulness of SGLT2i added to the HFrEF therapy.[21,22] However, the two trials have enrolled patients in stable clinical conditions and mainly in NYHA class II, although with high NP serum levels. Patients in NYHA class II were also those in whom the beneficial effects were more evident. In contrast, the Effect of Sotagliflozin on Cardiovascular Events in Patients with Type 2 Diabetes Post Worsening Heart Failure (SOLOIST-WHF) trial provided more data about the possible usefulness of SGLT2i in patients with features of AdvHF because they enrolled patients with T2DM with recent ADHF.[101] Moreover, some preliminary data about the use of SGLT2i in ADHF have shown the ability to increase urine output without concerns about their safety.[102]

From a practical point of view, SGLT2i are easy to introduce because of the once-daily single dose. However, some aspects related to SBP should be considered. In EMPEROR-reduced and DAPA-HF, an SBP greater than 95 to 100 mm Hg and the absence of history of hypotension were considered among the inclusion criteria. Moreover, in all trials, a reduction of SBP was observed after SGLT2i initiation as well as a slightly higher incidence of hypotension and dehydration than placebo (**Table 2**), particularly in patients with high loop diuretic dose.[103] Interestingly, dapagliflozin was also associated with a reduced need for loop diuretic dose increase. Considering these data, in patients with AdvHF with history of hypotension and/or with SBP between 90 and 95 mm Hg, SGLT2i should be cautiously introduced with a close follow-up and, eventually, a reduction of loop diuretics dose. The other aspect that should be considered is represented by the changes of renal function. In DAPA-HF the GFR should be >30 mL/min/1.73 m²,[22] and in EMPEROR-reduced greater than 25 mL/min/1.73 m².[23] In both trials, an initial small decline of GFR was observed, thus suggesting the need of a monitoring of renal function after SGLT2i introduction. However, note that the initial

Table 2
Clinical characteristics and adverse events of the main trials evaluating type 2 sodium-glucose cotransporter

	DAPA-HF[22]		EMPEROR-Reduced[23]		SOLOIST-WHF[101]	
	Dapaglifozin	Placebo	Empaglifozin	Placebo	Sotaglifozin	Placebo
Number of patients	2373	2371	1863	1867	608	614
Age (years)	62.2 ± 11.0	66.5 ± 10.8	67.2 ± 10.8	66.5 ± 11.2	69	70
Male (%)	76.2	77.0	76.5	75.6	67.4	65.1
Type 2 diabetes (%)	42		48.9		100	
NYHA class, (%)						
I	-	-	-	-	2.5	
II	67.7	67.4	75.1	75.0	46.1	
III	31.5	31.7	24.4	24.4	46.7	
IV	0.8	1.0	0.5	0.6	4.7	
LVEF (%)	31.2 ± 6.7	30.9 ± 6.9	27.7 ± 6.0	27.2 ± 6.1	35	35
GFR (ml/min *1.73 m2)	66.0 ± 19.6	65.5 ± 19.3	61.8 ± 21.7	62.2 ± 21.5	49.2	50.5
Median NT-proBNP	1428	1446	1887	1926	1816.8	1741.0
Therapy (%)						
ACEi/ARBs	-	-	70.5	68.9	-	-
ACEi	56.1	56.1	-	-	41.8	39.3
ARBs	28.4	26.7	-	-	40.3	44.0
ARNI	10.5	10.9	18.3	20.7	15.3	18.2
Beta-blockers	96.0	96.2	94.7	94.7	92.8	91.4
MRA	71.5	70.6	70.1	72.6	66.3	62.7
Adverse events (%)						
Volume depletion	7.5	6.8	10.6	9.9	9.4	8.8
Hypoglicemia	0.2	0.2	1.4	1.5	4.3	2.8
Worsening renal function	6.5 [a]	7.2 [a]	1.6 [b]	3.1 [b]	11.6	12.3
Withdrawal	10.5	10.9	16.3	18.0	4.8	3.8
Urinary tract infection	0.5	0.7	4.9	4.5	4.8	5.1

ACEi, ACE inhibitors; ARBs: Angiotensin II receptor blockers; GFR, glomerular filtration rate; LVEF, left ventricular ejection fraction; MRA, mineralcorticoid receptor antagonists; NT-proBNP, amino-terminal brain natriuretic peptide; PARADIGM-HF, Efficacy and Safety of LCZ696 Compared to Enalapril on Morbidity and Mortality of Patients With Chronic Heart Failure; PIONEERHF, Comparison of Sacubitril/Valsartan Versus Enalapril on Effect on NT-proBNP in Patients Stabilized From an Acute Heart Failure Episode; TRANSITION-HF, Initiation of sacubitril/valsartan in haemodynamically stabilised heart failure patients in hospital or early after discharge.

[a] Worsening renal function is a composite outcome of a reduction of 50% or more in the eGFR sustained for at least 28 days, end-stage renal disease, or death from renal causes. End-stage renal disease was defined as an eGFR of less than 15 mL/min/1.73 m^2 that was sustained for at least 28 days, long-term dialysis treatment (sustained for $\geq$28 days), or kidney transplant. Serious adverse events of acute kidney injury were reported in 23 patients (1.0%) in the dapagliflozin group and in 46 (1.9%) in the placebo group ($P = .007$).

[b] The composite renal outcome includes chronic dialysis or renal transplant or a sustained reduction of 40% or more in the eGFR or a sustained eGFR of less than 15 mL/min/1.73 m^2 in patients with a baseline eGFR of 30 mL/min/1.73 m^2 or more or a sustained eGFR of less than 10 mL/min/1.73 m^2 in those with a baseline eGFR of less than 30 mL/min/1.73 m^2.

decline was followed by a renal protection. Moreover, SGLT2i could also continue to exert a nephroprotective effect in patients with a marked reduction of GFR.[23,50]

SUMMARY

Disease-modifier drugs play a key role in improving survival of patients with HFrEF. Although their early use maximizes their beneficial effects to be maximized, these drugs could still improve prognosis of patients with AdvHF. However, because of the clinical features characterizing AdvHF, their optimal use can be challenging. The continuous medical effort to prescribe, introduce, reintroduce, or uptitrate disease-modifying drugs according to patients' conditions is mandatory as well as the empowerment and self-management of the patients and care givers. In addition, in AdvHF, the attempt of introducing the novel classes of disease-modifier drugs completes the strategies to ensure the best treatment of patients.

CLINICS CARE POINTS

- In patients with clinical features of AdvHF, revise medical therapy. All classes of disease-modifiers drugs, if not contraindicated, should be prescribed at the maximum tolerated dose.
- Consider the introduction of the novel classes of disease-modifier drugs if still not present.
- In the case of HF hospitalization, before discharge or early after, introduce, continue, or uptitrate optimal medical therapy.
- In the context of a dedicated management program, educate the patients to self-management of drug doses according to blood pressure monitoring. Monitor renal dysfunction and electrolyte disorders and modify the dose of disease-modifying drugs accordingly.

DISCLOSURE

M. Iacoviello received honoraria as a consultant in advisory boards from Astra Zeneca, Boehringer Ingelheim, Lilly, Merk Serono, Novartis, Vifor Pharma. The other authors have no disclosures. This review was not supported by external funding.

SUPPLEMENTARY DATA

Supplementary data related to this article can be found online at https://doi.org/10.1016/j.hfc.2021.05.002.

REFERENCES

1. Ponikowski P, Voors AA, Anker SD, et al. 2016 ESC guidelines for the diagnosis and treatment of acute and chronic heart failure: the task force for the diagnosis and treatment of acute and chronic heart failure of the European Society of Cardiology (ESC) Developed with the special contribution of the Heart Failure Association (HFA) of the ESC. Eur Heart J 2016;37:2129–200.
2. Garg R, Yusuf S. Overview of randomized trials of angiotensin-converting enzyme inhibitors on mortality and morbidity in patients with heart failure. Collaborative Group on ACE Inhibitor Trials. JAMA 1995;273:1450–6.
3. Hjalmarson A, Goldstein S, Fagerberg B, et al. Effects of controlled-release metoprolol on total mortality, hospitalizations, and well-being in patients with heart failure: the Metoprolol CR/XL Randomized Intervention Trial in congestive heart failure (MERIT-HF). MERIT-HF Study Group. JAMA 2000; 283:1295–302.
4. Packer M, Coats AJ, Fowler MB, et al. Effect of carvedilol on survival in severe chronic heart failure. N Engl J Med 2001;344:1651–8.
5. Packer M, Bristow MR, Cohn JN, et al. The effect of carvedilol on morbidity and mortality in patients with chronic heart failure. U.S. Carvedilol Heart Failure Study Group. N Engl J Med 1996;334: 1349–55.
6. Effect of metoprolol CR/XL in chronic heart failure: metoprolol CR/XL Randomised Intervention Trial in Congestive Heart Failure (MERIT-HF). Lancet 1999;353:2001–7.
7. Packer M, Fowler MB, Roecker EB, et al. Effect of carvedilol on the morbidity of patients with severe chronic heart failure: results of the carvedilol prospective randomized cumulative survival (COPERNICUS) study. Circulation 2002;106(17):2194–9.
8. CIBIS-II Investigators and Committees. The Cardiac Insufficiency Bisoprolol Study II (CIBIS-II): a randomised trial. Lancet 1999;353:9–13.
9. Flather MD, Shibata MC, Coats AJS, et al. Randomized trial to determine the effect of nebivolol on mortality and cardiovascular hospital admission in elderly patients with heart failure (SENIORS). Eur Heart J 2005;26:215–25.
10. Pitt B, Zannad F, Remme WJ, et al. The effect of spironolactone on morbidity and mortality in patients with severe heart failure. Randomized Aldactone Evaluation Study Investigators. N Engl J Med 1999;341:709–17.
11. Zannad F, McMurray JJ, Krum H, et al. Eplerenone in patients with systolic heart failure and mild symptoms. N Engl J Med 2011;364:11–21.
12. Mann DL. Mechanisms and models in heart failure: a combinatorial approach. Circulation 1999;100: 999–1008.
13. Braunwald E. Heart failure. JACC Heart Fail 2013; 1:1–20.
14. Yancy CW, Jessup M, Bozkurt B, et al. 2017 ACC/AHA/HFSA focused update of the 2013 ACCF/AHA guideline for the management of heart failure: a report of the American College of Cardiology/American Heart Association Task Force on Clinical Practice Guidelines and the Heart Failure Society of America. Circulation 2017;136:e137–61.
15. Crespo-Leiro MG, Metra M, Lund LH, et al. Advanced heart failure: a position statement of

the Heart Failure Association of the European Society of Cardiology. Eur J Heart Fail 2018;20: 1505–35.

16. Yancy CW, Jessup M, Bozkurt B, et al. 2013 ACCF/AHA guideline for the management of heart failure: executive summary: a report of the American College of Cardiology Foundation/American Heart Association Task Force on practice guidelines. Circulation 2013;128:1810–52.

17. Fang JC, Ewald GA, Allen LA, et al. Advanced (stage D) heart failure: a statement from the Heart Failure Society of America Guidelines Committee. J Card Fail 2015;21:519–34.

18. Maggioni AP, Dahlström U, Filippatos, et al. EUR-Observational Research Programme: regional differences and 1-year follow-up results of the Heart Failure Pilot Survey (ESC-HF Pilot). Eur J Heart Fail 2013;15:808–17.

19. Wu JR, Moser DK, Lennie TA, et al. Medication adherence in patients who have heart failure: a review of the literature. Nurs Clin North Am 2008;43: 133–53, vii–viii.

20. McMurray JJ, Packer M, Desai AS, et al. Angiotensin-neprilysin inhibition versus enalapril in heart failure. N Engl J Med 2014;371:993–1004.

21. Velazquez EJ, Morrow DA, DeVore AD, et al. Angiotensin-neprilysin inhibition in acute decompensated heart failure. N Engl J Med 2019;380: 539–48.

22. McMurray JJV, Solomon SD, Inzucchi SE, et al. Dapagliflozin in patients with heart failure and reduced ejection fraction. N Engl J Med 2019; 381:1995–2008.

23. Packer M, Butler J, Filippatos GS, et al. Evaluation of the effect of sodium-glucose co-transporter 2 inhibition with empagliflozin on morbidity and mortality of patients with chronic heart failure and a reduced ejection fraction: rationale for and design of the EMPEROR-Reduced trial. Eur J Heart Fail 2019;21:1270–8.

24. Han J, Chung F, Nguyen QL, et al. Evaluation of patients with heart failure to determine eligibility for treatment with Sacubitril/Valsartan: insights from a veterans administration healthcare system. Pharmacotherapy 2019;39:1053–9.

25. Longato E, Di Camillo B, Sparacino G, et al. Cardiovascular outcomes of type 2 diabetic patients treated with SGLT-2 inhibitors versus GLP-1 receptor agonists in real-life. BMJ Open Diabetes Res Care 2020;8:e001451.

26. CONSENSUS Trial Study Group. Effects of enalapril on mortality in severe congestive heart failure. Results of the Cooperative North Scandinavian Enalapril Survival Study (CONSENSUS). N Engl J Med 1987;316:1429–35.

27. SOLVD Investigators, Yusuf S, Pitt B, Davis CE, et al. Effect of enalapril on mortality and the development of heart failure in asymptomatic patients with reduced left ventricular ejection fractions. N Engl J Med 1992;327:685–91.

28. SOLVD Investigators, Yusuf S, Pitt B, Davis CE, et al. Effect of enalapril on survival in patients with reduced left ventricular ejection fractions and congestive heart failure. N Engl J Med 1991;325: 293–302.

29. Granger CB, McMurray JJ, Yusuf S, et al. Effects of candesartan in patients with chronic heart failure and reduced left-ventricular systolic function intolerant to angiotensin-converting-enzyme inhibitors: the CHARM-Alternative trial. Lancet 2003;362: 772–6.

30. Buggey J, Mentz RJ, DeVore AD, et al. Angiotensin receptor neprilysin inhibition in heart failure: mechanistic action and clinical impact. J Card Fail 2015; 21:741–50.

31. Díez J. Chronic heart failure as a state of reduced effectiveness of the natriuretic peptide system: implications for therapy. Eur J Heart Fail 2017;19: 167–76.

32. Miller WL, Phelps MA, Wood CM, et al. Comparison of mass spectrometry and clinical assay measurements of circulating fragments of B-type natriuretic peptide in patients with chronic heart failure. Circ Heart Fail 2011;4:355–60.

33. Bayés-Genís A, Barallat J, Galán A, et al. Soluble neprilysin is predictive of cardiovascular death and heart failure hospitalization in heart failure patients. J Am Coll Cardiol 2015;65(7): 657–65.

34. Nougué H, Pezel T, Picard F, et al. Effects of sacubitril/valsartan on neprilysin targets and the metabolism of natriuretic peptides in chronic heart failure: a mechanistic clinical study. Eur J Heart Fail 2019;21:598–605.

35. Januzzi JL, Butler J, Fombu E, et al. Rationale and methods of the prospective study of biomarkers, symptom improvement, and ventricular remodeling during Sacubitril/Valsartan Therapy for Heart Failure (PROVE-HF). Am Heart J 2018;199:130–6.

36. Desai AS, Solomon SD, Shah AM, et al. Effect of sacubitril-valsartan vs enalapril on aortic stiffness in patients with heart failure and reduced ejection fraction: a randomized clinical trial. JAMA 2019; 322:1–10.

37. Aimo A, Gaggin HK, Barison A, et al. Imaging, biomarker, and clinical predictors of cardiac remodeling in heart failure with reduced ejection fraction. JACC Heart Fail 2019;7:782–94.

38. Lupón J, Gavidia-Bovadilla G, Ferrer E, et al. Dynamic trajectories of left ventricular ejection fraction in heart failure. J Am Coll Cardiol 2018;72: 591–601.

39. Jong P, Yusuf S, Rousseau MF, et al. Effect of enalapril on 12-year survival and life expectancy in

patients with left ventricular systolic dysfunction: a follow-up study. Lancet 2003;361:1843–8.

40. Zinman B, Wanner C, Lachin JM, et al. Empagliflozin, Cardiovascular Outcomes, and Mortality in Type 2 Diabetes. N Engl J Med 2015;373:2117–28.

41. Perkovic V, de Zeeuw D, Mahaffey KW, et al. Canagliflozin and renal outcomes in type 2 diabetes: results from the CANVAS Program randomised clinical trials. Lancet Diabetes Endocrinol 2018;6: 691–704.

42. Perkovic V, Jardine MJ, Neal B, et al. Canagliflozin and renal outcomes in type 2 diabetes and nephropathy. N Engl J Med 2019;380:2295–306.

43. Wiviott SD, Raz I, Bonaca MP, et al. Dapagliflozin and cardiovascular outcomes in type 2 diabetes. N Engl J Med 2019;380:347–57.

44. Verma S, McMurray JJV. SGLT2 inhibitors and mechanisms of cardiovascular benefit: a state-of-the-art review. Diabetologia 2018;61:2108–17.

45. Seferović PM, Fragasso G, Petrie M, et al. Sodium-glucose co-transporter 2 inhibitors in heart failure: beyond glycaemic control. A position paper of the Heart Failure Association of the European Society of Cardiology. Eur J Heart Fail 2020;22: 1495–503.

46. Hallow KM, Helmlinger G, Greasley PJ, et al. Why do SGLT2 inhibitors reduce heart failure hospitalization? A differential volume regulation hypothesis. Diabetes Obes Metab 2018;20(3):479–87.

47. Griffin M, Rao VS, Ivey-Miranda J, et al. Empagliflozin in heart failure: diuretic and cardiorenal effects. Circulation 2020;142:1028–39.

48. Mordi NA, Mordi IR, Singh JS, et al. Renal and cardiovascular effects of SGLT2 inhibition in combination with loop diuretics in patients with type 2 diabetes and chronic heart failure: the RECEDE-CHF Trial. Circulation 2020;142:1713–24.

49. DeFronzo RA, Norton L, Abdul-Ghani M. Renal, metabolic and cardiovascular considerations of SGLT2 inhibition. Nat Rev Nephrol 2017;13:11–26.

50. Heerspink HJL, Stefánsson BV, Correa-Rotter R, et al. Dapagliflozin in patients with chronic kidney disease. N Engl J Med 2020;383:1436–46.

51. Inzucchi SE, Zinman B, Fitchett D, et al. How does empagliflozin reduce cardiovascular mortality? insights from a mediation analysis of the EMPA-REG OUTCOME trial. Diabetes Care 2018;41: 356–63.

52. Ferrannini E, Baldi S, Frascerra S, et al. Shift to fatty substrate utilization in response to sodium-glucose cotransporter 2 inhibition in subjects without diabetes and patients with type 2 diabetes. Diabetes 2016;65:1190–5.

53. Heerspink HJL, Perco P, Mulder S, et al. Canagliflozin reduces inflammation and fibrosis biomarkers: a potential mechanism of action for beneficial effects of SGLT2 inhibitors in diabetic kidney disease. Diabetologia 2019;62:1154–66.

54. Vaduganathan M, Claggett BL, Jhund PS, et al. Estimating lifetime benefits of comprehensive disease-modifying pharmacological therapies in patients with heart failure with reduced ejection fraction: a comparative analysis of three randomised controlled trials. Lancet 2020;396: 121–8.

55. Tavazzi L, Senni M, Metra M, et al. Multicenter prospective observational study on acute and chronic heart failure: one-year follow-up results of IN-HF (Italian Network on Heart Failure) outcome registry. Circ Heart Fail 2013;6:473–81.

56. Bhagat AA, Greene SJ, Vaduganathan M, et al. Initiation, continuation, switching, and withdrawal of heart failure medical therapies during hospitalization. JACC Heart Fail 2019;7:1–12.

57. Oliva F, Mortara A, Cacciatore G, et al. IN-HF Outcome Investigators. Acute heart failure patient profiles, management and in-hospital outcome: results of the Italian Registry on Heart Failure Outcome. Eur J Heart Fail 2012;14:1208–17.

58. Böhm M, Young R, Jhund PS, et al. Systolic blood pressure, cardiovascular outcomes and efficacy and safety of sacubitril/valsartan (LCZ696) in patients with chronic heart failure and reduced ejection fraction: results from PARADIGM-HF. Eur Heart J 2017;38:1132–43.

59. Ruggenenti P, Fassi A, Ilieva AP, et al. Preventing microalbuminuria in type 2 diabetes. N Engl J Med 2004;351:1941–51.

60. Brenner BM, Cooper ME, de Zeeuw D, et al. Effects of losartan on renal and cardiovascular outcomes in patients with type 2 diabetes and nephropathy. N Engl J Med 2001;345:861–9.

61. Remuzzi G, Ruggenenti P, Perna A, et al. Continuum of renoprotection with losartan at all stages of type 2 diabetic nephropathy: a post hoc analysis of the RENAAL trial results. J Am Soc Nephrol 2004;15:3117–25.

62. Damman K, Gori M, Claggett B, et al. Renal effects and associated outcomes during angiotensin-neprilysin inhibition in heart failure. JACC Heart Fail 2018;6:489–98.

63. Metra M, Cotter G, Gheorghiade M, et al. The role of the kidney in heart failure. Eur Heart J 2012;33: 2135–42.

64. Merril AJ. Edema and decreased renal blood flow in patients with chronic congestive heart failure; evidence of forward failure as the primary cause of edema. J Clin Invest 1946;25:389–400.

65. Ruggenenti P, Remuzzi G. Worsening kidney function in decompensated heart failure: treat the heart, don't mind the kidney. Eur Heart J 2011;32:2476–8.

66. Ljungman S, Laragh JH, Cody RJ. Role of the kidney in congestive heart failure. Relationship of

cardiac index to kidney function. Drugs 1990; 39(Suppl 4):10–21 [discussion 22-4].

67. Damman K, Navis G, Smilde TD, et al. Decreased cardiac output, venous congestion and the association with renal impairment in patients with cardiac dysfunction. Eur J Heart Fail 2007;9:872–8.

68. Beldhuis IE, Streng KW, Ter Maaten JM, et al. Renin-angiotensin system inhibition, worsening renal function, and outcome in heart failure patients with reduced and preserved ejection fraction: a meta-analysis of published study data. Circ Heart Fail 2017;10:e003588.

69. Damman K, Tang WH, Felker GM, et al. Current evidence on treatment of patients with chronic systolic heart failure and renal insufficiency: practical considerations from published data. J Am Coll Cardiol 2014;63:853–71.

70. Epstein M, Reaven NL, Funk SE, et al. Evaluation of the treatment gap between clinical guidelines and the utilization of renin-angiotensin-aldosterone system inhibitors. Am J Manag Care 2015;21: S212–20.

71. Rosano GMC, Tamargo J, Kjeldsen KP, et al. Expert consensus document on the management of hyperkalaemia in patients with cardiovascular disease treated with renin angiotensin aldosterone system inhibitors: coordinated by the Working Group on Cardiovascular Pharmacotherapy of the European Society of Cardiology. Eur Heart J Cardiovasc Pharmacother 2018;4:180–8.

72. Verhestraeten C, Heggermont WA, Maris M. Clinical inertia in the treatment of heart failure: a major issue to tackle. Heart Fail Rev. 2020 May 30.

73. Osterberg L, Blaschke T. Adherence to medication. N Engl J Med 2005;353:487–97.

74. Ho PM, Bryson CL, Rumsfeld JS. Medication adherence: its importance in cardiovascular outcomes. Circulation 2009;119:3028–35.

75. Schou M, Gislason G, Videbaek L, et al. Effect of extended follow-up in a specialized heart failure clinic on adherence to guideline recommended therapy: NorthStar Adherence Study. Eur J Heart Fail 2014;16:1249–55.

76. Packer M, McMurray JJ, Desai AS, et al. Angiotensin receptor neprilysin inhibition compared with enalapril on the risk of clinical progression in surviving patients with heart failure. Circulation 2015;131:54–61.

77. Desai AS, Claggett BL, Packer M, et al. Influence of Sacubitril/Valsartan (LCZ696) on 30-day readmission after heart failure hospitalization. J Am Coll Cardiol 2016;68:241–8.

78. Solomon SD, Claggett B, Packer M, et al. Efficacy of Sacubitril/Valsartan relative to a prior decompensation: the PARADIGM-HF trial. JACC Heart Fail 2016;4:816–22.

79. DeVore AD, Braunwald E, Morrow DA, et al. Initiation of angiotensin-neprilysin inhibition after acute decompensated heart failure: secondary analysis of the open-label extension of the PIONEER-HF trial. JAMA Cardiol 2020;5:202–7.

80. Khan Z, Gholkar G, Tolia S, et al. Effect of sacubitril/valsartan on cardiac filling pressures in patients with left ventricular systolic dysfunction. Int J Cardiol 2018;271:169–73.

81. Cacciatore F, Amarelli C, Maiello C, et al. Effect of Sacubitril-Valsartan in reducing depression in patients with advanced heart failure. J Affect Disord 2020;272:132–7.

82. Wachter R, Senni M, Belohlavek J, et al. Initiation of sacubitril/valsartan in haemodynamically stabilised heart failure patients in hospital or early after discharge: primary results of the randomised TRANSITION study. Eur J Heart Fail 2019;21: 998–1007.

83. Senni M, McMurray JJ, Wachter R, et al. Initiating sacubitril/valsartan (LCZ696) in heart failure: results of TITRATION, a double-blind, randomized comparison of two uptitration regimens. Eur J Heart Fail 2016;18:1193–202.

84. Vardeny O, Claggett B, Kachadourian J, et al. Reduced loop diuretic use in patients taking sacubitril/valsartan compared with enalapril: the PARADIGM-HF trial. Eur J Heart Fail 2019;21: 337–41.

85. Ter Maaten JM. Unravelling the effect of sacubitril/valsartan on loop diuretic dosing. Eur J Heart Fail 2019;21:342–4.

86. Ushijima K, Ando H, Arakawa Y, et al. Prevention against renal damage in rats with subtotal nephrectomy by sacubitril/valsartan (LCZ696), a dual-acting angiotensin receptor-neprilysin inhibitor. Pharmacol Res Perspect 2017;5:e00336.

87. Ayalasomayajula SP, Langenickel TH, Jordaan P, et al. Effect of renal function on the pharmacokinetics of LCZ696 (sacubitril/valsartan), an angiotensin receptor neprilysin inhibitor. Eur J Clin Pharmacol 2016;72:1065–73.

88. Haynes R, Judge PK, Staplin N, et al. Effects of Sacubitril/Valsartan versus irbesartan in patients with chronic kidney disease. Circulation 2018;138: 1505–14.

89. Desai AS, Vardeny O, Claggett B, et al. Reduced risk of hyperkalemia during treatment of heart failure with mineralocorticoid receptor antagonists by use of sacubitril/valsartan compared with enalapril: a secondary analysis of the PARADIGM-HF trial. JAMA Cardiol 2017;2:79–85.

90. Pitt B, Pedro Ferreira J, Zannad F. Mineralocorticoid receptor antagonists in patients with heart failure: current experience and future perspectives. Eur Heart J Cardiovasc Pharmacother 2017;3: 48–57.

91. DeMarco VG, Habibi J, Jia G, et al. Low-dose mineralocorticoid receptor blockade prevents western diet-induced arterial stiffening in female mice. Hypertension 2015;66:99–107.

92. McKelvie RS, Yusuf S, Pericak D, et al. Comparison of candesartan, enalapril, and their combination in congestive heart failure: randomized evaluation of strategies for left ventricular dysfunction (RE-SOLVD) pilot study. The RESOLVD Pilot Study Investigators. Circulation 1999;100:1056–64.

93. Vardeny O, Wu DH, Desai A, et al. Influence of baseline and worsening renal function on efficacy of spironolactone in patients With severe heart failure: insights from RALES (Randomized Aldactone Evaluation Study). J Am Coll Cardiol 2012;60:2082–9.

94. Vardeny O, Claggett B, Anand I, et al. Incidence, predictors, and outcomes related to hypo- and hyperkalemia in patients with severe heart failure treated with a mineralocorticoid receptor antagonist. Circ Heart Fail 2014;7:573–9.

95. Lisi F, Parisi G, Gioia MI, et al. Mineralcorticoid receptor antagonist withdrawal for hyperkalemia and mortality in patients with heart failure. Cardiorenal Med 2020;10:145–53.

96. Volterrani M, Perrone V, Sangiorgi D, et al. Effects of hyperkalaemia and non-adherence to renin-angiotensin-aldosterone system inhibitor therapy in patients with heart failure in Italy: a propensity-matched study. Eur J Heart Fail 2020;22:2049–55.

97. O'Connor CM, Gattis WA, Zannad F, et al. Beta-blocker therapy in advanced heart failure: clinical characteristics and long-term outcomes. Eur J Heart Fail 1999;1(1):81–8.

98. Reil JC, Böhm M. BEAUTIFUL results–the slower, the better? Lancet 2008;372:779–80.

99. Swedberg K, Komajda M, Böhm M, et al. Ivabradine and outcomes in chronic heart failure (SHIFT): a randomised placebo-controlled study. Lancet 2010;376:875–85.

100. De Ferrari GM, Mazzuero A, Agnesina L, et al. Favourable effects of heart rate reduction with intravenous administration of ivabradine in patients with advanced heart failure. Eur J Heart Fail 2008;10:550–5.

101. Bhatt DL, Szarek M, Steg PG, et al. Sotagliflozin in patients with diabetes and recent worsening heart failure. N Engl J Med 2021.

102. Damman K, Beusekamp JC, Boorsma EM, et al. Randomized, double-blind, placebo-controlled, multicentre pilot study on the effects of empagliflozin on clinical outcomes in patients with acute decompensated heart failure (EMPA-RESPONSE-AHF). Eur J Heart Fail 2020;22:713–22.

103. Jackson AM, Dewan P, Anand IS, et al. Dapagliflozin and diuretic use in patients with heart failure and reduced ejection fraction in DAPA-HF. Circulation 2020;142:1040–54.

Congestion in Patients with Advanced Heart Failure: Assessment and Treatment

Carlo Mario Lombardi, MD[a], Giuliana Cimino, MD[a], Pierpaolo Pellicori, PhD[b],
Andrea Bonelli, MD[a], Riccardo Maria Inciardi, MD[a], Matteo Pagnesi, MD[a],
Daniela Tomasoni, MD[a], Alice Ravera, MD[a], Marianna Adamo, MD[a],
Valentina Carubelli, PhD[a], Marco Metra, MD[a,*]

KEYWORDS

• Congestion • Heart failure • Diuretics • Organ dysfunction

KEY POINTS

- Congestion is a frequent finding in patients with advanced heart failure and is associated with the development of multiorgan complications and adverse outcomes.
- Early identification, prevention, and treatment of congestion remain a primary goal in the treatment of advanced heart failure.
- High doses of loop diuretics are associated with a worse prognosis.
- The assessment and the effective reduction of congestion with intensive medical or device therapy can improve symptoms and survival in patients with advanced heart failure.

INTRODUCTION

Heart failure (HF) is a progressive disease characterized by worsening symptoms, unplanned hospital admissions due to acute decompensation, development of multiorgan complications, and shortened life span.[1,2] According to the updated recommendations from the HF Association (HFA) of the European Society of Cardiology (ESC),[3] all patients with HF might progress to advanced HF, regardless of their left ventricular ejection fraction.[4] Advanced HF should be diagnosed in those with severe and persistent symptoms [New York Heart Association class III or IV], severe cardiac dysfunction, and impaired exercise tolerance (ie, 6 min walking test distance (<300 m)) who require frequent intravenous diuretics or inotropes.[5]

It has been suggested that up to 10% of the HF population might have advanced heart failure, but the true prevalence of this severe form of the disease remains to be determined.[6,7]

More than 90% of patients admitted to hospital with worsening HF[4,8,9] have signs and symptoms attributable to fluid overload or congestion. Congestion can deteriorate cardiac function and cause injury, impairment, and ultimately, the failure of extracardiac organs (lungs, brain, kidneys, intestine, liver), eventually leading to poor quality of life and an increased risk of early death. Thus, prevention, identification, and management of congestion and of its cardiac and extracardiac complications have evolved as therapeutic targets of interest in advanced HF.[10–12]

CONGESTION AND ORGAN DYSFUNCTION IN ADVANCED HEART FAILURE
Effects on Heart

Congestion increases preload, which leads to increased left ventricular wall stress and adverse

[a] Cardiology Unit, Department of Medical and Surgical Specialties, Radiological Sciences, and Public Health, University of Brescia, Brescia, Italy; [b] Robertson Institute of Biostatistics and Clinical Trials Unit, University of Glasgow, Glasgow, UK
* Corresponding author.
E-mail address: metramarco@libero.it

Heart Failure Clin 17 (2021) 575–586
https://doi.org/10.1016/j.hfc.2021.05.003
1551-7136/21/© 2021 Elsevier Inc. All rights reserved.

cardiac remodeling, worsens mitral and tricuspid valve regurgitation, and causes a progressive decline in the overall myocardial performance.[13] As a consequence, atria, and ventricles increase the production of natriuretic peptides to prevent further cardiac deterioration.[14] Abnormal levels of cardiac troponin are also detectable in a large proportion of patients with advanced HF, especially with high-sensitivity assays, revealing myocyte injury even in the absence of substantial stenosis in the main coronary arteries.[15–17]

Effects on Lungs

A prolonged and sustained increase in left atrial pressure will eventually be transmitted back to the pulmonary capillaries and increase the filtration rate of fluids into the pulmonary interstitium, causing lung stiffness, and in most patients, exertional dyspnea. The lymphatic system regularly drains interstitial fluid, but when the interstitial pressure exceeds the pleural pressure and drainage capacity, fluids move into the pleural and intra-alveolar spaces, causing pleural effusion and alveolar edema and possibly leading to breathlessness at rest or orthopnea.[18] In patients with advanced HF, cardiopulmonary remodeling occurs and is characterized by impaired permeability of the vascular bed and pulmonary vasoconstriction, and ultimately, pulmonary hypertension[19] causing right ventricular strain and dysfunction.

Effects on Liver

Another consequence of long-standing cardiac dysfunction and congestion is hepatic vein hypertension and the potential development of ascites, anorexia, and abdominal pain that cause discomfort and worsen quality of life. Biochemical evidence of hepatic dysfunction is present in most patients with advanced HF,[20–22] and elevated levels of liver enzymes foretell a poor prognosis.[23] In the setting of systemic congestion, cholestasis is usually observed, with elevation of alkaline phosphatase, bilirubin, and γ-glutamyltransferase (GGT),[22–24] that should be distinguished from acute centrilobular necrosis associated with hypoperfusion.[23] Hypoxic liver injury is the most common cause of a substantial increase in aminotransferase levels in the hospital.[25] It occurs in 5% to 10% of patients with critical illness and is a strong risk factor for mortality in the intensive care unit.[26,27] Hepatic dysfunction is frequently associated with renal dysfunction in advanced HF, with synergistic prognostic implications.[28–31]

Effects on Kidneys

Cardiorenal syndrome refers to the pathophysiological interplay between the heart and kidneys. Several observational studies showed that venous congestion is a stronger predictor of worsening renal function than cardiac output or mean arterial pressure in patients with advanced HF.[32–35] Elevated central venous pressure may worsen renal function through several different mechanisms, including pressure-induced reduction in renal blood flow, renal hypoxia, increased interstitial pressure, and interstitial fibrosis.[36] Other factors, such as inflammation (tissue damage, infection), nephrotoxic medication or contrast agents, low cardiac output,[37] and elevated intra-abdominal pressure[38] might further deteriorate renal function.

The presence of chronic renal dysfunction is the strongest risk factor for the development of in-hospital acute kidney injury,[39] suggesting that underlying severity of kidney disease is an important determinant of kidney reserve and the response to diuretic treatment. In patients hospitalized with HF, small absolute increases in serum creatinine (0.3 mg/dL) or cystatin C (0.3 mg/L) predict an adverse prognosis.[40–44] However, patients who experience transient worsening of renal function in conjunction with clinical improvement may have "pseudo-worsening renal function" and not be at increased risk for adverse events.[44] Pseudo-worsening renal function is mostly the result of changes in intraglomerular hemodynamics rather than renal injury. Although aggressive fluid removal is related to deterioration in renal function and hemoconcentration, the latter is associated with improved survival in advanced HF.[45] Clearly, the clinical scenario (worse or improved) must be considered when interpreting changes in renal function. Thus, some degree of worsening renal function is acceptable while effective decongestion is ongoing, but unfortunately, it is very difficult to predict the renal response to decongestion. In a recent consensus paper from the HFA-ESC on diuretic use, it has been proposed to investigate whether spot urinary sodium might guide diuretic therapy in the first phases of acute decompensation.[46] Preliminary experience suggests that low urinary sodium excretion during the first 6 h after initiation of loop diuretic therapy is associated with lower urine output on the first day and with all-cause mortality.[47]

Effects on Brain

A complex relationship exists between advanced HF, congestion, and cerebral dysfunction. Patients with advanced HF can frequently exhibit symptoms of cerebral dysfunction such as cognitive impairment, anxiety, depression, and delirium,[48] the occurrence of which is associated with adverse outcomes.[49,50] Hypoxemia and hypoperfusion are key drivers of cerebral dysfunction in advanced HF, but a silent, or clinically overt, cerebral infarction, or cardiac embolism in the context of a low cardiac output or atrial arrhythmia, autonomic imbalance, and hypotension, might cause additional brain injury. Central or peripheral neurologic damage might impair breathing and vascular responses, perpetuating a vicious circle. Conditions associated with advanced HF, such as old age, social isolation, sleep disturbances, and low adherence to medications, might additionally impair cognitive function, increase anxiety, and worsen congestion and symptoms of depression.[51]

Effects on Bowel

Elevated right atrial pressure and right ventricular dysfunction lead to progressive volume overload with systemic congestion,[52,53] a process that does not spare the intestine. Bowel edema might alter gut permeability, and disrupt the immunologic colonic barrier, leading to a state of bacterial-derived systemic inflammation.[52,54,55] Moreover, visceral venous congestion might contribute to the progression of cardiac dysfunction via additional mechanisms that include an increased intestinal sodium absorption[56] and reduced bioavailability of HF medications.[57] Not surprisingly, Intestinal edema has some clinical important clinical consequences,[58] from malabsorption[59] and loss of proteins, to phases of dyschezia and diarrhea,[60] malnutrition,[61] and finally, weight loss and cardiac cachexia,[62] with negative repercussions on quality of life and long-term outcomes.[52]

ASSESSMENT OF CONGESTION IN ADVANCED HEART FAILURE

At each stage of an HF patient's journey, specific assessment tools are used to qualify and quantify congestion to support treatment decisions.

Often, it is difficult to assess, especially when symptoms are mild. Imaging tools and biological tests are useful in ascertaining and quantifying congestion, despite not all are appropriate for use in all stages of patient management.

Biomarkers of Congestion in Advanced Heart Failure

In consideration of the pathophysiologic complexity and the need for improved diagnosis and prognostication, it is no surprise that the biomarker field in HF has exploded in recent years and yielded a plethora of novel tools that facilitate the identification of those with congestion,[63] and perhaps their management, with more precision (**Table 1**).

Natriuretic Peptides

The system of natriuretic peptides (NPs) counteracts the cardiovascular and renal effects related to the activation of the renin–angiotensin–aldosterone system(RAAS).[64] It consists of 3 structurally similar peptides with cardiorenal protective properties: NP atrial (ANP), NP type B (BNP), and NP type C (CNP).[65] ANP and BNP are mainly expressed in heart tissue and are released by cardiomyocytes in response to mechanical strain.[64] All NPs are synthesized as prehormones. In the case of HF, as the filling pressure of the left ventricle (LV) increases, the lengthening of the heart fibers causes the secretion of NP precursors. These undergo the proteolytic action of specific proteases resulting in the synthesis of biologically active derivatives, which in turn interact with

Table 1 Biomarkers in *advanced heart failure*	
Biomarkers in Advanced Heart Failure	**Increased Values**
BNP	>100 pg/mL
NT-proBNP	>300 pg/mL
MR-proANP	>120 pg/mL
MR-proADM	>0.52 nmol/L
High-sensitivity TroponinT	>14 ng/L
Creatinine	> 0.95 mg/dL in women; >1.17 mg/dL in men
Cystatin C	> 0.95 mg/L
Blood Urea Nitrogen	>48 mg/dL
Alanine transaminase	>45 U/L in women; >55 U/L in men
Aspartate transaminase	>43 U/L in women; >48 U/L in men
Alkaline phosphatase	>220 U/L
Total bilirubin	> 1 mg/dL
Cancer Antigen 125 (CA-125)	> 35 units/mL

Abbreviations: BNP, brain natriuretic peptide; MR-proADM, Midregional proadrenomedullin; MR-proANP, Mild Regional pro-Atrial Natriuretic Peptide; NT-pro, BNP, N-terminal, pro-B type natriuretic peptide.

specific receptors for NP (PNR-A, PNR-B, and PNR-C).[65]

One of the most recognized effects of NPs is vasodilation,[66] but they also promote the excretion of water and sodium by inhibiting the reabsorption of sodium in the proximal and distal tubule, also preventing the reduction of glomerular filtration by regulating tubule-glomerular feedback. NPs inhibit renin secretion, thereby inhibiting the renin–angiotensin system (RAS). They reduce the secretion of aldosterone by the adrenal cortex. In addition to the direct effects on the kidney, the inhibitory action of NPs on the RAAS and sympathetic nervous system contributes to their natriuretic, diuretic, and hemodynamic effects (**Fig. 1**). NPs are cleared from the circulation via 2 mechanisms: binding to PNR-C and internalization of the complex or inactivation by enzymatic degradation by neprilysin (NEP).[65] The latter has a high affinity for ANP and CNP and a lower affinity for BNP, which is much more resistant to hydrolysis.[66] It should be remembered that NEP does not hydrolyze N terminal (NT)-proBNP, a biomarker of the stress of the left ventricular wall, which therefore remains a useful indicator of the therapeutic and prognostic effect of NEP inhibition.[67,68] Assessment of natriuretic peptide levels is central for diagnosis and prognosis in HF care, but strategies of treatment guided by serial NPs measurements yielded mixed results.[69,70]

Midregional Proadrenomedullin

A promising biomarker that reflects congestion in advanced HF is the biologically active form of adrenomedullin (ADM).[71–74]

First isolated from human pheochromocytoma, a cancer of the adrenal medulla,[75] from which it takes its name, ADM is a 52-amino acid ringed vasodilatory peptide hormone with natriuretic, vasodilatory, and hypotensive effects mediated by cyclic adenosine monophosphate (cAMP), nitric oxide, and renal prostaglandin systems.[76]

The ADM gene encodes a preprohormone, which after cleavage, generates a pro-ADM peptide, which by proteolytic fragmentation becomes a glycine-extended, inactive ADM. This is enzymatically converted to bio-ADM. Secretion of ADM has been demonstrated from endothelial cells, cardiac myocytes, vascular smooth muscle cells, and leukocytes. ADM is cleared by neutral endopeptidase and through binding with its receptors. It has been hypothesized that ADM plays an essential role in maintaining endothelial barrier function, and disruption hereof results in vascular leakage and systemic and pulmonary edema.[77–80]

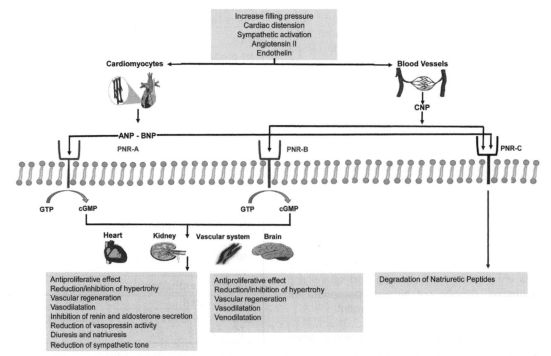

Fig. 1. Effects of natriuretic peptides (NPs). NP, natriuretic peptide; ANP, atrial natriuretic peptides; BNP, brain natriuretic peptide; CNP, natriuretic peptide C; PNR, peptide natriuretic receptor A-B-C; GTP, guanosine triphosphate; cGMP, cyclic guanosine monophosphate.

ADM production is stimulated by volume overload; thus, increased plasma levels of ADM reflect intravascular or tissue congestion.[81] Increasing levels of MR-proADM levels are associated with worsening LV systolic function, high comorbidity burden, suboptimal doses of HF medications, and a lower likelihood of LV reverse remodeling. MR-proADM improves prediction even in models corrected by NPs.[82,83]

Carbohydrate Antigen-125

Carbohydrate antigen (CA)-125 is a glycoprotein secreted from ovarian cancer and lymphomatous cells in a process stimulated by inflammatory activation.[84–86] CA-125 is expressed on cells that derive from the coelom, the embryonic mesoderm cavity that gives rise in humans to the pleural, pericardial, and peritoneal cavities.[87] The proposed physiologic function of the glycoprotein is to protect the luminal surfaces from physical stress via lubrication and hydration. The protein is released from cell surfaces into the blood, pleural, and ascitic fluids and thus can be easily measured.

In addition to CA-125 being traditionally used as a marker for ovarian cancer monitoring and risk stratification, elevated levels are also found in patients with HF,[88] perhaps reflecting the activation of mesothelial cells in response to hemodynamic and inflammatory stress due to congestion.[86,87]

In patients discharged from an episode of acute HF, temporal changes in CA-125 correlate with clinical status and prognosis.[89] Compared with standard care, in the CHANCE-HF trial, CA-125–guided diuretic therapy reduced the risk of HF readmissions and deaths at 1 year.[90,91]

ROLE OF ECHOCARDIOGRAPHY, LUNG ULTRASOUNDS, AND RIGHT HEART CATHETERIZATION TO ASSESS CONGESTION IN ADVANCED HEART FAILURE

In assessing and grading congestion in advanced HF, physical examination and chest x-ray have limited accuracy in detecting congestion.

An echocardiogram is mandatory in patients hospitalized with advanced HF to assess left ventricular ejection fraction and diastolic function, to exclude clinically important valvular regurgitation or stenosis or the presence of pleural or pericardial effusion, and to estimate right atrial pressure and intravascular volume from the inferior vena cava (IVC) diameter. Observational studies suggest that serial assessment of the IVC diameter might be useful to monitor response to diuretic therapy in hospitalized patients with HF and that a

persistently dilated inferior vena cava at hospital discharge identifies those more likely to deteriorate quickly.[92] Ongoing randomized controlled trials will clarify whether an assessment of IVC by ultrasound might guide treatment in advanced HF and improve decongestion.[93] Other ultrasound methods for quantification of congestion in the lungs (ie, B-lines), kidneys, and jugular vein exist, but additional research is required to demonstrate their utility in this setting.[94] Among them, the number of B-lines has been reported to correlate with pulmonary wedge pressure, as well as with parameters of diastolic and systolic dysfunction.[95] Recently, some authors demonstrated that tailored lung ultrasound-guided diuretic therapy significantly reduced a composite outcome of the urgent visit, hospitalization for worsening HF, and death.[96]

In patients with advanced HF right heart catheterization should predict postdischarge outcome and represents the gold standard to quantify hemodynamics, but it should be reserved only for candidates for advanced mechanical therapies or heart transplantation or when diagnostic doubts persist.[97]

HOW TO TREAT CONGESTION IN ADVANCED HEART FAILURE

Advanced heart failure is often the final stage of the progression of chronic HF. Typically, in this situation, episodes of cardiac decompensations are frequent despite optimized evidence-based therapy and the use of aggressive oral diuretic therapy. For a small subset of patients with advanced disease, for instance, those relatively young with few or no comorbidities, timely referral for long-term mechanical circulatory support devices or heart transplantation is the goal for treatment. However, for the vast majority, short-term therapies are the only available resource to overcome systemic and pulmonary congestion, end-organ damage, and cardiac dysfunction.[3]

High-ceiling diuretics acting on the loop of Henle are the cornerstone for the relief of signs and symptoms of fluid retention, but they might perpetuate the same pathophysiologic processes that contribute to the progression of HF.[98] Although observational studies reported a strong association between the use of loop diuretics, especially in higher doses, and mortality,[99,100] this association is more likely to reflect the severity of congestion rather than their deleterious effects on cardiac function.[98] The use of sequential nephron blockade (NBD) for patients who respond poorly to a loop diuretic with the addition of a thiazide might produce a potent diuresis but increases the risk of hypokalemia[101]; combining high doses of aldosterone antagonists might correct hypokalemia[102] but offers no other advantages to usual care in those hospitalized.[3,103] In the recently reported SOLOIST-WHF trial that enrolled many patients hospitalized with severe HF and type II diabetes, a combination of sotagliflozin, a dual sodium–glucose cotransporter-2 and 1 inhibitor, with a loop diuretics was safe, and compared with loop diuretic alone, led to a lower number of deaths from cardiovascular causes and hospitalizations and urgent visits for HF.[104] Another large trial is currently ongoing to test whether adding acetazolamide to a loop diuretic improves decongestion and clinical outcomes in patients with advanced HF.[105]

Vasopressin and adenosine-A1 receptor antagonists, exogenous NPs, and low-dose dopamine might decrease short-term fluid overload but failed to improve long-term outcomes in clinical trials.[106–108] Therefore, the use of continuous intravenous infusion of vasopressor and inotropes is not routinely recommended by guidelines, but it might be reserved to selected cases, especially as a bridge to surgical therapies, while tolvaptan might be considered to increase urine output when hyponatremia occurs.[109] Repeated doses of levosimendan might be beneficial to improve decongestion and prevent cardiac deterioration,[110] whereas agents with inotropic properties, such as digoxin, might enhance diuresis and control ventricular rate in those congested with atrial fibrillation. Recently, a large phase III trial called GALACTIC-HF showed that another oral inotrope, omecamtiv mecarbil, significantly reduced the incidence of heart failure event or death from cardiovascular causes in outpatients or inpatients with symptomatic heart failure with reduced ejection fraction.[111] Patients treated with omecamtiv mecarbil had a significant reduction (10%) in the NT-proBNP level at 24 weeks, suggesting a direct effect against congestion.

Ultrafiltration (UF),[4,112] which uses a semipermeable membrane to remove fluid, is an alternative decongestive therapy that might be used especially in case of diuretic resistance and kidney dysfunction. Compared with using loop diuretics, ultrafiltration does not cause substantial neurohormonal activation and allows precise control of the rate and amount of fluid removal. Moreover, ultrafiltration reduces the risk of hypokalemia and hypomagnesemia and may restore diuretic responsiveness. However, UF is invasive and necessitates of an extracorporeal circuit, a peripheral or central venous catheter, and in addition, anticoagulant therapy.[113] UF has been evaluated in several trials, and results are promising[114–118]; however, the rate of UF-related complications still causes concern.[113] Use of intermittent peritoneal dialysis might be reserved for patients with advanced and refractory congestive HF in a domiciliary context.[119]

SUMMARY

Congestion is a classic feature of advanced HF and is associated with the development of multiorgan complications and adverse outcomes, but its assessment and management are still a major challenge for the modern HF physician. Therefore, further research is needed to improve diagnosis and quantification of congestion and to identify the best therapeutic strategies that might improve the clinical status, well-being, and it is hoped, long-term outcomes of patients with advanced HF.

CLINICS CARE POINTS

- In the evaluation of congestion, perform a complete clinical examination and integrate it with echocardiographic and biochemical data.
- Avoid using high doses of loop diuretics if they are not needed.
- Uses a precision approach that accounts for multiorgan involvement and personalizes congestion treatment based on patient characteristics.

DISCLOSURE STATEMENT

All other authors declare that they have no known competing financial interests or personal relationships that could have appeared to influence the work reported in this paper. Marco Metra reports personal consulting honoraria from Bayer, Novartis, Fresenius, Servier, and Windtree Therapeutics for participation to advisory board meetings and executive committees of clinical trials; Valentina Carubelli received consulting honoraria from CVie Therapeutics Limited, Servier, and Windtree Therapeutics. All the other authors have nothing to disclose.

REFERENCES

1. Metra M, Teerlink JR. Heart failure. Lancet 2017; 390(10106):1981–95. https://doi.org/10.1016/S0140-6736(17)31071-1.

2. Tomasoni D, Lombardi CM, Sbolli M, et al. Acute heart failure: more questions than answers. Prog Cardiovasc Dis 2020;63(5):599–606. https://doi.org/10.1016/j.pcad.2020.04.007.

3. Crespo-Leiro MG, Metra M, Lund LH, et al. Advanced heart failure: a position statement of the Heart Failure Association of the European Society of Cardiology. Eur J Heart Fail 2018;20(11):1505–35. https://doi.org/10.1002/ejhf.1236.

4. Ponikowski P, Voors AA, Anker SD, et al. 2016 ESC guidelines for the diagnosis and treatment of acute and chronic heart failure. Rev Esp Cardiol (Engl Ed) 2016;69(12):1167. https://doi.org/10.1016/j.rec.2016.11.005. English, Spanish.

5. Metra M, Dinatolo E, Dasseni N. The New Heart Failure Association definition of advanced heart failure. Card Fail Rev 2019;5(1):5–8. https://doi.org/10.15420/cfr.2018.43.1.

6. Bjork JB, Alton KK, Georgiopoulou VV, et al. Defining advanced heart failure: a systematic review of criteria used in clinical trials. J Card Fail 2016;22(7):569–77. https://doi.org/10.1016/j.cardfail.2016.03.003.

7. Fang JC, Ewald GA, Allen LA, et al. Advanced (stage D) heart failure: a statement from the Heart Failure Society of America Guidelines Committee. J Card Fail 2015;21(6):519–34. https://doi.org/10.1016/j.cardfail.2015.04.013.

8. Rudiger A, Harjola VP, Müller A, et al. Acute heart failure: clinical presentation, one-year mortality and prognostic factors. Eur J Heart Fail 2005;7(4):662–70. https://doi.org/10.1016/j.ejheart.2005.01.014.

9. Nieminen MS, Brutsaert D, Dickstein K, et al. Euro-Heart Failure Survey II (EHFS II): a survey on hospitalized acute heart failure patients: description of population. Eur Heart J 2006;27(22):2725–36. https://doi.org/10.1093/eurheartj/ehl193.

10. Mebazaa A, Longrois D, Metra M, et al. Agents with vasodilator properties in acute heart failure: how to design successful trials. Eur J Heart Fail 2015;17(7):652–64. https://doi.org/10.1002/ejhf.294.

11. Platz E, Jhund PS, Girerd N, et al. Expert consensus document: reporting checklist for quantification of pulmonary congestion by lung ultrasound in heart failure. Eur J Heart Fail 2019;21(7):844–51. https://doi.org/10.1002/ejhf.1499.

12. Metra M, Dasseni N, Lombardi C. Assessment of congestion in acute heart failure: when simplicity does not go along with accuracy. J Card Fail 2018;24(9):550–2. https://doi.org/10.1016/j.cardfail.2018.08.004.

13. Parrinello G, Greene SJ, Torres D, et al. Editorial expression of concern: water and sodium in heart failure: a spotlight on congestion. Heart Fail Rev 2021. https://doi.org/10.1007/s10741-021-10113-w.

14. Volpe M, Carnovali M, Mastromarino V. The natriuretic peptides system in the pathophysiology of heart failure: from molecular basis to treatment. Clin Sci (Lond) 2016;130(2):57–77. https://doi.org/10.1042/CS20150469.

15. Januzzi JL Jr, Filippatos G, Nieminen M, et al. Troponin elevation in patients with heart failure: on behalf of the third universal definition of myocardial infarction global task force: heart failure section. Eur Heart J 2012;33(18):2265–71. https://doi.org/10.1093/eurheartj/ehs191.

16. Collins SP, Jenkins CA, Harrell FE Jr, et al. Identification of emergency department patients with acute heart failure at low risk for 30-day adverse events: the STRATIFY decision tool. JACC Heart Fail 2015;3(10):737–47. https://doi.org/10.1016/j.jchf.2015.05.007.

17. Thygesen K. 'Ten Commandments' for the fourth universal definition of myocardial infarction 2018. Eur Heart J 2019;40(3):226. https://doi.org/10.1093/eurheartj/ehy856.

18. Dobbe L, Rahman R, Elmassry M, et al. Cardiogenic pulmonary edema. Am J Med Sci 2019;358(6):389–97. https://doi.org/10.1016/j.amjms.2019.09.011.

19. Rosenkranz S, Gibbs JS, Wachter R, et al. Left ventricular heart failure and pulmonary hypertension. Eur Heart J 2016;37(12):942–54. https://doi.org/10.1093/eurheartj/ehv512.

20. Ambrosy AP, Vaduganathan M, Huffman MD, et al. Clinical course and predictive value of liver function tests in patients hospitalized for worsening heart failure with reduced ejection fraction: an analysis of the EVEREST trial. Eur J Heart Fail 2012;14(3):302–11. https://doi.org/10.1093/eurjhf/hfs007.

21. Biegus J, Hillege HL, Postmus D, et al. Abnormal liver function tests in acute heart failure: relationship with clinical characteristics and outcome in the PROTECT study. Eur J Heart Fail 2016;18(7):830–9. https://doi.org/10.1002/ejhf.532.

22. Auer J. What does the liver tell us about the failing heart? Eur Heart J 2013;34(10):711–4. https://doi.org/10.1093/eurheartj/ehs440.

23. Møller S, Bernardi M. Interactions of the heart and the liver. Eur Heart J 2013;34(36):2804–11. https://doi.org/10.1093/eurheartj/eht246.

24. Samsky MD, Patel CB, DeWald TA, et al. Cardiohepatic interactions in heart failure: an overview and clinical implications. J Am Coll Cardiol 2013;61(24):2397–405. https://doi.org/10.1016/j.jacc.2013.03.042.

25. Whitehead MW, Hawkes ND, Hainsworth I, et al. A prospective study of the causes of notably raised aspartate aminotransferase of liver origin. Gut 1999;45(1):129–33. https://doi.org/10.1136/gut.45.1.129.

26. Fuhrmann V, Kneidinger N, Herkner H, et al. Hypoxic hepatitis: underlying conditions and risk factors for mortality in critically ill patients. Intensive Care Med 2009;35(8):1397–405. https://doi.org/10.1007/s00134-009-1508-2.

27. Fuhrmann V, Kneidinger N, Herkner H, et al. Impact of hypoxic hepatitis on mortality in the intensive care unit. Intensive Care Med 2011;37(8):1302–10. https://doi.org/10.1007/s00134-011-2248-7.

28. Waseem N, Chen PH. Hypoxic hepatitis: a review and clinical update. J Clin Transl Hepatol 2016;4(3):263–8. https://doi.org/10.14218/JCTH.2016.00022.

29. Kim MS, Kato TS, Farr M, et al. Hepatic dysfunction in ambulatory patients with heart failure: application of the MELD scoring system for outcome prediction. J Am Coll Cardiol 2013;61(22):2253–61. https://doi.org/10.1016/j.jacc.2012.12.056.

30. Poelzl G, Ess M, Von der Heidt A, et al. Concomitant renal and hepatic dysfunctions in chronic heart failure: clinical implications and prognostic significance. Eur J Intern Med 2013;24(2):177–82. https://doi.org/10.1016/j.ejim.2012.11.009.

31. Parissis JT, Farmakis D, Andreoli C, et al. Cardio-reno-hepatic interactions in acute heart failure: the role of γ-glutamyl transferase. Int J Cardiol 2014;173(3):556–7. https://doi.org/10.1016/j.ijcard.2014.03.127.

32. Mullens W, Abrahams Z, Francis GS, et al. Importance of venous congestion for worsening of renal function in advanced decompensated heart failure. J Am Coll Cardiol 2009;53(7):589–96. https://doi.org/10.1016/j.jacc.2008.05.068.

33. Nohria A, Tsang SW, Fang JC, et al. Clinical assessment identifies hemodynamic profiles that predict outcomes in patients admitted with heart failure. J Am Coll Cardiol 2003;41(10):1797–804. https://doi.org/10.1016/s0735-1097(03)00309-7.

34. Mullens W, Nijst P. Cardiac output and renal dysfunction: definitely more than impaired flow. J Am Coll Cardiol 2016;67(19):2209–12. https://doi.org/10.1016/j.jacc.2016.03.537.

35. Palazzuoli A, Lombardi C, Ruocco G, et al. Chronic kidney disease and worsening renal function in acute heart failure: different phenotypes with similar prognostic impact? Eur Heart J Acute Cardiovasc Care 2016;5(8):534–48. https://doi.org/10.1177/2048872615589511.

36. Legrand M, Mebazaa A, Ronco C, et al. When cardiac failure, kidney dysfunction, and kidney injury intersect in acute conditions: the case of cardiorenal syndrome. Crit Care Med 2014;42(9):2109–17. https://doi.org/10.1097/CCM.0000000000000404.

37. Ishihara S, Gayat E, Sato N, et al. Similar hemodynamic decongestion with vasodilators and inotropes: systematic review, meta-analysis, and meta-regression of 35 studies on acute heart failure. Clin Res Cardiol 2016;105(12):971–80. https://doi.org/10.1007/s00392-016-1009-6.

38. Mullens W, Abrahams Z, Skouri HN, et al. Elevated intra-abdominal pressure in acute decompensated heart failure: a potential contributor to worsening renal function? J Am Coll Cardiol 2008;51(3):300–6. https://doi.org/10.1016/j.jacc.2007.09.043.

39. Hsu CY, Ordoñez JD, Chertow GM, et al. The risk of acute renal failure in patients with chronic kidney disease. Kidney Int 2008;74(1):101–7. https://doi.org/10.1038/ki.2008.107.

40. Metra M, Cotter G, Davison BA, et al. Effect of serelaxin on cardiac, renal, and hepatic biomarkers in the Relaxin in Acute Heart Failure (RELAX-AHF) development program: correlation with outcomes. J Am Coll Cardiol 2013;61(2):196–206. https://doi.org/10.1016/j.jacc.2012.11.005.

41. Damman K, Valente MA, Voors AA, et al. Renal impairment, worsening renal function, and outcome in patients with heart failure: an updated meta-analysis. Eur Heart J 2014;35(7):455–69. https://doi.org/10.1093/eurheartj/eht386.

42. Metra M, Nodari S, Parrinello G, et al. Worsening renal function in patients hospitalised for acute heart failure: clinical implications and prognostic significance. Eur J Heart Fail 2008;10(2):188–95. https://doi.org/10.1016/j.ejheart.2008.01.011.

43. Damman K, Tang WH, Testani JM, et al. Terminology and definition of changes renal function in heart failure. Eur Heart J 2014;35(48):3413–6. https://doi.org/10.1093/eurheartj/ehu320.

44. Damman K, Testani JM. The kidney in heart failure: an update. Eur Heart J 2015;36(23):1437–44. https://doi.org/10.1093/eurheartj/ehv010.

45. Testani JM, Chen J, McCauley BD, et al. Potential effects of aggressive decongestion during the treatment of decompensated heart failure on renal function and survival. Circulation 2010;122(3):265–72. https://doi.org/10.1161/CIRCULATIONAHA.109.933275.

46. Mullens W, Damman K, Harjola VP, et al. The use of diuretics in heart failure with congestion - a position statement from the Heart Failure Association of the European Society of Cardiology. Eur J Heart Fail 2019;21(2):137–55. https://doi.org/10.1002/ejhf.1369.

47. Damman K, Ter Maaten JM, Coster JE, et al. Clinical importance of urinary sodium excretion in acute heart failure. Eur J Heart Fail 2020;22(8):1438–47. https://doi.org/10.1002/ejhf.1753.

48. Levin SN, Hajduk AM, McManus DD, et al. Cognitive status in patients hospitalized with acute decompensated heart failure. Am Heart J 2014;168(6):917–23. https://doi.org/10.1016/j.ahj.2014.08.008.

49. Inouye SK, Rushing JT, Foreman MD, et al. Does delirium contribute to poor hospital outcomes? A three-site epidemiologic study. J Gen Intern Med 1998;13(4):234–42. https://doi.org/10.1046/j.1525-1497.1998.00073.x.

50. Sokoreli I, Pauws SC, Steyerberg EW, et al. Prognostic value of psychosocial factors for first and recurrent hospitalizations and mortality in heart failure patients: insights from the OPERA-HF study. Eur J Heart Fail 2018;20(4):689–96. https://doi.org/10.1002/ejhf.1112.

51. Kindermann I, Fischer D, Karbach J, et al. Cognitive function in patients with decompensated heart failure: the Cognitive Impairment in Heart Failure (CogImpair-HF) study. Eur J Heart Fail 2012;14(4):404–13. https://doi.org/10.1093/eurjhf/hfs015.

52. Ikeda Y, Ishii S, Yazaki M, et al. Portal congestion and intestinal edema in hospitalized patients with heart failure. Heart Vessels 2018;33(7):740–51. https://doi.org/10.1007/s00380-018-1117-5.

53. Polsinelli VB, Sinha A, Shah SJ. Visceral congestion in heart failure: right ventricular dysfunction, splanchnic hemodynamics, and the intestinal microenvironment. Curr Heart Fail Rep 2017;14(6):519–28. https://doi.org/10.1007/s11897-017-0370-8.

54. Verbrugge FH, Dupont M, Steels P, et al. Abdominal contributions to cardiorenal dysfunction in congestive heart failure. J Am Coll Cardiol 2013;62(6):485–95. https://doi.org/10.1016/j.jacc.2013.04.070.

55. Pasini E, Aquilani R, Testa C, et al. Pathogenic gut flora in patients with chronic heart failure. JACC Heart Fail 2016;4(3):220–7. https://doi.org/10.1016/j.jchf.2015.10.009.

56. Polsinelli VB, Marteau L, Shah SJ. The role of splanchnic congestion and the intestinal microenvironment in the pathogenesis of advanced heart failure. Curr Opin Support Palliat Care 2019;13(1):24–30. https://doi.org/10.1097/SPC.0000000000000414.

57. Sundaram V, Fang JC. Gastrointestinal and liver issues in heart failure. Circulation 2016;133(17):1696–703. https://doi.org/10.1161/CIRCULATIONAHA.115.020894.

58. Peacock WF, Costanzo MR, De Marco T, et al. Impact of intravenous loop diuretics on outcomes of patients hospitalized with acute decompensated heart failure: insights from the ADHERE registry. Cardiology 2009;113(1):12–9. https://doi.org/10.1159/000164149.

59. Arutyunov GP, Kostyukevich OI, Serov RA, et al. Collagen accumulation and dysfunctional mucosal barrier of the small intestine in patients with chronic heart failure. Int J Cardiol 2008;125(2):240–5. https://doi.org/10.1016/j.ijcard.2007.11.103.

60. Ohman L, Simrén M. Intestinal microbiota and its role in irritable bowel syndrome (IBS). Curr Gastroenterol Rep 2013;15(5):323. https://doi.org/10.1007/s11894-013-0323-7.

61. Sze S, Pellicori P, Zhang J, et al. Malnutrition, congestion and mortality in ambulatory patients with heart failure. Heart 2019;105(4):297–306. https://doi.org/10.1136/heartjnl-2018-313312.

62. Anker SD, Negassa A, Coats AJ, et al. Prognostic importance of weight loss in chronic heart failure and the effect of treatment with angiotensin-converting-enzyme inhibitors: an observational study. Lancet 2003;361(9363):1077–83. https://doi.org/10.1016/S0140-6736(03)12892-9.

63. Ahmad T, Fiuzat M, Pencina MJ, et al. Charting a roadmap for heart failure biomarker studies. JACC Heart Fail 2014;2(5):477–88. https://doi.org/10.1016/j.jchf.2014.02.005.

64. Nathisuwan S, Talbert RL. A review of vasopeptidase inhibitors: a new modality in the treatment of hypertension and chronic heart failure. Pharmacotherapy 2002;22(1):27–42. https://doi.org/10.1592/phco.22.1.27.33502.

65. Levin ER, Gardner DG, Samson WK. Natriuretic peptides. N Engl J Med 1998;339(5):321–8. https://doi.org/10.1056/NEJM199807303390507.

66. Marcus LS, Hart D, Packer M, et al. Hemodynamic and renal excretory effects of human brain natriuretic peptide infusion in patients with congestive heart failure. A double-blind, placebo-controlled, randomized crossover trial. Circulation 1996;94(12):3184–9. https://doi.org/10.1161/01.cir.94.12.3184.

67. Solomon SD, Zile M, Pieske B, et al. Prospective comparison of ARNI with ARB on Management of heart failUre with preserved ejectioN fracTion (PARAMOUNT) Investigators. The angiotensin receptor neprilysin inhibitor LCZ696 in heart failure with preserved ejection fraction: a phase 2 double-blind randomised controlled trial. Lancet 2012;380(9851):1387–95. https://doi.org/10.1016/S0140-6736(12)61227-6.

68. Sauer AJ, Cole R, Jensen BC, et al. Practical guidance on the use of sacubitril/valsartan for heart failure. Heart Fail Rev 2019;24(2):167–76. https://doi.org/10.1007/s10741-018-9757-1.

69. Troughton RW, Frampton CM, Brunner-La Rocca HP, et al. Effect of B-type natriuretic peptide-guided treatment of chronic heart failure on total mortality and hospitalization: an individual patient meta-analysis. Eur Heart J 2014;35(23):1559–67. https://doi.org/10.1093/eurheartj/ehu090.

70. Felker GM, Anstrom KJ, Adams KF, et al. Effect of natriuretic peptide-guided therapy on hospitalization or cardiovascular mortality in high-risk patients with heart failure and reduced ejection fraction: a

randomized clinical trial. JAMA 2017;318(8): 713–20. https://doi.org/10.1001/jama.2017.10565.

71. Nishikimi T, Saito Y, Kitamura K, et al. Increased plasma levels of adrenomedullin in patients with heart failure. J Am Coll Cardiol 1995;26(6): 1424–31. https://doi.org/10.1016/0735-1097(95) 00338-X.

72. Jougasaki M, Wei CM, McKinley LJ, et al. Elevation of circulating and ventricular adrenomedullin in human congestive heart failure. Circulation 1995; 92(3):286–9. https://doi.org/10.1161/01.cir.92.3. 286.

73. Self WH, Storrow AB, Hartmann O, et al. Plasma bioactive adrenomedullin as a prognostic biomarker in acute heart failure. Am J Emerg Med 2016;34(2):257–62. https://doi.org/10.1016/j.ajem. 2015.10.033.

74. Kremer D, Ter Maaten JM, Voors AA. Bio-adrenomedullin as a potential quick, reliable, and objective marker of congestion in heart failure. Eur J Heart Fail 2018;20(9):1363–5. https://doi.org/10. 1002/ejhf.1245.

75. Kitamura K, Kangawa K, Kawamoto M, et al. Adrenomedullin: a novel hypotensive peptide isolated from human pheochromocytoma. 1993. Biochem Biophys Res Commun 2012;425(3):548–55. https://doi.org/10.1016/j.bbrc.2012.08.022.

76. Nadar SK, Shaikh MM. Biomarkers in routine heart failure clinical care. Card Fail Rev 2019;5(1):50–6. https://doi.org/10.15420/cfr.2018.27.2.

77. Temmesfeld-Wollbrück B, Hocke AC, Suttorp N, et al. Adrenomedullin and endothelial barrier function. Thromb Haemost 2007;98(5):944–51. https:// doi.org/10.1160/th07-02-0128.

78. Koyama T, Ochoa-Callejero L, Sakurai T, et al. Vascular endothelial adrenomedullin-RAMP2 system is essential for vascular integrity and organ homeostasis. Circulation 2013;127(7):842–53. https:// doi.org/10.1161/CIRCULATIONAHA.112.000756.

79. Voors AA, Kremer D, Geven C, et al. Adrenomedullin in heart failure: pathophysiology and therapeutic application. Eur J Heart Fail 2019;21(2):163–71. https://doi.org/10.1002/ejhf.1366.

80. Pandhi P, Ter Maaten JM, Emmens JE, et al. Clinical value of pre-discharge bio-adrenomedullin as a marker of residual congestion and high risk of heart failure hospital readmission. Eur J Heart Fail 2020;22(4):683–91. https://doi.org/10.1002/ejhf. 1693.

81. Hirano S, Imamura T, Matsuo T, et al. Differential responses of circulating and tissue adrenomedullin and gene expression to volume overload. J Card Fail 2000;6(2):120–9. https://doi.org/10.1054/jcaf. 2000.7277.

82. Morbach C, Marx A, Kaspar M, et al. Prognostic potential of midregional pro-adrenomedullin following decompensation for systolic heart failure:

comparison with cardiac natriuretic peptides. Eur J Heart Fail 2017;19(9):1166–75. https://doi.org/10. 1002/ejhf.859.

83. Ter Maaten JM, Kremer D, Demissei BG, et al. Bio-adrenomedullin as a marker of congestion in patients with new-onset and worsening heart failure. Eur J Heart Fail 2019;21(6):732–43. https://doi. org/10.1002/ejhf.1437.

84. Bottoni P, Scatena R. The role of CA 125 as tumor marker: biochemical and clinical aspects. Adv Exp Med Biol 2015;867:229–44. https://doi.org/10. 1007/978-94-017-7215-0_14.

85. Marth C, Zeimet AG, Widschwendter M, et al. Regulation of CA 125 expression in cultured human carcinoma cells. Int J Biol Markers 1998;13(4): 207–9.

86. Zeimet AG, Offner FA, Marth C, et al. Modulation of CA-125 release by inflammatory cytokines in human peritoneal mesothelial and ovarian cancer cells. Anticancer Res 1997;17(4B):3129–31.

87. Zeillemaker AM, Verbrugh HA, Hoynck van Papendrecht AA, et al. CA 125 secretion by peritoneal mesothelial cells. J Clin Pathol 1994;47(3): 263–5. https://doi.org/10.1136/jcp.47.3.263.

88. Llàcer P, Bayés-Genís A, Núñez J. Carbohydrate antigen 125 in heart failure. New era in the monitoring and control of treatment. Med Clin (Barc) 2019;152(7):266–73. https://doi.org/10.1016/j. medcli.2018.08.020. English, Spanish.

89. Núñez J, Núñez E, Sanchis J, et al. Antigen carbohydrate 125 and brain natriuretic peptide serial measurements for risk stratification following an episode of acute heart failure. Int J Cardiol 2012; 159(1):21–8. https://doi.org/10.1016/j.ijcard.2011. 02.001.

90. D'Aloia A, Vizzardi E, Metra M. Can carbohydrate antigen-125 be a new biomarker to guide heart failure treatment?: The CHANCE-HF trial. JACC Heart Fail 2016;4(11):844–6. https://doi.org/10.1016/j. jchf.2016.09.001.

91. Núñez J, Llàcer P, Bertomeu-González V, et al. Carbohydrate antigen-125-guided therapy in acute heart failure: CHANCE-HF: a randomized study. JACC Heart Fail 2016;4(11):833–43. https://doi. org/10.1016/j.jchf.2016.06.007.

92. Goonewardena SN, Gemignani A, Ronan A, et al. Comparison of hand-carried ultrasound assessment of the inferior vena cava and N-terminal pro-brain natriuretic peptide for predicting readmission after hospitalization for acute decompensated heart failure. JACC Cardiovasc Imaging 2008; 1(5):595–601. https://doi.org/10.1016/j.jcmg.2008. 06.005.

93. Jobs A, Vonthein R, König IR, et al. Inferior vena cava ultrasound in acute decompensated heart failure: design rationale of the CAVA-ADHF-

DZHK10 trial. ESC Heart Fail 2020;7(3):973–83. https://doi.org/10.1002/ehf2.12598.

94. Pellicori P, Platz E, Dauw J, et al. Ultrasound imaging of congestion in heart failure: examinations beyond the heart. Eur J Heart Fail 2021;23(5): 703–12. https://doi.org/10.1002/ejhf.2032.

95. Agricola E, Bove T, Oppizzi M, et al. "Ultrasound comet-tail images": a marker of pulmonary edema: a comparative study with wedge pressure and extravascular lung water. Chest 2005;127(5): 1690–5. https://doi.org/10.1378/chest.127.5.1690.

96. Rivas-Lasarte M, Álvarez-García J, Fernández-Martínez J, et al. Lung ultrasound-guided treatment in ambulatory patients with heart failure: a randomized controlled clinical trial (LUS-HF study). Eur J Heart Fail 2019;21(12):1605–13. https://doi.org/10.1002/ejhf.1604.

97. Cooper LB, Mentz RJ, Stevens SR, et al. Hemodynamic predictors of heart failure morbidity and mortality: fluid or flow? J Card Fail 2016;22(3):182–9. https://doi.org/10.1016/j.cardfail.2015.11.012.

98. Pellicori P, Cleland JG, Zhang J, et al. Cardiac dysfunction, congestion and loop diuretics: their relationship to prognosis in heart failure. Cardiovasc Drugs Ther 2016;30(6):599–609. https://doi.org/10.1007/s10557-016-6697-7.

99. Domanski M, Norman J, Pitt B, et al. Diuretic use, progressive heart failure, and death in patients in the Studies of Left Ventricular Dysfunction (SOLVD). J Am Coll Cardiol 2003;42(4):705–8. https://doi.org/10.1016/s0735-1097(03)00765-4.

100. Neuberg GW, Miller AB, O'Connor CM, et al. Diuretic resistance predicts mortality in patients with advanced heart failure. Am Heart J 2002; 144(1):31–8. https://doi.org/10.1067/mhj.2002.123144.

101. Rosenberg J, Gustafsson F, Galatius S, et al. Combination therapy with metolazone and loop diuretics in outpatients with refractory heart failure: an observational study and review of the literature. Cardiovasc Drugs Ther 2005;19(4):301–6. https://doi.org/10.1007/s10557-005-3350-2.

102. Butler J, Anstrom KJ, Felker GM, et al. Efficacy and safety of spironolactone in acute heart failure: the ATHENA-HF randomized clinical trial. JAMA Cardiol 2017;2(9):950–8. https://doi.org/10.1001/jamacardio.2017.2198.

103. Costanzo MR, Cozzolino M, Aspromonte N, et al. Extracorporeal ultrafiltration in heart failure and cardio-renal syndromes. Semin Nephrol 2012;32(1): 100–11. https://doi.org/10.1016/j.semnephrol.2011.11.013.

104. Bhatt DL, Szarek M, Steg PG, et al. Sotagliflozin in patients with diabetes and recent worsening heart failure. N Engl J Med 2021;384(2):117–28. https://doi.org/10.1056/NEJMoa2030183.

105. Mullens W, Verbrugge FH, Nijst P, et al. Rationale and design of the ADVOR (Acetazolamide in decompensated heart failure with volume overload) trial. Eur J Heart Fail 2018;20(11):1591–600. https://doi.org/10.1002/ejhf.1307.

106. Konstam MA, Gheorghiade M, Burnett JC Jr, et al, Efficacy of Vasopressin Antagonism in Heart Failure Outcome Study With Tolvaptan (EVEREST) Investigators. Effects of oral tolvaptan in patients hospitalized for worsening heart failure: the EVEREST outcome trial. JAMA 2007;297(12):1319–31. https://doi.org/10.1001/jama.297.12.1319.

107. Massie BM, O'Connor CM, Metra M, et al. Rolofylline, an adenosine A1-receptor antagonist, in acute heart failure. N Engl J Med 2010;363(15):1419–28. https://doi.org/10.1056/NEJMoa0912613.

108. O'Connor CM, Starling RC, Hernandez AF, et al. Effect of nesiritide in patients with acute decompensated heart failure. N Engl J Med 2011;365(1): 32–43. https://doi.org/10.1056/NEJMoa1100171.

109. Cox ZL, Hung R, Lenihan DJ, et al. Diuretic strategies for loop diuretic resistance in acute heart failure: the 3T trial. JACC Heart Fail 2020;8(3):157–68. https://doi.org/10.1016/j.jchf.2019.09.012.

110. Comín-Colet J, Manito N, Segovia-Cubero J, et al. Efficacy and safety of intermittent intravenous outpatient administration of levosimendan in patients with advanced heart failure: the LION-HEART multicentre randomised trial. Eur J Heart Fail 2018; 20(7):1128–36. https://doi.org/10.1002/ejhf.1145.

111. Teerlink JR, Diaz R, Felker GM, et al. Cardiac myosin activation with omecamtiv mecarbil in systolic heart failure. N Engl J Med 2021;384(2): 105–16. https://doi.org/10.1056/NEJMoa2025797.

112. Yancy CW, Jessup M, Bozkurt B, et al. 2013 ACCF/AHA guideline for the management of heart failure: executive summary: a report of the American College of Cardiology Foundation/American Heart Association Task Force on practice guidelines. Circulation 2013;128(16):1810–52. https://doi.org/10.1161/CIR.0b013e31829e8807.

113. Costanzo MR. The cardiorenal syndrome in heart failure. Heart Fail Clin 2020;16(1):81–97. https://doi.org/10.1016/j.hfc.2019.08.010.

114. Costanzo MR, Guglin ME, Saltzberg MT, et al. Ultrafiltration versus intravenous diuretics for patients hospitalized for acute decompensated heart failure. J Am Coll Cardiol 2007;49(6):675–83. https://doi.org/10.1016/j.jacc.2006.07.073.

115. Grodin JL, Carter S, Bart BA, et al. Direct comparison of ultrafiltration to pharmacological decongestion in heart failure: a per-protocol analysis of CARRESS-HF. Eur J Heart Fail 2018;20(7): 1148–56. https://doi.org/10.1002/ejhf.1158.

116. Marenzi G, Muratori M, Cosentino ER, et al. Continuous ultrafiltration for congestive heart failure: the CUORE trial. J Card Fail 2014;20(5):378.e1–9.

117. Costanzo MR, Negoianu D, Jaski BE, et al. Aqua-pheresis versus intravenous diuretics and hospital-izations for heart failure. JACC Heart Fail 2016;4(2): 95–105. https://doi.org/10.1016/j.jchf.2015.08.005.

118. Hu J, Wan Q, Zhang Y, et al. Efficacy and safety of early ultrafiltration in patients with acute decom-pensated heart failure with volume overload: a prospective, randomized, controlled clinical trial. BMC Cardiovasc Disord 2020;20(1):447. https://doi.org/10.1186/s12872-020-01733-5.

119. Daugirdas JT, Blake PG, Ing TS, et al. Handbook of dialysis. 3rd edition. Philadelphia: Lippincott Wil-liams and Wilkins; 2001. p. 333–42.

Inotropes in Patients with Advanced Heart Failure
Not Only Palliative Care

Daniele Masarone, MD, PhD[a],*, Enrico Melillo, MD[a], Rita Gravino, MD[a],
Vittoria Errigo, MD[a], Maria Luigia Martucci, MD[a], Angelo Caiazzo, MD[b],
Andrea Petraio, MD[b], Gerhard Pölzl, MD[c], Giuseppe Pacileo, MD[a]

KEYWORDS

- Advanced heart failure • Inotropes • Inodilators • Levosimendan • Left ventricular assist device
- Heart transplant

KEY POINTS

- Inotropes are medications that remain a cornerstone for improving cardiac contractility and stabilizing hemodynamics in patients with advanced heart failure (HF).
- The intermittent use of classical inotropes (dobutamine, enoximone) in patients with advanced HF alleviates symptoms and improves the quality of life; however, serious safety issues have been raised with these drugs.
- Levosimendan may be the inotrope of choice for repeated administration for patients with advanced HF considering both the long-lasting effect of its active metabolite OR-1896 and its safety profile.
- Repeated infusion of levosimendan reduces hospitalizations (a key factor of quality of life) and perhaps even improves the overall prognosis of the disease.
- Repeated infusion of levosimendan is a therapeutic approach for selected patients with advanced HF, especially patients ineligible to left ventricular assist device or heart transplantation (destination therapy) or as a bridge to these long-term therapeutic options.

INTRODUCTION

Although improvements in pharmacologic and nonpharmacologic therapies have resulted in a better prognosis in patients with chronic heart failure (HF), between 1% and 10% of these patients progress to an advanced stage of the disease.[1]

Patients with advanced HF have a hemodynamic profile characterized by a low cardiac output[2] and high left ventricular filling pressures[3] and a clinical course characterized by high mortality and frequent rehospitalization despite optimal medical therapy.[4]

The term inotrope is derived from Greek words ἴς (ís, meaning "sinew," "tendon," "strength," or "force") and τρόπος (trópos, meaning "turn," "direction," or "way") and has been widely used for several years to describe drugs that directly improve the contractile function of the heart.

Inotropes are the drugs of choice in patients with acute HF with hypoperfusion; however, recently, their use is also extending to patients with advanced HF to preserve end-organ perfusion, acting as a "bridge" to heart transplantation or long-term mechanical circulatory support[5–7] (left ventricular assist device [LVAD]) or "palliative"

[a] Heart Failure Unit, Department of Cardiology, AORN dei Colli-Monaldi Hospital, Via Leonardo Bianchi 1, Naples 80100, Italy; [b] Heart Transplant Unit, Department of Cardiac Surgery and Transplant, AORN dei Colli-Monaldi Hospital, Naples 80100, Italy; [c] Department of Internal Medicine III, Cardiology and Angiology, Medical University of Innsbruck, Christoph-Probst-Platz, Innrain 52, 6020 Innsbruck, Austria
* Corresponding author.
E-mail address: daniele.masarone@ospedalideicolli.it

therapy for patients in whom the aforementioned treatment modalities are unfeasible (destination therapy).[8,9]

In this review, we summarize the pharmacology of inotropes and the evidence for their use in patients with advanced HF to provide a practical guide for physicians involved in these patients' care.

CLASSIFICATION OF INOTROPES

The term inotropic is an umbrella term encompassing numerous drugs with different mechanisms of action that share the ability to improve cardiac contractility (**Table 1**).

According to Feldman's classification, inotropic drugs can be divided into four categories according to their mechanisms of action[10]:

- Class I: drugs that increase the intracellular levels of cyclic adenosine monophosphate (cAMP) by stimulating beta-adrenergic receptors (dopamine and dobutamine) or inhibiting phosphodiesterase (milrinone and enoximone).
- Class II: drugs that affect the sarcolemmal ion pumps and channels (digoxin).
- Class III: drugs that increase the sensitivity of the contractile proteins to calcium. At this time, no inotropes of this type are available or under clinical investigation.
- Class IV: drugs with multiple mechanisms of action, such as levosimendan, which increases the regulatory site's affinity on troponin C for calcium and open adenosine triphosphate (ATP)-dependent potassium

channels in vascular smooth muscles and mitochondria.

CLINICAL PHARMACOLOGY OF INOTROPES

This section will summarize the pharmacologic characteristics of inotropes to better understand their proper use in patients with advanced HF.

B-Agonists

These drugs activate membrane-bound G-protein–coupled adrenergic receptors that stimulate adenylyl cyclase to transform ATP into cAMP.[11,12]

Protein kinase A activated by cAMP phosphorylates multiple downstream targets, including phospholamban (which increases sarcoplasmic reticulum calcium uptake by sarco-endoplasmic reticulum calcium ATPase 2a), ryanodine receptors (which then release more calcium during depolarization), and troponin C (which facilitates actin exposure for myosin). These calcium-mediated effects increase cardiac contractility.[13]

However, these drugs increase heart rate[14] and alter myocardial relaxation,[15] ultimately increasing myocardial oxygen consumption.[16]

Different β-agonists have different pharmacologic properties because of their different affinities to β-1 receptors and their action on other receptors.

Dopamine is an endogenous molecule. At low doses (0.5–2.5 µg/kg/min), dopamine causes renal and splanchnic vasodilation and increases renal blood flow, regardless of myocardial effects, by activating dopaminergic receptors 1 and 2.[17,18] At moderate doses (3–5 µg/kg/min), it mainly exerts inotropic and chronotropic positive effects

Table 1 Pharmacology of inotropes			
Pharmacologic Agent	**Mechanism of Action**	**Hemodynamic Effects**	**Dose**
Dopamine	DR>β1>α	Increase CO/CI Increase PVR/SVR Increase HR	No bolus dosing Infusion dose: 1–20 µg/kg/min
Dobutamine	β1>β2>α	Increase CO/CI Reduce PVR/SVR Increase HR	No bolus dosing Infusion dose: 2–20 µg/kg/min
Milrinone/Enoximone	PD3 inhibitors	Increase CO/CI Reduce PVR/SVR	Loading dose 20–50 µg/kg/min Infusion dose: 0.2–0.75 µg/kg/min
Levosimendan	Calcium sensitizer	Increase CO/CI Reduce PVR/SVR	No bolus dosing Infusion dose: 0.05–0.2 µg/kg/min

Abbreviations: CI, cardiac index; CO, cardiac output; DR, dopaminergic receptors; HR, heart rate; PVR, pulmonary vascular resistance; SVR, systemic vascular resistance.

through β-1 receptors,[19] whereas at higher doses (>5 μg/kg/min), dopamine causes vasoconstriction by stimulating adrenergic α-1 receptors.[20]

Dobutamine is a synthetic analog of dopamine that predominantly exerts an inotropic action with a weak chronotropic activity.[21]

At low doses (<5 μg/kg/min), dobutamine induces vasodilation and slight inotropic effects[22]; for this reason, it can lower the mean arterial pressure with consequent systemic hypoperfusion. At higher doses (>10 μg/kg/min), dobutamine exerts inotropic, chronotropic, and weak vasoconstriction action.[23,24]

Phosphodiesterase III Inhibitors

Milrinone and enoximone exert their pharmacologic action by inhibiting phosphodiesterase III (an enzyme of the sarcoplasmic reticulum responsible for the degradation of cAMP) with a consequent increase in intracellular cAMP concentration,[25,26] which in turn increases the intracellular concentration of calcium.

In addition to their inotropic effect, phosphodiesterase III inhibitors cause peripheral and pulmonary vasodilation (through an effect on vascular smooth muscle cells), reducing systemic and pulmonary pressures and resistance.[27]

However, the prolonged and continuous use of these drugs induces tolerance to their effect and, in the long term, increases vascular resistance in end-organs.[28]

Levosimendan

Levosimendan is a calcium sensitizer drug with a triple mechanism of action (**Fig. 1**).

Levosimendan's inotropic effects are related to its direct bond with troponin C that selectively increases troponin C's affinity to calcium in a concentration-dependent manner[29]; therefore, its inotropic action does not disturb myocardial relaxation or myocardial oxygen consumption–supply balance.[30]

Moreover, levosimendan causes vasodilation by activating ATP-sensitive potassium channels in smooth vascular muscle cells[31]; this effect also causes vasodilatation of afferent arterioles in the glomeruli, increasing renal blood flow, and reducing renal vein pressure (because of a functional improvement of the right ventricle with a significant reduction in right-sided pressures), which, thus, lead to a better renal function in patients with HF.[32]

In addition to these positive hemodynamic outcomes, levosimendan has important pleiotropic effects (**Fig. 2**), including protection of myocardial, renal, and liver cells from ischemia–reperfusion injury, and anti-inflammatory and antioxidant effects; these properties, mainly related to the activation of ATP-sensitive potassium channels in the mitochondria,[33,34] possibly make levosimendan an "organ protective" inodilator.[35,36]

Another particular feature of levosimendan is its prolonged action compared with other inotropic drugs, which lasts for several days after infusion.

In fact, the long half-life of its active metabolite OR-1896 (approximately 80 h) results in a persistence of the pharmacologic effect for about 10 to 14 days.[37]

Although no dosage adjustment is required in patients with renal dysfunction, patients with moderate-to-severe chronic kidney disease (ie, estimated glomerular filtration rate < 59 mL/min/1.73 m^2) have difficulty eliminating the drug, thus extending its half-life up to 1.5 times, further prolonging the drug's action.

Choice of Inotropes

All aforementioned inotropic agents, in addition to increasing cardiac contractility, have vasoactive properties, causing both vasoconstriction as in the case of dopamine and high-dose dobutamine and vasodilation as in the case of low-dose dobutamine, phosphodiesterase III inhibitors, and levosimendan (the latter two, in particular, thanks to their dual mechanism of action, are called inodilators).[38,39]

These peculiar pharmacologic actions should be considered when choosing between the different inotropes for patients. Inodilators are the drugs of choice in patients who have peripheral vasoconstriction, also, since its inotropic effect is independent of the beta-adrenergic stimulation, they are the drug of choice in patients under chronic beta-blockade.[40]

A third and more specific indication for the use of an inodilator over another inotrope are type II pulmonary hypertension, in fact, both milrinone and levosimendan have documented vasodilatory effect on the pulmonary vasculature.[41] Patients with advanced HF often have concomitant renal and/or hepatic failure. In the case of chronic kidney disease with severe reduction of glomerular filtration rate (ie, estimated glomerular filtration rate < 30 mL/kg/min), the choice of inotropes should be based on the half-life of the drugs. Dobutamine is the agent with the shortest half-life (2 minutes), therefore is the drug of choice.[42] However, it should be noted that in patients with acute cardiorenal syndrome, levosimendan represents the drug of choice as it increases renal perfusion and reduces venous congestion more efficiently than other inotropes.

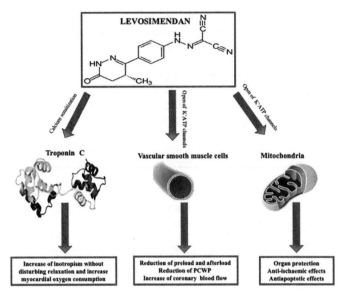

Fig. **1.** Mechanism of action of levosimendan.

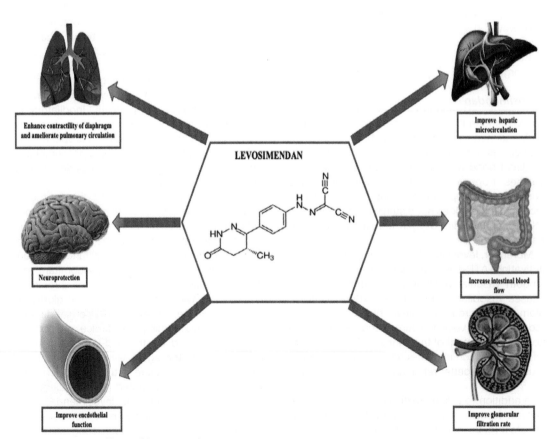

Fig. 2. Pleiotropic effects of levosimendan.

For patients with chronic liver disease, dobutamine is also the first choice because of the prevalent renal elimination. However, similarly to the cardiorenal syndrome indications, levosimendan has better supporting evidence in ameliorate liver function tests compared with dobutamine in people with acute cardiohepatic dysfunction.[43] Inotropes carry a non-negligible risk of major adverse events. Dopamine can induce tachyarrhythmias, especially at high doses.[44] Dobutamine, in addition to tachyarrhythmias, at low doses can cause hypotension due to vasodilation.[45] Moreover, phosphodiesterase III inhibitors cause tachyarrhythmias and severe arterial hypotension,[46] particularly in patients with a reduced glomerular filtration rate, and, therefore, should be avoided in patients with moderate-to-severe chronic kidney disease. Levosimendan can cause arrhythmias and hypotension. The most common arrhythmia is atrial fibrillation. The arrhythmogenic effect of the levosimendan is less pronounced than those of other inotropes because of the avoidance of calcium overload in cardiomyocytes.[47] Besides, limited data show that the hypotensive effect of levosimendan may not require an increase of vasopressors in cardiogenic shock as in the case of phosphodiesterase III inhibitors.[48] Both adverse events can be avoided or limited if no loading dose is administered.[49]

INOTROPES IN ADVANCED HEART FAILURE

Patients with advanced HF account for 1% to 10% of all patients with HF, a prevalence that is bound to increase with the increase in the population with HF and the improvement in pharmacologic and nonpharmacologic therapies leading to increased survival.[4]

Patients with advanced HF suffer from severe and persistent symptoms, often not responding disease-modifying drugs, a marked limitation of functional capacity and poor quality of life.[50]

In addition, these patients present with progressive deterioration of several organs (particularly the kidneys and liver) and frequent HF relapses that often require hospitalization.[51] As advanced HF is a persistent condition that worsens over time, permanent solutions such as LVAD[52,53] or heart transplantation[54,55] are required. In this context, periodic infusion of inotropes can be a useful therapy either as a "bridge" to transplant or LVAD or as a palliative therapy if these solutions are unfeasible for the patient's age or clinical characteristics.[56,57]

In small studies, pulsed infusions of classical inotropes (ie, dobutamine and milrinone) are associated with improvement in hemodynamic parameters and quality of life in patients with advanced HF. However, because of the adverse effects described earlier, serious safety issues have been raised with these drugs.[58]

Therefore, levosimendan seems to be the drug of choice, considering both the long-lasting effect of its active metabolite OR-1896 that facilitates the use of levosimendan as an intermittent infusion at low doses and its safety profile.[48,59]

In addition, as patients with advanced HF frequently have comorbidities, the pleiotropic effects of levosimendan may also be useful in the management of these conditions.

REPETITIVE INFUSION OF LEVOSIMENDAN IN PATIENTS WITH ADVANCED HEART FAILURE

The goals of advanced HF therapy include hemodynamic stabilization and improvement of symptoms, quality of life, and functional capacity. Furthermore, the reduction of hospitalizations for HF is another key objective, both as a desirable result in itself and as a way to avoid the increased mortality accompanying hospitalization.

All aforementioned pharmacologic properties of levosimendan, especially the persistence of its metabolism-mediated effect, make it suitable for intermittent use in managing advanced HF as destination therapy or as a "bridge" to advanced therapy (i.e., LVAD or heart transplantation).

Repetitive Infusion of Levosimendan as Destination Therapy in Patients with Advanced Heart Failure

Initial observations have provided encouraging evidence showing that levosimendan infusions result in hemodynamic,[60] neurohormonal,[61] and inflammatory cytokine[62] improvements in patients with chronic advanced HF.

Following these preliminary study, numerous clinical trials and real-world experiences have shown that the repeated use of levosimendan at fixed intervals is safe and effective in patients with advanced HF, alleviating clinical symptoms, reducing hospitalizations, and improving the quality of life (**Table 2**).

In addition, a recent meta-analysis of 7 randomized trials, involving 438 patients who received intermittent infusions of levosimendan and followed up for 8 months, has shown that levosimendan significantly reduced hospitalizations and mortality.[63]

Most studies have involved the administration of levosimendan every 4 weeks for 24 hours.

However, in the Levorep study, the safety and efficacy of pulsed infusions of levosimendan (every

Table 2
Summary of the clinical studies on repetitive infusion of levosimendan in patients with advanced heart failure

Study	N° of Patients Enrolled	Levosimendan Dose	Infusion Duration	Infusion Frequency	End-Points
Efficacy and safety of intermittent, long-term, concomitant dobutamine and levosimendan infusions in severe heart failure refractory to dobutamine alone[60]	36	Bolus dosing (6 mg/kg) Infusion rate (0.2 mcg/kg/min)	24 h	2 wk	45 d survival rate
Effects of serial levosimendan infusions on left ventricular performance and plasma biomarkers of myocardial injury and neurohormonal and immune activation in patients with advanced heart failure[77]	25	Bolus dosing (6 mg/kg) Infusion rate (0.1–0.4 mcg/kg/min)	24 h	3 wk	Left ventricular dimension and volumes, left ventricular ejection fraction. Plasma levels of • C reactive protein • Troponin T • Interleukin-6 • N Terminal Pro Brian Natriuretic Peptide
A 6-mo follow-up of intermittent levosimendan administration effect on systolic function, specific activity questionnaire, and arrhythmia in advanced heart failure[78]	50	Bolus dosing (6 mg/kg) Infusion rate (0.1–0.2 mcg/kg/min)	24 h	30 d	Left ventricular dimension and volumes, left ventricular ejection fraction, pulmonary artery systolic pressure, degree of mitral regurgitation. Symptoms and quality of life
Assessment of quality of life using 3 different activity questionnaires in heart failure patients after monthly, intermittent administration of levosimendan during 6 mo[79]	20	No bolus dosing Infusion rate (0.1 mcg/kg/min)	24 h	30 d	Left ventricular ejection fraction Quality of life
Intermittent levosimendan infusions in advanced heart failure: favorable effects on left	33	No bolus dosing Infusion rate (0.1–0.4 mcg/kg/min)	24 h	30 d	Left ventricular diastolic volume, degree of mitral regurgitation, pulmonary artery systolic pressure, E/

(continued on next page)

Table 2
(continued)

Study	N° of Patients Enrolled	Levosimendan Dose	Infusion Duration	Infusion Frequency	End-Points
ventricular function, neurohormonal balance, and 1-y survival[80]					e' ratio. Non- invasive (impedance cardiography) cardiac index and systemic vascular resistance
Levosimendan and prostaglandin E1 for uptitration of beta-blockade in patients with refractory, advanced chronic heart failure[81]	75	Bolus dosing (12 mg/kg) Infusion rate (0.1 mg/kg/min)	24 h	4 wk	Left ventricular ejection fraction Brian Natriuretic Peptide plasma levels β-blockers dose
Efficacy and safety of the pulsed infusions of levosimendan in outpatients with advanced heart failure (LevoRep) study: a multicenter randomized Trial[64]	120	No bolus dosing Infusion rate (0.2 mcg/kg/min)	6 h	2 wk	Distance covered at 6 min walking distance test Quality of life
Multicenter, double-blind, randomized, a placebo-controlled trial evaluating the efficacy and safety of intermittent levosimendan in outpatients with advanced chronic heart failure: the LION Heart Study[65]	69	No bolus dosing Infusion rate (0.2 mcg/kg/min)	6 h	2 wk	Plasma level of N-Terminal Pro Brain Natriuretic Peptide Heart failure-related hospital admission
Scheduled intermittent inotropes for Ambulatory Advanced Heart Failure. The RELEVANT-HF multicenter collaboration[82]	185	No bolus dosing Infusion rate (0.05–0.2mcg/kg/min)	24 h	3–4 wk	Heart failure-related hospital admission Heart failure-related hospital admission duration days
Efficacy and safety of repeated infusion of levosimendan in outpatients with advanced heart failure: a real-world experience[66]	15	No bolus dosing Infusion rate (0.2 mcg/kg/min)	6–8 h	2 wk	Heart failure-related hospital admission Quality of life Distance covered at 6 min walking distance test Appropriate ICD discharge

2 weeks for 6 hours) was evaluated in 120 outpatients with advanced HF.

In this trial, levosimendan administration did not reach the primary end-point (simultaneous improvement in exercise capacity and quality of life).[64]

More recently, the LION-HEART study has investigated the efficacy and safety of levosimendan in outpatients with advanced HF with an administration schedule that essentially replicated the Levorep study (every 2 weeks for 6 hours at an infusion rate of 0.2 mg/kg/min).

In this small pivotal study, 69 patients with advanced HF were randomized into two groups—scheduled ambulatory infusion of levosimendan (48 patients) or placebo (21 patients)—at 25 weeks of follow-up for levosimendan infusion, reduced plasma concentrations of N-terminal (NT)-prohormone brain natriuretic peptide, and hospitalization for HF.[65]

Following the publication of the LION-HEART study, our group evaluated the effectiveness of repeated infusions of levosimendan in outpatients with advanced HF and confirmed that levosimendan reduced hospitalizations and improved both distance covered in the 6-minute walking test and the quality of life without a significant increase in arrhythmic burden evaluated with periodic controls of the implantable cardioverter–defibrillator.[66]

A trial is currently in progress to verify the effectiveness of repetitive administrations of levosimendan in outpatients with advanced HF; the aim of the Repetitive Levosimendan Infusion for Patients With Advanced Chronic Heart Failure (LEODOR) trial (NCT03437226) is to evaluate the efficacy and safety of two intermittent schedules of levosimendan therapy (6-hour continuous infusion at a rate of 0.2 mg/kg/min every 2 weeks or 24-hour continuous infusion at a rate of 0.1 mg/kg/min every 3 weeks) in terms of efficacy and safety.[67]

Pending the results of this trial, we believe, based on our experience and data in the literature as well, that fixed-time infusions of levosimendan are a well-tolerated and useful therapy in selected patients with advanced HF.[68]

Repetitive Infusion of Levosimendan as a Bridge to Left Ventricular Assist Device

Intermediate-term or long-term mechanical circulatory support using intracorporeal LVAD is increasingly used for managing advanced HF either as a bridge-to-transplant or as a destination therapy with the intent of lifetime support.[69]

In patients with social or psychological temporary contraindication to LVAD (ie, lack of an adequate support system and lack of acceptance

of the device), repetitive infusion of levosimendan may be a useful option as a "bridge" to decision therapy.[70]

In addition, in a small trial, preoperative infusion of levosimendan before LVAD implantation is associated with better hemodynamic performance of the right ventricle and better clinical outcomes.[71,72]

Repetitive Infusion of Levosimendan as a Bridge to Transplantation

Heart transplantation remains the gold standard therapy for selected patients, resulting in demonstrable improvements in the quality of life, functional status, and longevity over conventional therapy.[73–75]

However, the scarcity of organs continues to limit the number of transplantations performed each year, increasing the waiting time for a compatible and suitable heart.[50]

Recently, Ponz de Antonio and colleagues have shown that in a population of 11 patients waiting for heart transplantation, a fixed-time scheduled infusion of levosimendan (infusion of 6 hours every 2 months at a dose of 0.1–0.2 mg/kg/min, according to the patient's blood pressure) reduces the rehospitalization rate and the need for urgent transplantation (22% of the patients who underwent repeated infusion of levosimendan needed an emergency heart transplant compared with the emergency transplant rates of 64% and 44% in European and Spanish registries, respectively, in 2017).[76]

Based on these preliminary data and our experience, we believe that repeated infusion of levosimendan may be a suitable therapeutic option in patients on the elective waiting list for heart transplantation (i.e., stages 5 and 6 of the United Network of Organ Sharing Allocation System).

SUMMARY

Inotropes increase cardiac output by improving cardiac contractility through several mechanisms of action; however, they have variable vasodilator or vasoconstrictor effects depending on the drug and dose used.

In patients with advanced HF, inotropes are an important therapeutic option as they could improve the hemodynamic profile and quality of life and alleviate symptoms of these patients.

In addition, repeated infusions of levosimendan, a drug preferred for repeated use over others because of the long half-life of its active metabolite and its pleiotropic effects, reduce hospitalizations (a key factor in the quality of life) and perhaps even improve the overall prognosis of the disease.

Evidence from properly powered randomized clinical trials is awaited to confirm the use of levosimendan as destination therapy or as a bridge to long-term therapeutic options such as LVAD or heart transplantation.

CLINICS CARE POINTS

- Patients with advanced heart failure have a pathophysiology characterized by persistent hypoperfusion and increased left ventricular filling pressure that results in the severe reduction in functional capacity and the frequent hospitalizations that such patients present.

- Inotropes are the drugs of choice in patients with acute HF with hypoperfusion; however, recently, their use is also extending to patients with advanced HF to preserve end-organ perfusion, acting as a "bridge" to heart transplantation or long-term mechanical circulatory support.

- Pulsed infusions of classical inotropes (ie, dobutamine and milrinone) are associated with improvement in hemodynamic parameters and quality of life in patients with advanced heart failure. However, because of the adverse effects of these drugs, serious safety issues have been raised.

- Levosimendan is a calcium-sensitizing inodilators with a triple mechanism of action, whose infusion results in hemodynamic, neurohormonal, and inflammatory cytokine improvements in patients with chronic advanced HF.

- In addition, levosimendan has important pleiotropic effects, including protection of myocardial, renal, and liver cells from ischemia–reperfusion injury, and anti-inflammatory and antioxidant effects; these properties possibly make levosimendan an "organ protective" inodilator.

- In clinical trials and real-world evidence, infusion of levosimendan at fixed intervals is safe and effective in patients with advanced HF, alleviating clinical symptoms, reducing hospitalizations, and improving the quality of life.

- Therefore, the use of repeated doses of levosimendan could represent the therapy of choice as a bridge to transplant/left ventricular assist device implantation or as palliative therapy in patients with advanced heart failure.

DISCLOSURE

The authors have nothing to disclose.

REFERENCES

1. Crespo-Leiro MG, Metra M, Lund LH, et al. Advanced heart failure: a position statement of the Heart Failure Association of the European Society of Cardiology. Eur J Heart Fail 2018;20:1505–35.
2. Jain CC, Borlaug BA. Hemodynamic assessment in heart failure. Catheter Cardiovasc Interv 2020;95:420–8.
3. Borlaug BA, Kass DA. Invasive hemodynamic assessment in heart failure. Cardiol Clin 2011;29:269–80.
4. Chaudhry SP, Stewart GC. Advanced Heart Failure: Prevalence, Natural History, and Prognosis. Heart Failure Clin 2016;12:323–33.
5. Nizamic T, Murad MH, Allen LA, et al. Ambulatory Inotrope Infusions in Advanced Heart Failure: A Systematic Review and Meta-Analysis. JACC Heart Fail 2018;6:757–67.
6. Jiménez J, Jara J, Bednar B, et al. Long-term (> 8 weeks) home inotropic therapy as destination therapy in patients with advanced heart failure or as bridge to heart transplantation. Int J Cardiol 2005;99:47–50.
7. Farmakis D, Agostoni P, Baholli L, et al. A pragmatic approach to using inotropes for the management of acute and advanced heart failure: An expert panel consensus. Int J Cardiol 2019;297:83–90.
8. Wordingham SE, McIlvennan CK, Dionne-Odom JN, et al. Complex Care Options for Patients With Advanced Heart Failure Approaching End of Life. Curr Heart Fail Rep 2016;13:20–9.
9. Whellan DJ, Goodlin SJ, Dickinson MG, et al. End-of-life care in patients with heart failure. J Card Fail 2014;20:121–34.
10. Feldman AM. Classification of positive inotropic agents. J Am Coll Cardiol 1993;22:1223–7.
11. Stiles GL, Caron MG, Lefkowitz RJ. Beta-adrenergic receptors: biochemical mechanisms of physiological regulation. Physiol Rev 1984;64:661–743.
12. Lowes BD, Simon MA, Tsvetkova TO, et al. Inotropes in the beta-blocker era. Clin Cardiol 2000;23:11–6.
13. Colucci WS, Wright RF, Braunwald E. New positive inotropic agents in the treatment of heart failure: Mechanisms of action and recent clinical developments. II. N Engl J Med 1986;314:349–58.
14. Felker GM, O'Connor CM. Rational use of inotropic therapy in heart failure. Curr Cardiol Rep 2001;3:108–13.
15. Carroll JD, Lang RM, Neumann AL, et al. The differential effects of positive inotropic and vasodilator therapy on diastolic properties in patients with

congestive cardiomyopathy. Circulation 1986;74: 815–25.

16. DeWitt ES, Black KJ, Thiagarajan RR, et al. Effects of commonly used inotropes on myocardial function and oxygen consumption under constant ventricular loading conditions. J Appl Phys 1985 2016;121:7–14.

17. Power DA, Duggan J, Brady HR. Renal-dose (low-dose) dopamine for the treatment of sepsis-related and other forms of acute renal failure: ineffective and probably dangerous. Clin Exp Pharmacol Physiol Suppl 1999;26:S23–8.

18. Torres-Courchoud I, Chen HH. Is there still a role for low-dose dopamine use in acute heart failure? Curr Opin Crit Care 2014;20:467–71.

19. van Veldhuisen DJ, Girbes AR, de Graeff PA, et al. Effects of dopaminergic agents on cardiac and renal function in normal man and in patients with congestive heart failure. Int J Cardiol 1992;37:293–300.

20. Allwood MJ, Cobbold AF, Ginsburg J. Peripheral vascular effects of noradrenaline, isopropylnoradrenaline and dopamine. Br Med Bull 1963;19:132–6.

21. Dubin A, Lattanzio B, Gatti L. The spectrum of cardiovascular effects of dobutamine - from healthy subjects to septic shock patients. Espectro dos efeitos cardiovasculares da dobutamina - de voluntários saudáveis a pacientes em choque séptico. Rev Bras Ter Intensiva 2017;29:490–8.

22. Mikulic E, Cohn JN, Franciosa JA. Comparative hemodynamic effects of inotropic and vasodilator drugs in severe heart failure. Circulation 1977;56: 528–33.

23. Ruffolo RR Jr. The pharmacology of dobutamine. Am J Med Sci 1987;294:244–8.

24. Ginwalla M, Tofovic DS. Current Status of Inotropes in Heart Failure. Heart Failure Clin 2018;14(4): 601–16.

25. Boswell-Smith V, Spina D, Page CP. Phosphodiesterase inhibitors. Br J Pharmacol 2006;147:252–7.

26. Augoustides JG, Riha H. Recent progress in heart failure treatment and heart transplantation. J Cardiothorac Vasc Anesth 2009;23:738–48.

27. Pagel PS, Hettrick DA, Warltier DC. Influence of levosimendan, pimobendan, and milrinone on the regional distribution of cardiac output in anaesthetized dogs. Br J Pharmacol 1996;119:609–15.

28. Colucci WS. Cardiovascular effects of milrinone. Am Heart J 1991;121:1945–7.

29. Papp Z, Agostoni P, Alvarez J, et al. Levosimendan Efficacy and Safety: 20 Years of SIMDAX in Clinical Use. J Cardiovasc Pharmacol 2020;76:4–22.

30. Kurdi M, Pollesello P, Booz GW. Levosimendan Comes of Age: 20 Years of Clinical Use. J Cardiovasc Pharmacol 2020;76:1–3.

31. Nieminen MS, Fruhwald S, Heunks LM, et al. Levosimendan: current data, clinical use and future development. Heart Lung Vessel 2013;5:227–45.

32. Yilmaz MB, Grossini E, Silva Cardoso JC, et al. Renal effects of levosimendan: a consensus report. Cardiovasc Drugs Ther 2013;27:581–90.

33. Farmakis D, Alvarez J, Gal TB, et al. Levosimendan beyond inotropy and acute heart failure: Evidence of pleiotropic effects on the heart and other organs: An expert panel position paper. Int J Cardiol 2016;222: 303–12.

34. Parissis JT, Andreadou I, Bistola V, et al. Novel biologic mechanisms of levosimendan and its Effect on the failing heart. Expert Opin Investig Drugs 2008;17:1143–50.

35. Grossini E, Pollesello P, Bellofatto K, et al. Protective effects elicited by levosimendan against liver ischemia/reperfusion injury in anesthetized rats. Liver Transpl 2014;20:361–75.

36. Grossini E, Molinari C, Pollesello P, et al. Levosimendan protection against kidney ischemia/reperfusion injuries in anesthetized pigs. J Pharmacol Exp Ther 2012;342:376–88.

37. Pathak A, Lebrin M, Vaccaro A, et al. Pharmacology of levosimendan: inotropic, vasodilatory and cardioprotective effects. J Clin Pharm Ther 2013;38:341–9.

38. Dei Cas L, Metra M, Visioli O. Clinical pharmacology of inodilators. J Cardiovasc Pharmacol 1989;14: S60–71.

39. Maack C, Eschenhagen T, Hamdani N, et al. Treatments targeting inotropy. Eur Heart J 2019;40: 3626–44.

40. Francis GS, Bartos JA, Adatya S. Inotropes J Am Coll Cardiol 2014;63:2069–78.

41. Hansen MS, Andersen A, Nielsen-Kudsk JE. Levosimendan in pulmonary hypertension and right heart failure. Pulm Circ 2018;8:1225–32.

42. Parissis JT, Farmakis D, Nieminen M. Classical inotropes and new cardiac enhancers. Heart Fail Rev 2007;12:149–56.

43. Heringlake M, Alvarez J, Bettex D, et al. An update on levosimendan in acute cardiac care: applications and recommendations for optimal efficacy and safety. Expert Rev Cardiovasc Ther 2021;19(4): 325–35.

44. Velasco M, Luchsinger A. Dopamine: pharmacologic and therapeutic aspects. Am J Ther 1998;5: 37–43.

45. Lindenfeld J, Lowes BD, Bristow MR. Hypotension with dobutamine: beta-adrenergic antagonist selectivity at low doses of carvedilol. Ann Pharmacother 1999;33:1266–9.

46. Cruickshank JM. Phosphodiesterase III inhibitors: long-term risks and short-term benefits. Cardiovasc Drugs Ther 1993;7:655–60.

47. Packer M, Colucci W, Fisher L, et al. Effect of levosimendan on the short-term clinical course of patients with acutely decompensated heart failure. JACC Heart Fail 2013;1:103–11.

48. Farmakis D, Agostoni P, Baholli L, et al. A pragmatic approach to the use of inotropes for the management of acute and advanced heart failure: An expert panel consensus. Int J Cardiol 2019; 297:83–90.

49. De Luca L, Colucci WS, Nieminen MS, et al. Evidence-based use of levosimendan in different clinical settings. Eur Heart J 2006;27:1908–20.

50. Truby LK, Rogers JG. Advanced Heart Failure: Epidemiology, Diagnosis, and Therapeutic Approaches. JACC Heart Fail 2020;8:523–36.

51. Cheshire C, Bhagra CJ, Bhagra SK. A review of the management of patients with advanced heart failure in the intensive care unit. Ann Transl Med 2020;8: 828–35.

52. Miller RJH, Teuteberg JJ, Hunt SA. Innovations in Ventricular Assist Devices for End-Stage Heart Failure. Annu Rev Med 2019;70:33–44.

53. Vieira JL, Ventura HO, Mehra MR. Mechanical circulatory support devices in advanced heart failure: 2020 and beyond. Prog Cardiovasc Dis 2020;63: 630–9.

54. Miller L, Birks E, Guglin M, et al. Use of Ventricular Assist Devices and Heart Transplantation for Advanced Heart Failure. Circ Res 2019;124: 1658–78.

55. Guglin M, Zucker MJ, Borlaug BA, et al. Evaluation for Heart Transplantation and LVAD Implantation: JACC Council Perspectives. J Am Coll Cardiol 2020;75:1471–87.

56. Graffagnino JP, Avant LC, Calkins BC, et al. Home Therapies in Advanced Heart Failure: Inotropes and Diuretics. Curr Heart Fail Rep 2020;17:314–23.

57. Chuzi S, Allen LA, Dunlay SM, et al. Palliative Inotrope Therapy: A Narrative Review. JAMA Cardiol 2019;4:815–22.

58. Altenberger J, Pölzl G. Repetitive levosimendan for a LION's heart? Eur J Heart Fail 2018;20(7):1137–8.

59. Bouchez S, Fedele F, Giannakoulas G, et al. Levosimendan in Acute and Advanced Heart Failure: an Expert Perspective on Posology and Therapeutic Application. Cardiovasc Drugs Ther 2018;32: 617–24.

60. Nanas JS, Papazoglou P, Tsagalou EP. Efficacy and safety of intermittent, long-term, concomitant dobutamine and Levosimendan infusion in severe heart failure refractory to dobutamine alone. Am J Cardiol 2005;95:768–71.

61. Nieminen MS, Akkila J, Hasenfuss G, et al. Hemodynamic and neurohumoral effects of continuous infusion of levosimendan in patients with congestive heart failure. J Am Coll Cardiol 2000;36:1903–12.

62. Parissis JT, Adamopoulos S, Antoniades C, et al. Effects of levosimendan on circulating pro-inflammatory cytokines and soluble apoptosis mediators in patients with decompensated advanced heart failure. Am J Cardiol 2004;93:1309–12.

63. Silvetti S, Belletti A, Fontana A, et al. Rehospitalization after intermittent levosimendan treatment in advanced heart failure patients: a meta-analysis of randomized trials. ESC Heart Fail 2017;4:595–604.

64. Altenberger J, Parissis JT, Costard-Jaeckle A, et al. Efficacy and safety of the pulsed infusions of levosimendan in outpatients with advanced heart failure (LevoRep) study: a multicentre randomized trial. Eur J Heart Fail 2014;16:898–906.

65. Comín-Colet J, Manito N, Segovia-Cubero J, et al. Efficacy and safety of intermittent intravenous outpatient administration of levosimendan in patients with advanced heart failure: the LION-HEART multicentre randomised trial. Eur J Heart Fail 2018;20:1128–36.

66. Masarone D, Valente F, Verrengia M, et al. Efficacy and safety of repeated infusion of levosimendan in outpatients with advanced heart failure: a real-world experience. J Cardiovasc Med (Hagerstown) 2020;21:919–21.

67. Pölzl G, Allipour Birgani S, Comín-Colet J, et al. Repetitive levosimendan infusions for patients with advanced chronic heart failure in the vulnerable post-discharge period. ESC Heart Fail 2019;6(1): 174–81.

68. Masarone D, Pacileo G. Repeated infusion of levosimendan in outpatients with advanced heart failure: to cure sometimes, to relieve often, and to comfort always. J Cardiovasc Med (Hagerstown) 2021; 22(2):150.

69. Han JJ, Acker MA, Atluri P. Left ventricular assist devices. Circulation 2018;138:2841–51.

70. Cholley B, Levy B, Fellahi JL, et al. Levosimendan in the light of the results of the recent randomized controlled trials: an expert opinion paper. Crit Care 2019;23:38–392.

71. Sponga S, Ivanitskaia E, Potapov E, et al. Preoperative treatment with levosimendan in candidates for mechanical circulatory support. ASAIO J 2012;58: 6–11.

72. Theiss HD, Grabmaier U, Kreissl N, et al. Preconditioning with levosimendan before implantation of left ventricular assist devices. Artif Organs 2014;38: 231–4.

73. Fang JC, Ewald GA, Allen LA, et al. Advanced (stage D) heart failure: a statement from the Heart Failure Society of America Guidelines Committee. J Card Fail 2015;21:519–34.

74. Yancy CW, Jessup M, Bozkurt B, et al. 2017 ACC/AHA/HFSA focused update of the 2013 ACCF/AHA guideline for the management of heart failure: a report of the American College of Cardiology/American Heart Association Task Force on Clinical Practice Guidelines and the Heart Failure Society of America. J Am Coll Cardiol 2017;70:776–803.

75. Ponikowski P, Voors AA, Anker SD, et al. 2016 ESC Guidelines for the diagnosis and treatment of acute

and chronic heart failure: The Task Force for the diagnosis and treatment of acute and chronic heart failure of the European Society of Cardiology (ESC). Developed with the special contribution of the Heart Failure Association (HFA) of the ESC. Eur J Heart Fail 2016;18:891–975.

76. Ponz de Antonio I, de Juan Bagudá JS, Rodríguez Chaverri A, et al. Levosimendan as bridge to transplant in patients with advanced heart failure. Rev Esp Cardiol (Engl Ed) 2020;73:422–4.

77. Parissis JT, Adamopoulos S, Farmakis D, et al. Effects of serial levosimendan infusions on left ventricular performance and plasma biomarkers of myocardial injury and neurohormonal and immune activation in patients with advanced heart failure [published correction appears in Heart. 2009 Jan; 95(1):84]. Heart 2006;92(12):1768–72.

78. Mavrogeni S, Giamouzis G, Papadopoulou E, et al. A 6-month follow-up of intermittent levosimendan administration effect on systolic function, specific activity questionnaire, and arrhythmia in advanced heart failure. J Card Fail 2007;13:556–9.

79. Papadopoulou EF, Mavrogeni SI, Dritsas A, et al. Assessment of quality of life using three activity questionnaires in heart failure patients after monthly, intermittent administration of levosimendan during a six-month period. Hellenic J Cardiol 2009;50: 269–74.

80. Malfatto G, Della Rosa F, Villani A, et al. Intermittent levosimendan infusions in advanced heart failure: favourable effects on left ventricular function, neurohormonal balance, and one-year survival. J Cardiovasc Pharmacol 2012;60:450–5.

81. Berger R, Moertl D, Huelsmann M, et al. Levosimendan and prostaglandin E1 for uptitration of beta-blockade in patients with refractory, advanced chronic heart failure. Eur J Heart Fail 2007;9:202–8.

82. Oliva F, Perna E, Marini M, et al. Scheduled intermittent inotropes for Ambulatory Advanced Heart Failure. The RELEVANT-HF multicentre collaboration. Int J Cardiol 2018;272:255–9.

Cardiac Resynchronization Therapy and Cardiac Contractility Modulation in Patients with Advanced Heart Failure
How to Select the Right Candidate?

William T. Abraham, MD

KEYWORDS

- Cardiac contractility modulation • Cardiac resynchronization therapy • Heart failure
- Heart failure with reduced ejection fraction • Heart failure with mildly reduced ejection fraction

KEY POINTS

- Cardiac resynchronization therapy (CRT) is a well-accepted treatment of patients with heart failure with LVEF of 35% or less and a wide QRS complex.
- Treatment options for patients with heart failure, left ventricular ejection fraction (LVEF) greater than or equal to 25 to less than or equal to 45%, and QRS <130 milliseconds are limited.
- Cardiac contractility modulation, delivered by the Optimizer Smart System, is a device-based therapy that is indicated for use in this patient population. It has been approved by the FDA since 2019.
- The implantation procedure is similar to that of other CRM devices.
- The safety and efficacy of this device and procedure have been investigated and confirmed in several clinical studies, and more clinical testing is currently ongoing.

INTRODUCTION

Heart failure represents a major and growing public health concern. In the United States, approximately 6.5 million Americans have heart failure and about 960,000 new cases are diagnosed each year.[1] Worldwide, the prevalence of heart failure is estimated to be about 60 million people.[2] Heart failure results in substantial morbidity and mortality, and from a patient-centered view, it is associated with substantial reduction in physical, social, and emotional functioning.[1,3] For example, about 75% of patients with heart failure find it difficult to carry out usual activities, despite treatment with guideline-directed medical therapy (GDMT).[4,5] Thus, improving heart failure symptoms, quality of life, and physical activity continues to be an unmet medical need in patients with heart failure. This article discusses two forms of electrical therapy for the failing heart, cardiac resynchronization therapy (CRT) and cardiac contractility modulation (CCM), which improve heart failure symptoms, quality of life, and physical activity in patients with wide and narrow QRS complexes, respectively. In the case of CRT, reductions in heart failure morbidity and mortality have also been shown; with CCM, the evidence is suggestive of a similar impact.

CARDIAC RESYNCHRONIZATION THERAPY

CRT is a well-established device treatment of heart failure, first approved by the US Food and Drug Administration (FDA) in 2001. The evidence

Division of Cardiovascular Medicine, 473 West 12th Avenue, Suite 200, Columbus, OH 43065, USA
E-mail address: William.Abraham@osumc.edu

Heart Failure Clin 17 (2021) 599–606
https://doi.org/10.1016/j.hfc.2021.05.005
1551-7136/21/© 2021 Elsevier Inc. All rights reserved.

supporting its use is extensively reviewed elsewhere[6–8] and briefly summarized here. More than 8500 New York Heart Association (NYHA) functional class II, III, and ambulatory IV patients with heart failure with reduced ejection fraction (HFrEF) and a wide QRS (≥120 or 130 milliseconds) have been evaluated in landmark randomized controlled trials of CRT.[9–15] In NYHA functional class III and ambulatory IV patients, CRT improves quality of life, functional status, and exercise capacity, and also reduces morbidity and mortality. In NYHA functional class II patients, CRT reduces morbidity and mortality. Regardless of NYHA functional class, CRT also improves cardiac structure and function (also known as reverse remodeling) and reduces secondary mitral regurgitation.[16] These improvements in clinical and patient-centered outcomes occur most prominently in patients with left bundle branch block (LBBB) and a wide QRS of 150 milliseconds or greater, although they may also be seen in patients with LBBB and narrower QRS durations (120–149 milliseconds).[17]

In contrast, patients with a narrow QRS (<120–130 milliseconds) do not benefit from CRT. In the Echocardiographic-CRT (Echo-CRT) trial,[18] 809 NYHA functional class III or IV HFrEF patients with a QRS less than 130 milliseconds and echocardiographic evidence of left ventricular dyssynchrony were randomized in a double-blind manner to receive active CRT (device implanted and CRT turned on) or no CRT (device implanted and CRT turned off). In these patients, CRT did not reduce the primary end point of death or hospitalization for heart failure and was associated with a statistically significant increase in mortality. Rather than being beneficial, CRT is harmful in HFrEF patients with narrow QRS.

Considering the totality of data on CRT, guidelines recommend its use based on several factors, including QRS morphology and duration. There is one clear class I recommendation for CRT: CRT is indicated for patients who have left ventricular ejection fraction (LVEF) less than or equal to 35%, sinus rhythm, LBBB with a QRS duration greater than or equal to 150 milliseconds, and NYHA functional class II, III, or ambulatory IV symptoms on GDMT. The other more nuanced recommendations for CRT are explicitly stated in the US and European heart failure guidelines.[4,5] Of particular note, there is one strong contraindication to the use of CRT and that is in patients with narrow QRS complexes, based on the results of the Echo-CRT trial. In sum, CRT should be considered in NYHA functional class II, III, and ambulatory IV HFrEF patients (LVEF ≤35%) with LBBB or dependence on ventricular pacing, receiving optimally tolerated GDMT, and it should

not be used in patients with narrow QRS. Based on these criteria, only about 20% of patients with heart failure are eligible for CRT.[19] An emerging alternative for some patients who are not indicated for CRT is CCM.

CARDIAC CONTRACTILITY MODULATION

Patients who do not qualify for CRT and who have an LVEF ranging from 25% to 45% are eligible for CCM. The remainder of this article focuses on this newer form of electrical therapy for heart failure. So, what is CCM? CCM is an innovative device-based therapy that delivers electrical signals to the ventricular myocardium during the absolute refractory period of the heart. In selected patients, randomized controlled trials have shown that CCM therapy is safe and effective in improving heart failure symptoms, quality of life, functional status, and exercise capacity.[20–22]

Cardiac Contractility Modulation Signals and Signal Delivery

CCM signals are nonexcitatory high current (7.5 V at >20 millisecond duration) electrical impulses (**Fig. 1**). These signals are timed to occur during the absolute refractory period of the myocyte's action potential. These impulses activate intracellular mechanisms that favorably alter myocardial gene expression, protein levels, and phosphorylation to enhance calcium delivery, which in turn increases myocardial contractility.[23–25] The improvement in contractility occurs with no increase in myocardial oxygen consumption, so that the efficiency of the heart as a pump is improved.[26] Other contributory mechanisms of CCM action may include a favorable effect on autonomic balance.[27]

CCM signals are delivered to the interventricular septum using an implanted pulse generator and two standard pacing leads, via the Optimizer System (Marlton, NJ) (**Fig. 2**). The system has had several different iterations since being first available in 2002, with the latest being the Optimizer Smart System (as of 2021).[28,29] The three-lead version of the Optimizer System received FDA approval March 2019, and the two-lead system pictured received FDA approval in October 2019 and CE Mark in 2016. The CCM device is physically similar to other implantable cardiac devices, such as a pacemaker or defibrillator, with a pulse generator and intracardiac leads. Implantation of the Optimizer system is also similar to other cardiac implantable electronic devices and is generally performed by cardiac electrophysiologists or other physicians skilled in the implantation of cardiac pacemakers and defibrillators. Importantly

A Cardiac contractility modulation implanted intracardiac device

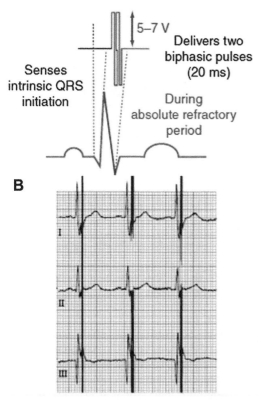

B

Electrocardiogram with CCM stimuli timed during refractory period

Fig. 1. CCM stimulation. (*A*) CCM implanted intracardiac device senses the intrinsic QRS initiation and then delivers two biphasic pulses of 5–7 V over a total of 20 ms during the absolute refractory period. (*B*) Electrocardiogram leads I, II, and III from a patient with an implanted CCM device demonstrating the CCM stimuli timed during the refractory period. (*From* Campbell CM, Kahwash R, Abraham WT. Optimizer Smart in the treatment of moderate-to-severe chronic heart failure. Future Cardiol. 2020 Jan;16(1):13-25; with permission.)

and necessarily, given the large amount of current delivered, the generator of the Optimizer system has a rechargeable battery. The patient can recharge the battery at home, with recommendations that it be done on a weekly basis. This advance is in contrast to other implantable cardiac devices that require periodic generator replacement procedures at the end of battery life. Because battery longevity for the current Optimizer Smart is about 15-years, device replacement procedures may not be necessary.

Clinical Trials of Cardiac Contractility Modulation

The last few decades have seen much research on CCM therapy, beginning with bench testing, animal testing, and then progressing to clinical trials. Each of the Optimizer system generations has been tested in clinical patient populations. In addition to safety and effectiveness studies starting in 2006, there have been several major clinical trials that compared the effectiveness of the Optimizer Smart System plus optimally tolerated GDMT with GDMT alone. These landmark trials of CCM are summarized next.

FIX-CHF-4 trial

The FIX-CHF-4 trial was a randomized, double-blind, crossover study conducted in Europe and published in 2008.[20] Inclusion criteria included patents with symptomatic heart failure (NYHA functional class $\geq$II), LVEF less than or equal to 35%, and peak Vo_2 between 10 and 20 mL/kg/min. Patients were required to be on GDMT including a diuretic, a β-blocker, and an angiotensin-converting enzyme inhibitor or angiotensin-receptor blocker. Preexisting implantable cardioverter-defibrillator (ICD) or pacemaker was allowed. Exclusion criteria included CRT device, atrial fibrillation, or greater than or equal to 8900 premature ventricular contractions (PVCs) on a 24-hour Holter monitor. There were 164 patients enrolled in this study who received CCM device implantation. Half of the patients were randomized to have the device turned on for 3 months and then off for 3 months. The other half of the patients had the device turned off for 3 months and then on for 3 months. At study initiation, and again at 3- and 6-month postimplantation, the enrolled patients were assessed by 6-minute hall walk test (6MWT), peak Vo_2, and Minnesota Living with Heart Failure quality of life Questionnaire (MLHFQ). The coprimary end points were improvements in peak Vo_2 and MLHFQ. A comparison of values at the end of active treatment periods versus the end of sham treatment periods demonstrated statistically significant improvement in peak Vo_2 and MLHFQ (P = .03 for each parameter). Patients during active CCM therapy showed a between-group improvement in peak Vo_2 of 0.99 mL/kg/min compared with patients whose device was turned off. Importantly, there was no significant difference in adverse events (AEs) between either group. Also, there was no change in ICD firing, arrhythmia burden, or PVCs as measured by Holter monitor. This trial demonstrated the preliminary safety and effectiveness of CCM as a treatment of heart failure.

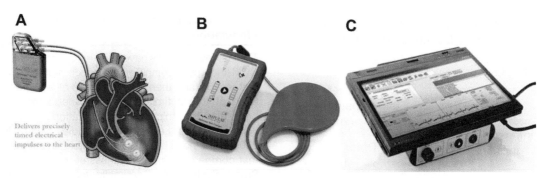

Fig. 2. Optimizer system. Current Optimizer System devices (*A-C*) with transcutaneous home charger (*B*), Optimizer Smart implantable CCM pulse generator with intracardiac leads (*A*), and wireless programmer (*C*). (*Courtesy of* Impulse Dynamics, Marlton, NJ; with permission.)

FIX-HF-5 trial

The pivotal FIX-HF-5 trial, published in 2011, evaluated the safety and clinical benefits of CCM plus GDMT versus GDMT alone, in a large randomized, controlled, unblinded patient cohort.[21] An unblinded trial design was chosen primarily as the optimal way to ensure device safety over the 1-year time frame. In total, there were 428 patients recruited for this study. Inclusion criteria were similar to the FIX-CHF-4 trial, except NYHA class was limited to III or IV, LVEF less than or equal to 35%, and peak V_{O_2} greater than or equal to 9 mL/kg/min. The study's primary clinical end point was greater than or equal to 20% improvement in ventilatory anaerobic threshold (VAT). VAT is considered to be an unbiased measure of exercise tolerance that is not subject to the placebo effect, but it also had not been measured as a primary end point in any prior large-scale heart failure studies. Before implantation, and at 3 and 6 months, the enrolled patients were assessed by 6MWT, VAT, peak V_{O_2}, echocardiogram, and MLHFQ.

VAT, although objective, is plagued by interobserver variability. Indeed, 30% of patients in this study had indeterminate values and thus, FIX-HF-5 did not meet its primary end point. However, the secondary end points were achieved with improved peak V_{O_2} (by 0.65 mL/kg/min; $P = .024$), and improved MLHFQ (by −9.7 points; $P<.0001$), compared with GDMT alone. The study met the primary safety end point for CCM of noninferiority of all-cause mortality and hospitalizations compared with GDMT alone. Importantly, a prespecified subgroup analysis of the FIX-HF-5 trial showed that clinical benefits were more pronounced in patients with higher range LVEF ($\geq$25%).[30] For example, peak V_{O_2} improved by 1.31 mL/kg/min ($P = .001$) in the CCM group, compared with GDMT alone. Also, of note, although the inclusion criteria required an LVEF

of less than or equal to 35%, the echocardiogram core laboratory found that a sizable portion of the enrolled patients actually had ejection fractions up to 45%. Serendipitously, these patients showed an even more robust response to CCM therapy. This finding informed decisions about inclusion criteria in future trials.

FIX-HF-5C trial

The FIX-HF-5C confirmatory study was based on the FIX-HF-5 study and the subgroup analysis cited previously. It was published in 2018,[22] and was designed to address CCM benefits found in the subgroup that emerged as the best responders in the FIX-HF-5 study: specifically, those patients with mild-to-moderate reduction in LVEF (25%–45%). Inclusion criteria were similar to previous studies: NYHA class III or ambulatory IV symptoms despite GDMT, LVEF ranging from 25% to 45%, and normal sinus rhythm with QRS less than or equal to 130 milliseconds. Patients with LVEF less than 35% were required to have an ICD. A total of 160 patients were enrolled in the United States and in the European Union in a randomized, unblinded fashion. Patients were randomized to continued GDMT alone (n = 86) or CCM plus GDMT (n = 74). Patients were assessed with peak V_{O_2} (the primary end point), MLHFQ score, NYHA functional class, and 6MWT. Assessments were completed at baseline and then at 3 and 6 months following implantation of the three-lead Optimizer IV CE system.

The FIX-HF-5C study met its primary end point with a peak V_{O_2} difference between groups of 0.84 mL/kg/min (95% Bayesian credible interval, 0.123–1.552; posterior probability, 0.989) favoring CCM. Statistically significant differences were also seen in quality of life by MLHFQ with a −11.7-point improvement ($P<.001$) favoring CCM. Patients with CCM were 5.97 times more likely to improve by at least one NYHA functional class, compared with GDMT alone (P<.001). The average 6MWT improved by 43 m (P = .02), with CCM compared with control subjects. In a prespecified subgroup analysis based on LVEF (25%–34% vs 35%–45%), HFrEF and HFmrEF patients benefitted equally from CCM (interaction P values for peak V_{O_2}, MLHFQ, and NYHA all demonstrating no difference in response between subgroups), although numerically HFmrEF patients demonstrated a larger CCM treatment effect. Furthermore, a post hoc analysis demonstrated that the composite end point of cardiovascular death and heart failure hospitalization was lower in the CCM group with a greater than 70% event rate reduction from 10.8% to 2.9%. This difference was almost completely driven by reduction in heart failure hospitalizations and requires confirmation in future studies. The FIX-HF-5C authors concluded that CCM improved exercise tolerance and quality of life when compared with OMT and led to fewer hospitalizations. Based on the FIX-HF-5C trial, the FDA approved the three-lead Optimizer system in March 2019.

FIX-HF-5-C2 trial

The FIX-HF-5C2 (two-lead) study was a multicenter, prospective, single-arm treatment-only confirmatory study of the two-lead configuration of the Optimizer Smart System.[31] Use of the two-lead system was made possible by the development of a wavefront conduction velocity algorithm that took advantage of differences in conduction velocity between impulses traveling through the His-Purkinje system (supraventricular) and those traveling via ventricular myocardium (ventricular). In addition to eliminating the need for the atrial sensing lead (and its associated complications), this algorithm opened up the possibility of delivering CCM therapy to patients in atrial fibrillation, and 15% of enrolled patients indeed had atrial fibrillation. The study was designed to evaluate improvement in exercise time quantified by peak V_{O_2}.

Subjects who received the Optimizer Smart System two-lead configuration under the FIX-HF-5C2 protocol were compared with subjects in the control group of the FIX-HF-5C protocol with respect to peak V_{O_2} mean change at 24 weeks from baseline. Safety was assessed by the number of subjects experiencing an Optimizer device- or procedure-related complication through the 24-week follow-up period, as determined by an independent events adjudication committee.

There were no unanticipated adverse device effects or deaths reported in the FIX-HF-5C2 study. There was a total of 13 AEs reported in nine subjects: six nonserious AEs in four subjects and seven serious AEs in five subjects. None of the

AEs were attributed to the Optimizer device and only one AE was reported as "possibly" related to the Optimizer implant procedure (worsening heart failure serious AE occurring 4 days after implant). No Optimizer lead or ICD lead-related AEs were reported. The between-group peak V_{O_2} difference of 1.73 mL/kg/min was statistically significantly superior and the two-lead system received FDA approval in October 2019.

Effect of Cardiac Contractility Modulation on Long-Term Outcomes

Although randomized clinical trials have suggested improvement in heart failure morbidity end points, CCM survival benefits and long-term sustainability of clinical effects have remained not fully addressed in a prospective fashion, because of the short-term follow-up of prior randomized clinical trials. Both retrospective and prospective observational studies start to address these questions. A retrospective study of 68 patients with a CCM device and mean follow-up of 4.5 years demonstrated lower mortality rates than predicted by the Seattle Heart Failure Model (SHFM).[32] The Kaplan–Meier analysis of mortality rate was 14.2% at 5 years versus that predicted by SHFM of 27.7%. In a single-center retrospective study, 81 patients with CCM sustained improvements in ejection fraction, quality of life (MLHFQ), symptoms (eg, fatigue, shortness of breath), and exercise tolerance through an average of 3-year follow-up.[33] These patients had mortality rates lower than predicted by the Meta-Analysis Global Group in Chronic heart failure score. However, there was not a significant change in peak V_{O_2}.

The largest study to date to address long-term outcomes is the CCM-REG$_{25-45}$. CCM-REG$_{25-45}$ was a multicenter prospective observational registry designed to address long-term (3-year) mortality of patients who received CCM as part of routine clinical indication in Europe compared with the predicted mortality assessed by the SHFM. A total of 140 patients were enrolled in the overall cohort, 83 patients in a CCM-REG$_{25-34}$ subgroup and 57 patients in a CCM-REG$_{34-45}$ subgroup. Patients were well treated in accordance with GDMT standards at the time of enrollment (>90% received renin-angiotensin-aldosterone system inhibitors and β-blockers). The study showed that observed survival rates in the overall group (LVEF 25%–45%) and in the lower LVEF group (25%–34%) were similar to predicted survival by the SHFM (P: NS for both). In the group with LVEF of 35% to 45%, observed survival was significantly higher than predicted survival by the SHFM (P = .046).

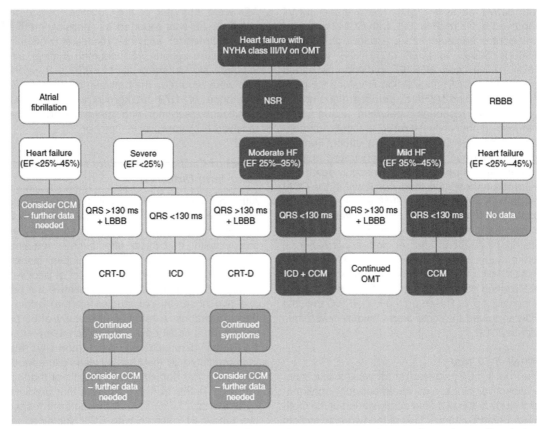

Fig. 3. Cardiac device–based therapy decision-making pathway. Decision-making pathway for cardiac device–based therapy for patients with heart failure based on LVEF and electrocardiogram characteristics. *Dark blue boxes* indicate randomized clinical trials and current indications for CCM. *Light blue boxes* are either based on registry trials or represent future directions for CCM. CRT indications also include NYHA functional class II patients. In the United States, CCM is indicated for NYHA functional class III patients. EF, ejection fraction; HF, heart failure; RBBB, right bundle branch block; NSR, normal sinus rhythm; OMT, optimal medical therapy. (*From* Campbell CM, Kahwash R, Abraham WT. Optimizer Smart in the treatment of moderate-to-severe chronic heart failure. Future Cardiol. 2020 Jan;16(1):13-25; with permission.)

The study also showed significant improvement in NYHA functional class and quality of life assessed by MLHFQ, and 70% to 80% reduction in heart failure hospitalization rate in the 2 years following CCM implant across all LVEF ranges. The study results provide further insight into the potential clinical benefits of CCM among patients selected in a practice setting and further support CCM as an effective therapy for heart failure.

Indication for Cardiac Contractility Modulation

According to the FDA indication statement "The OPTIMIZER Smart System, which delivers CCM therapy, is indicated to improve 6-minute hall walk distance, quality of life, and functional status of NYHA Class III heart failure patients who remain symptomatic despite guideline directed medical therapy, who are in normal sinus rhythm, are not indicated for CRT, and have an LVEF ranging from 25% to 45%."

PATIENT SELECTION FOR CARDIAC RESYNCHRONIZATION THERAPY AND CARDIAC CONTRACTILITY MODULATION

Fig. 3 presents a decision tree for the application of CRT and CCM therapies, with or without a concomitant ICD. At the present time, CCM targets patients without an indication for CRT. Thus, there is little overlap in the indications for these two forms of cardiac implantable electrical devices in the treatment of heart failure. One unique niche for CCM is in the HFmrEF patients with LVEF of 35% to 45%, where no other cardiac implantable electrical device is indicated. This, along with the possible greater benefit of CCM in this HFmrEF population, make it an ideal choice of device therapy for such patients.

CLINICS CARE POINTS

- For patients without a CRT indication, CCM is an emerging electrical therapy.

- Clinical efficacy was assessed in most trials at 24 weeks, although in practice, patients often report significant improvement in their functional abilities within 1 month.

- In the FIX-HF-5C trial, 82% of patients improved by one NYHA functional class and 43% improved by two NYHA functional classes. Importantly, no patients reported worsening of their NYHA status, and the nonresponder rate of 18% to 19% is roughly half of what has been seen with CRT in the last two decades.

- Patients are required to charge their device every week, and should create a set schedule so that the battery does not run out, because this device requires more energy than other cardiac implantable electrical devices (eg, pacemakers).

- More than 80% of patients require CCM and ICD therapies. A new iteration of the Optimizer device will incorporate these two therapies into one system with one implanted pulse generator, one pacemaker lead, and one ICD lead. The unique dual battery design will incorporate the rechargeable technology of the existing platform and will offer 20 years of longevity.

DISCLOSURE

Dr W.T. Abraham has received consulting fees from Impulse Dynamics. The author has no other relevant affiliations or financial involvement with any organization or entity with a financial interest in or financial conflict with the subject matter or materials discussed in the manuscript apart from those disclosed.

REFERENCES

1. Benjamin EJ, Blaha MJ, Chiuve SE, et al. Heart disease and stroke statistics-2017 update: a report from the American Heart Association. Circulation 2017;135:e146–603.

2. Lippi G, Sanchis-Gomar F. Global epidemiology and future trends of heart failure. AME Med 2020;5: 15–20.

3. Calvert MJ, Freemantle N, Cleland JG. The impact of chronic heart failure on health-related quality of life data acquired in the baseline phase of the CARE-HF study. Eur J Heart Fail 2005;7:243–51.

4. Yancy CW, Jessup M, Bozkurt B, et al. 2017 ACC/AHA/HFSA focused update of the 2013 ACCF/AHA guideline for the management of heart failure: a report of the American College of Cardiology/American Heart Association task force on clinical practice guidelines and the Heart Failure Society of America. Circulation 2017;136(6):e137–61.

5. Ponikowski P, Voors AA, Anker SD, et al. 2016 ESC Guidelines for the diagnosis and treatment of acute and chronic heart failure: the Task Force for the diagnosis and treatment of acute and chronic heart failure of the European Society of Cardiology (ESC). Developed with the special contribution of the Heart Failure Association (HFA) of the ESC. Eur J Heart Fail 2016;18:891–975.

6. Abraham WT, Hayes DL. Cardiac resynchronization therapy for heart failure. Circulation 2003;108(21): 2596–603.

7. Prinzen FW, Vernooy K, Auricchio A. Cardiac resynchronization therapy: state-of-the-art of current applications, guidelines, ongoing trials, and areas of controversy. Circulation 2013;128:2407–18.

8. Jaffe LM, Morin DP. Cardiac resynchronization therapy: history, present status, and future directions. Ochsner J 2014;14:596–607.

9. Cazeau S, Leclercq C, Lavergne T, et al, Multisite Stimulation in Cardiomyopathies (MUSTIC) Study Investigators. Effects of multisite biventricular pacing in patients with heart failure and intraventricular conduction delay. N Engl J Med 2001;344:873–80.

10. Abraham WT, Fisher WG, Smith AL, et al, MIRACLE Study Group. Multicenter InSync Randomized Clinical Evaluation. Cardiac resynchronization in chronic heart failure. N Engl J Med 2002;346:1845–53.

11. Bristow MR, Saxon LA, Boehmer J, et al, Comparison of Medical Therapy, Pacing, and Defibrillation in Heart Failure (COMPANION) Investigators. Cardiac-resynchronization therapy with or without an implantable defibrillator in advanced chronic heart failure. N Engl J Med 2004;350:2140–50.

12. Cleland JG, Daubert JC, Erdmann E, et al, Cardiac Resynchronization-Heart Failure (CARE-HF) Study Investigators. The effect of cardiac resynchronization on morbidity and mortality in heart failure. N Engl J Med 2005;352:1539–49.

13. Linde C, Abraham WT, Gold MR, et al, REVERSE (REsynchronization reVErses Remodeling in Systolic left vEntricular dysfunction) Study Group. Randomized trial of cardiac resynchronization in mildly symptomatic heart failure patients and in asymptomatic patients with left ventricular dysfunction and previous heart failure symptoms. J Am Coll Cardiol 2008;52:1834–43.

14. Moss AJ, Hall WJ, Cannom DS, et al, MADIT-CRT Trial Investigators. Cardiac-resynchronization

therapy for the prevention of heart-failure events. N Engl J Med 2009;361:1329–38.

15. Tang AS, Wells GA, Talajic M, et al, Resynchronization-Defibrillation for Ambulatory Heart Failure Trial Investigators. Cardiac-resynchronization therapy for mild-to-moderate heart failure. N Engl J Med 2010;363:2385–95.

16. St John Sutton MG, Plappert T, Abraham WT, et al, Multicenter InSync Randomized Clinical Evaluation (MIRACLE) Study Group. Effect of cardiac resynchronization therapy on left ventricular size and function in chronic heart failure. Circulation 2003;107: 1985–90.

17. Zareba W, Klein H, Cygankiewicz I, et al, MADIT-CRT Investigators. Effectiveness of cardiac resynchronization therapy by QRS morphology in the multicenter automatic defibrillator implantation trial-cardiac resynchronization therapy (MADIT-CRT). Circulation 2011;123:1061–72.

18. Ruschitzka F, Abraham WT, Singh JP, et al, EchoCRT Study Group. Cardiac-resynchronization therapy in heart failure with a narrow QRS complex. N Engl J Med 2013;369:1395–405.

19. Osmanska J, Hawkins NM, Toma M, et al. Eligibility for cardiac resynchronization therapy in patients hospitalized with heart failure. ESC Heart Fail 2018; 5:668–74.

20. Borggrefe MM, Lawo T, Butter C, et al. Randomized, double blind study of non-excitatory, cardiac contractility modulation electrical impulses for symptomatic heart failure. Eur Heart J 2008;29:1019–28.

21. Kadish A, Nademanee K, Volosin K, et al. A randomized controlled trial evaluating the safety and efficacy of cardiac contractility modulation in advanced heart failure. Am Heart J 2011;161: 329–37. e1-2.

22. Abraham WT, Kuck K-H, Goldsmith RL, et al. A randomized controlled trial to evaluate the safety and efficacy of cardiac contractility modulation. JACC Heart Fail 2018;6:874–83.

23. Brunckhorst CB, Shemer I, Mika Y, et al. Cardiac contractility modulation by non-excitatory currents: studies in isolated cardiac muscle. Eur J Heart Fail 2006;8:7–15.

24. Imai M, Rastogi S, Gupta RC, et al. Therapy with cardiac contractility modulation electrical signals improves left ventricular function and remodeling in dogs with chronic heart failure. J Am Coll Cardiol 2007;49:2120–8.

25. Butter C, Rastogi S, Minden HH, et al. Cardiac contractility modulation electrical signals improve myocardial gene expression in patients with heart failure. J Am Coll Cardiol 2008;51:1784–9.

26. Butter C, Wellnhofer E, Schlegl M, et al. Enhanced inotropic state of the failing left ventricle by cardiac contractility modulation electrical signals is not associated with increased myocardial oxygen consumption. J Card Fail 2007;13:137–42.

27. Tschöpe C, Kherad B, Klein O, et al. Cardiac contractility modulation: mechanisms of action in heart failure with reduced ejection fraction and beyond. Eur J Heart Fail 2019;21:14–22.

28. Kahwash R, Burkhoff D, Abraham WT. Cardiac contractility modulation in patients with advanced heart failure. Expert Rev Cardiovasc Ther 2013;11: 635–45.

29. Campbell CM, Kahwash R, Abraham WT. Optimizer Smart in the treatment of moderate-to-severe chronic heart failure. Future Cardiol 2019; 16:13–25.

30. Abraham WT, Nademanee K, Volosin K, et al. Subgroup analysis of a randomized controlled trial evaluating the safety and efficacy of cardiac contractility modulation in advanced heart failure. J Card Fail 2011;17:710–7.

31. Wiegn P, Chan R, Jost C, et al. Safety, performance, and efficacy of cardiac contractility modulation delivered by the 2-2ead OPTIMIZER SMART System. Circ Heart Fail 2020;13:e006512.

32. Kloppe A, Lawo T, Mijic D, et al. Long-term survival with cardiac contractility modulation in patients with NYHA II or III symptoms and normal QRS duration. Int J Cardiol 2016;209:291–5.

33. Kuschyk J, Roeger S, Schneider R, et al. Efficacy and survival in patients with cardiac contractility modulation: long-term single center experience in 81 patients. Int J Cardiol 2015;183:76–81.

Mitral and Tricuspid Valves Percutaneous Repair in Patients with Advanced Heart Failure: Panacea, or Pandora's Box?

Valeria Cammalleri, MD, PhD[a,b], Simona Mega, MD[a], Gian Paolo Ussia, MD[a], Francesco Grigioni, MD, PhD[a,*]

KEYWORDS

- Mitral regurgitation • MitraClip • Tricuspid regurgitation • Transcatheter mitral valve repair
- Transcatheter tricuspid valve repair • Transcatheter valve replacement • Advanced heart failure
- Heart failure with reduced ejection fraction

KEY POINTS

- In heart failure with reduced ejection fraction, the advent of transcatheter therapies to address secondary (functional) mitral and tricuspid regurgitation offers new and previously unimaginable therapeutic opportunities.
- Nowadays, MitraClip is becoming an established therapy for severe functional mitral regurgitation when not associated with end-stage left ventricular dysfunction.
- Edge-to-edge tricuspid repair is the most developed transcatheter option currently available for functional tricuspid regurgitation.
- Transcatheter annuloplasty and valve replacement for functional atrioventricular regurgitations are still under investigation.
- The future appears bright for transcatheter mitral and tricuspid therapies, albeit their definitive place in routine clinical practice and in therapeutic algorithms is yet to be refined.

INTRODUCTION

In heart failure with reduced ejection fraction (HFrEF), secondary (functional) mitral (FMR) and tricuspid regurgitation (FTR) are common and negatively contribute to symptoms and prognosis.[1,2] Two main mechanisms cause FMR. One mechanism is annular dilatation and/or loss of annular contraction; the second is restricted leaflets motion. Restricted leaflets motion occurs when left ventricular (LV) remodeling implies papillary muscle displacement causing chordal tethering.

Similarly to FMR, FTR occurs in the presence of a macroscopically normal valve apparatus and is due to the deformation of the valvular-ventricular complex.[3,4]

The cornerstone of treatment of FMR complicating HFrEF is guideline-directed medical treatment (GDMT) and—when applicable—cardiac resynchronization therapy (CRT).[5–9] In refractory HFrEF (stage D) patients without comorbidities, ventricular assist devices and heart transplantation have also to be considered.[7–9] A recent European position statement highlights the importance of a multidisciplinary approach for the management of FMR in HFrEF patients, starting from the diagnosis to multiple treatment options, including GDMT,

a Department of Cardiology, Policlinico Universitario Campus Bio-Medico, Via Álvaro del Portillo, 21, Roma 00128, Italy; b Department of Cardiology, Policlinico Universitario Tor Vergata, Viale Oxford 81, Roma 00133, Italy
* Corresponding author.
E-mail address: f.grigioni@unicampus.it

Heart Failure Clin 17 (2021) 607–618
https://doi.org/10.1016/j.hfc.2021.05.006
1551-7136/21/© 2021 Elsevier Inc. All rights reserved.

device therapy, and transcatheter repair in selected cases.[9]

FTR is usually treated medically, and conventional surgery is mostly considered in the presence of a correctable left heart disease.[5,6]

Nowadays, in this already composite clinical scenario, transcatheter mitral and tricuspid valve therapies are emerging as adjunctive and promising therapeutic opportunities for HFrEF.

PREVALENCE AND IMPACT OF SECONDARY (FUNCTIONAL) MITRAL REGURGITATION IN STAGE C-D HFrEF

In stage C-D HFrEF, grade $\geq$3+ FMR is common, with a reported prevalence ranging from 17% to 45% and increased morbidity and mortality.[10–15] Consequently, clinicians sought for therapies challenging FMR aiming at improving symptoms and prognosis. Established and evidence-based treatments for FMR complicating HFrEF, include GDMT and, when indicated, CRT. Besides improving FMR, both these approaches showed to correct ventricular remodeling and function, symptoms and survival.

By restoring a synchronous LV contraction, CRT improves leaflet tethering and closing forces of the mitral valve apparatus. Usually, the positive effects of CRT on FMR occurs within 3 to 6 months from implant.[14] However, only 50% of patients with FMR complicating HFrEF favorably respond to CRT. A positive response to CRT implantation is expected in the presence of an anteroseptal to posterior wall radial strain dyssynchrony more than 200 milliseconds, an end-systolic LV dimension indexed less than 29 mm/m^2, and in the absence of a scar at lead insertion.[16]

In patients treated with GDMT and if needed CRT, conventional surgery for FMR—although performed for many years—did not demonstrate to improve prognosis further. Open-heart surgery for FMR can be performed in experienced centers, but operative mortality is not negligible, and long-term results are varying and less reproducible when compared with primary (organic) degenerative mitral regurgitation (MR). Altogether, available data indicate that the full potential of conventional open-heart surgery for FMR remains to be defined.[5,6] Furthermore, FMR complicating HFrEF often presents with associated relevant comorbidities, eventually increasing the surgical risk and possibly leading to an inoperable condition.[17] Based on this scenario, transcatheter therapies for FMR have become the focus of an intensive clinical research because of their potentially low periprocedural risks and long-lasting results.

MITRAL VALVE PERCUTANEOUS REPAIR

Table 1 gives an overview of the most applied transcatheter techniques developed to address FMR.

The MitraClip system (Abbott Vascular, Abbott Park, IL, USA) represents the most widely applied device with broad experience and an extensive clinical data collection. The procedure mimics Alfieri's edge-to-edge surgical technique, using a transfemoral venous approach and transseptal puncture.[18] The first clinical data on this transcatheter technique derive from the randomized trial Endovascular Valve Edge-to-Edge Repair Study (EVEREST II). The EVEREST II for the first time demonstrated that transcatheter repair compared with conventional surgery although less effective in reducing MR, was associated with superior safety and similar improvement in clinical outcome.[19] The population initially enrolled in the EVEREST II was affected by degenerative MR, and only later patients with FMR were included. Consequently, the MitraClip system received US market approval in 2013 only for treating inoperable patients with primary severe MR. Conversely, in Europe, edge-to-edge repair was applied to treat FMR in high-risk and inoperable HFrEF patients as early as in 2008.[20–23] The approval in the USA for FMR was given in 2019 after the positive results of the COAPT trial.[24] Up to date, more than 90,000 patients with severe symptomatic MR were treated with the MitraClip system. MitraClip has currently evolved as an important nonsurgical treatment option for patients with symptomatic FMR who are at high surgical risk or judged inoperable after GDMT and CRT, if applicable. As a prerequisite, current guidelines recommend a reasonable life expectancy (>1 year) to avoid futility.[5,6] Still, 1-year rate of overall mortality in patients with functional MR undergoing percutaneous MV repair ranges between 18% and 29%.[23–26] The favorable safety profile of MitraClip shown in the EVEREST trials has been lately confirmed by prospective and retrospective registries enrolling elderly, high-risk patients, and those suffering from advanced HFrEF.[20–23,27,28] More recently, two landmark randomized trials compared for the first time MitraClip to GDMT in FMR complicating LV dysfunction: the COAPT (Cardiovascular Outcomes Assessment of the MitraClip Percutaneous Therapy for Heart Failure Patients With Functional Mitral Regurgitation) and the MITRA-FR (Multicenter Study of Percutaneous Mitral Valve Repair MitraClip Device in Patients With Severe Secondary Mitral Regurgitation).[24,25] Except for a valve area less than 4 cm^2 in COAPT, no specific mitral valve anatomic exclusion criteria

Table 1
Overview of percutaneous mitral valve repair devices that have already CE approval and devices with promising techniques

Repair Mode	Device	Description	Access	Clinical Experience
Leaflet repair	MitraClip (Abbot Vascular, USA)	Based on the "edge-to-edge" technique	TF-transseptal	>90,000 Impl CE approval FDA approval for DMR and FMR
	PASCAL (Edwards Lifesciences, Irvine, CA)	Based on the "edge-to-edge" technique Independent grasping of the leaflets	TF-transseptal	CE approval
Direct Annuloplasty	Cardioband (Edwards Lifesciences, Irvine, CA)	Implantation of an adjustable band to the posterior annulus	TF-transseptal	CE approval
	Mitralign (Mitralign, Inc.; Tewksbury, MA)	Anchoring on the hinge of the annulus Plication of the posterior annulus with 2 pairs of pledges Reducing MV annulus diameter	TF-transseptal	CE approval
	Arto system (MVRx, Inc.; San Mateo, USA)	Implantation of an atrial septal anchor and a coronary sinus anchor Cinching of the anchors leads to a reduction of AP diameter	TJ and TF-transseptal	Investigational
	Iris Device (Millipede Inc., USA)	Semirigid nitinol ring that is implanted in the mitral valve annulus	TF-transseptal	Investigational
Indirect Annuloplasty	Carillon (Cardiac Dimensions, USA)	Nitinol anchors placed in the distal and proximal coronary sinus Reduction of MV annulus diameter upon deployment of the device	TJ	CE approval
Chordal Replacement	NeoChord (NeoChord, USA)	Surgical off-pump procedure Implantation of artificial chords through a transapical access	TA	CE approval
	TSD-5 device (Harpoon Medical, Inc.)	Surgical off-pump procedure Implantation of artificial chords through a transapical access	TA	Ongoing CE approval study

Abbreviations: AP, anterior-posterior; DMR, degenerative mitral regurgitation; FMR, functional mitral regurgitation; MV, mitral valve; TA, transapical; TF, transfemoral; TJ, transjugular.

were applied to both trials. MITRA-FR had less strict clinical inclusion criteria than COAPT. Patients with nonambulatory NYHA class IV, LV end-systolic diameter above 70 mm, right-sided congestive HF with moderate or severe right ventricle (RV) dysfunction, estimated pulmonary artery pressure more than 70 mm Hg, chronic obstructive pulmonary disease with home oxygen therapy or chronic outpatient oral steroid use were excluded from COAPT but theoretically included in MITRA-FR. In COAPT, optimal medical therapy was strictly applied at the highest tolerable dosage before randomization and after randomization, no adjustment was intended. In MITRA-FR, optimization of medical therapy was allowed after randomization. Patients' recruitment was a major challenge in both trials (**Table 2**). The ratio between screened and randomized patients was much lower in MITRA-FR than in COAPT illustrated by the fact that of 15 patients screened, approximately 10 were randomized in MITRA-FR compared with only 6 in COAPT.

In terms of results, in the COAPT trial, MitraClip was superior to GDMT alone at 2 years in reducing mortality and rehospitalization. In the MITRA-FR trial, the mortality rate at 1 year and rehospitalization were similar in the 2 arms of treatment. Regarding safety and efficacy, the MITRA-FR trial was characterized by a higher complication rate and lower success rate than the COAPT. To understand the discrepancies between these trials, two key aspects regarding MR and LV dimension should be underscored besides inclusion criteria. There was a higher prevalence of patients with effective regurgitant orifice area (EROA) <30 mm^2 in MITRA-FR compared with the COAPT population. Moreover, MITRA-FR patients presented with more dilated ventricles at inclusion compared with COAPT patients (left ventricular end-diastolic volume (LVEDV) index 135 mL/m^2 in MITRA-FR versus 101 mL/m^2 in COAPT). Hence, MITRA-FR likely included patients with less severe MR and more enlarged LV diameters, whereas COAPT enrolled patients

Table 2
Key differences between the MITRA-FR and COAPT trials

Patient selection and trial design	• COAPT had stricter inclusion/exclusion criteria vs MITRA-FR with limits on LV size and excluded RHF, PH and untreated "clinically significant" CAD. • MITRA-FR patients typically had less severe MR, more LV dilatation, and more advanced HF compared with the patients in COAPT. • The mortality benefit in COAPT was mainly observed in the second year, potentially favoring the study with the longer follow-up duration.
Enrollment and medical therapy	• COAPT had a larger sample size of highly selected patients evaluated by a central eligibility committee. The percentage of patients enrolled but deemed not eligible for randomization was 32% in MITRA-FR and 61% in COAPT. • COAPT randomized patients on maximal tolerated GDMT including device therapy and coronary revascularization where appropriate (changes to GDMT discouraged following randomization). • In MITRA-FR, the local heart team enrolled patients (304) and GDMT could be uptitrated after randomization (there was no monitoring of medication alterations during follow-up). • GDMT adjustment as per real-world clinical practice may have reduced FMR thus diminishing the benefit of edge-to-edge repair in MITRA-FR.
Procedural safety and durability	• 8.5% complication rate in COAPT compared with 14.6% in MITRA-FR (should be interpreted with caution as the trials had different safety parameters). • Superior durability of MR reduction after MitraClip in COAPT (MR $\leq$ grade II in 94.8% of patients), follow-up echocardiographic data were incomplete in MITRA-FR (MR $\geq$ grade 2 in "at least" 48/132 patients).

Abbreviations: CAD, coronary artery disease; PH, pulmonary hypertension; RHF, right heart failure.

with more severe MR and less diseased ventricles.

Finally, the COAPT trial was larger in terms of the patient population enrolled and was designed to have a longer follow-up duration. Of note, recent data from the MITRA-FR trial showed a trend of reduced hospitalization for HF in the MitraClip arm at 2 years.[29]

TRANSCATHETER MITRAL VALVE REPLACEMENT

The field of transcatheter mitral valve replacement (TMVR) is still in its infancy, mainly limited by the high rate of screening failure due to an unsuitable anatomy. Two approaches are currently being investigated: the off-label use of transcatheter heart valves originally designed for the aortic position (mainly for valve-in-valve, valve-in-ring, and valve-in-mitral annular calcification) and the use of dedicated devices. Among the issues that still need to be addressed, obstruction of the LV outflow tract, valve thrombogenicity, and access route are probably the most salient.[30]

CONTROVERSIES

In general, identifying patients with HFrEF who may benefit from valve interventions and particularly from transcatheter FMR repair remains a subject of ongoing controversies.

In FMR complicating HFrEF, Grayburn PA et al.[31] suggested that physicians should determine whether the estimated degree of FMR is proportionate to the degree of ventricular dilatation (**Fig. 1**). This concept is based on the principle that EROA being an isolated measure of FMR severity does not consider the extent of LV remodeling. A patient whose FMR severity is consistent with the amount of LV dilatation would fall in the definition of "proportional" FMR. In these patients, a correction of the valvular lesion would bring little

or no improvement to a diseased ventricle affected by a nonsignificant amount of FMR-induced volume overload. Conversely, a patient might respond more favorably to FMR correction in the presence of a relatively large EROA associated with an only moderately dilated ventricle (disproportionate FMR). On the clinical ground, to assess FMR proportionality, some authors suggest focusing on the ratio of regurgitant volume to ventricular end-diastolic volume. This ratio may anticipate the extent of reverse remodeling occurring after FMR correction.[31] Similarly, regurgitant fraction, by including FMR severity, ventricular volumes and function could also provide valuable information.

This multiparametric approach according to some authors outperforms current guideline-based algorithms in identifying patients who may benefit most from intervention. The 2 recently published controlled randomized trials previously mentioned confirmed the rationale of this working hypothesis.[24,25] With this respect, MITRA-FR patients likely represented a cohort with "proportionate" FMR in whom transcatheter mitral repair was unlikely to alter prognosis. Conversely, the reduction of "disproportionate" MR in the COAPT interrupted the vicious cycle of adverse remodeling eventually resulting in a positive result of the trial. The overarching lesson from both trials is that FMR treatment can influence the outcome in HFrEF patients who remain symptomatic despite GDMT only when FMR independently contributes to disease progression. Conversely, FMR correction brings no improvement and is probably futile in patients in whom it represents a marker of an end-stage underlying ventricular dysfunction.

The divergent results of these two cornerstone trials draw attention to the immediate need for clinical parameters, but also for improved imaging techniques (advanced echocardiography, cardiac computed tomography, and magnetic resonance), including thresholds of MR severity, to identify

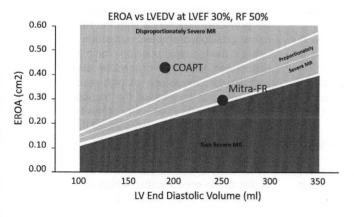

Fig. 1. Relationship between EROA and LVEDV. RF, regurgitant fraction. (*Adapted from* Grayburn PA, Sannino A, Packer M. Proportionate and disproportionate functional mitral regurgitation: a new conceptual framework that reconciles the results of the MITRA-FR and COAPT trials. JACC Cardiovasc Imaging 2019;12:353–62; with permission.)

better responders to transcatheter mitral repair, and exclude patients who are expected to derive little symptomatic benefit or improvement in quality of life. In this case, specialist palliative care should be offered.[9]

PREVALENCE AND IMPACT OF SECONDARY TR IN ADVANCED HEART FAILURE

The heterogeneity of etiologies associated with TR makes the evaluation of its prognostic impact and the therapeutic implications challenging to estimate. Clinical assessment of tricuspid valve disease is often difficult because of the absence of early clinical features, which can lead to a late referral of patients after a severe, long-lasting disease.

The prevalence of tricuspid valve disease is increasing steadily, with the most common form of the disease, TR, occurring in an estimated percentage of 65% to 85% of the European population.[32] Among patients referred for echocardiography, a diagnosis of moderate/severe TR is performed in about 16% of all comers, and among them, FTR comprises 85% to 90% of all severe TR.[33] FTR is produced mainly through two mechanisms variably associated. The first is valve tenting, caused by right ventricular enlargement and dysfunction. Right ventricular enlargement can represent an isolated disease or due to left heart diseases resulting in pulmonary hypertension. The second mechanism generating FTR is annular enlargement.[3] Once FTR is established, the progressive right ventricular remodeling and dysfunction resulting from the chronic volume overload causes papillary muscle displacement and leaflet tethering, which worsens TR and leads to further ventricular dilatation.[3]

The primary complication for TR is obviously right-sided heart failure (RHF), carrying an increased risk of end-organ dysfunction and atrial arrhythmias. Furthermore, the shifting of the interventricular septum toward the left side reduces LV preload and decreases systemic forward cardiac output.

With respect to the prognostic implication, moderate and severe TR is associated with a worse survival even when adjusted for systolic pulmonary artery pressure, and biventricular function.[34] One-year survival has been described approaching 90% in mild TR, 80% in moderate TR, and 65% in severe TR.[34]

Management of RHF implies managing the symptoms and treating the cause. Diuretics are the mainstay for symptomatic management in acute and chronic RHF; sodium and water restriction also improve volume overload symptoms.[35]

Reperfusion therapy and embolectomy are indicated in RHF patients presenting with pulmonary embolism. Similarly, percutaneous coronary intervention is recommended in patients with ongoing right ventricular ischemia.[35]

Despite being frequently observed on echocardiography, FTR is usually considered for conventional surgery only in the presence of an indication for left heart surgery.[5,6]

In isolate FTR, surgical intervention is usually evaluated when the patient is symptomatic, poorly responding to high dosage of diuretics and/or in the presence of progressive right ventricular dysfunction.[35,36] Typically, those are very high-risk patients with previous left-heart surgery. In this setting, operative mortality rate can be as high as 10% to 25%, and postoperative survival remains dismal.[37]

Based on this rationale, the evidence that surgical correction of isolated FTR improves survival or symptoms is still lacking.

Nowadays, transcatheter tricuspid valve intervention techniques by avoiding cardiopulmonary bypass, sternotomy and intubation, is perceived by the scientific community as a potential tool to improve survival in this group of patients. Research and industry are currently very active in this domain.

TRICUSPID VALVE PERCUTANEOUS REPAIR

Over the past decade, the evolving understanding of the complex anatomy and physiology of the tricuspid valve and the increasing evidence of the negative lasting impacts of untreated tricuspid disease led to an outburst of novel transcatheter tricuspid valve interventions.

As most procedures were adapted from left atrioventricular valve interventions, they follow similar underlying principles: edge-to-edge repair enhancing leaflet coaptation, annuloplasty aiming for annular size reduction and valve replacement. **Table 3** illustrates the results of transcatheter approaches dedicated to the tricuspid valve. A decade-long experience with the MitraClip in the mitral position prompted numerous operators to use it in the tricuspid position. The main difficulties associated with this procedure stem from the problematic acquisition of high-resolution echocardiographic images of the tricuspid valve, as well as the lack of versatility of the MitraClip system in the right atrium, because of the limited distance between the inferior vena cava and the tricuspid valvular plane. The best results appear to occur by attaching the anterior and/or posterior leaflet to the septal leaflet, which can also reduce annular dimensions without distorting the valve.[37]

Table 3
Short-term (in-hospital or 30-days) outcomes of transcatheter tricuspid valve intervention devices

	Trial/Study	Technical Success[a]	Mortality	TR Volume Reduction (mL)
TriAlign	SCOUT I[48] NCT02574650 SCOUT II is enrolling	12/15	0	−2.7 ± 39.5
TriCinch	Giannini and Colombo[37]	20/24	-	-
Cardioband	TRI-REPAIR[52] TriBAND ongoing NCT03779490	28/30	2/30	−35.6 ± 35.3
MitraClip and TriClip	Nickenig et al.[41] TRILUMINATE NCT03227757[36]	6/64 10/85	3/64 0	−26.4 ± 7.8 − 18.6 ± 21.2
FORMA	Perlman[47] SPACER enrolling NCT02787408		2/47	-

[a] No standardized definition for "technical success."

This zone is also easier to target because of the more favorable angle between inferior vena cava and valvular plane.[38] More than one clip is usually necessary to achieve a satisfactory result. The MitraClip in the setting of FTR showed encouraging results in terms of right ventricular reverse remodeling and improvement of cardiac output.[39–44] Furthermore, the MitraClip applied to patients with elevated liver enzymes due to congestion lead to a significant improvement.[45] The "TriClip" is essentially a modification of the MitraClip NT percutaneous delivery system and was investigated in the TRILUMINATE study.[42] This trial enrolled 85 patients with moderate or greater TR, NYHA class II or higher, systolic pulmonary artery pressure ≤60 mm Hg. The TriClip appeared to be safe and effective in reducing TR by at least one grade and was associated with clinical improvement after 6 months. More in detail, in the TRILUMINATE study, 4% of patients experienced a major adverse event at follow-up and all-cause mortality occurred in 5%. No periprocedural deaths, conversions to surgery, device embolization, myocardial infarctions, or strokes occurred.

The PASCAL device has also been successfully adapted from the mitral to the tricuspid position. Although the experience is limited, results are encouraging.[46,47] The Forma device (Edwards Lifesciences) has been created to reduce FTR by providing a new surface of coaptation for the leaflets. It consists of a foam-filled spacer inserted through the subclavian or the axillary vein, which is placed in the regurgitant orifice and anchored to the RV apex.[48] The ongoing SPACER study (NCT02787408) will provide more data on this device.

The TriAlign and TriCinch devices have been developed mimicking the surgical annuloplasty techniques.[49,50] The TriAlign device is a transcatheter suture annuloplasty technique performed transjugularly. An insulated radiofrequency wire is advanced into the RV to retrogradely cross the tricuspid annulus. Thereafter, two pledgets are placed at the posteroseptal and the anteroposterior commissures, which are then cinched to obliterate the posterior tricuspid leaflet, yielding a "bicuspidisation" of the tricuspid valve.[49] The TriCinch device is no longer available. It was delivered through the femoral vein. It presented an epicardial coil with 2 hemostasis seals implanted in the midanterior part of the tricuspid annulus. To maintain tension applied to the annulus, a nitinol stent, connected to the coil through a Dacron band was placed into the inferior vena cava. The clinical use of the TriCinch has only been described in small case series.[50–52] In the open-heart surgical setting, the ring annuloplasty technique is currently preferred by most teams and uses rigid or semirigid rings, planar or nonplanar to fit the tricuspid anatomy. The transcatheter equivalent ring annuloplasty can be performed with the Cardioband device, which was also used for mitral annuloplasty.[38] It consists of a flexible implant delivered through a flexible catheter. Multiple anchors are attached to the annulus, and once they are all fixed, tensions can be applied to reduce the dilated annulus to a physiologic size. The TrIcuspid Regurgitation RePAIr With CaRdioband Transcatheter System (TRI-REPAIR) study reported a technical success of 100% and a significant reduction in tricuspid annular septolateral diameter, and grade of TR at 6 months and 2 years of follow-up. The echocardiographic improvement was also associated with a symptomatic and functional benefit.[53,54]

Data from the real-world setting derives from the TriValve Registry, which is a large-scale international database collecting data on the different transcatheter tricuspid valve interventions.[41] The midterm results reported a procedural success rate of 72.8% with no difference among devices (66% MitraClip, 9% CAVI, 8% FORMA, 6% Trialign, 4% Cardioband, 4% TriCinch, 3% others). Procedural failure (residual TR ≥ grade 2+) was identified as a predictor of adverse outcomes. Periprocedural mortality was 0% and an adverse event occurred in 10.3% at 30-days follow-up.[41] A recently published propensity-matched case-control study comparing transcatheter valve therapy to medical treatment alone further supports transcatheter therapy.[51] In the 268 patients from the TriValve registry that were matched to patients medically managed, transcatheter tricuspid valve treatment was associated with a survival benefit (mortality 23 ± 3% vs 36 ± 3%, P = .001), as well as a reduction of rehospitalization for HF (26 ± 3% vs 47 ± 3% P<.0001) at 1-year follow-up.[55] Prospective randomized studies are needed to confirm these findings.

TRANSCATHETER TRICUSPID VALVE REPLACEMENT

Transcatheter tricuspid valve replacement is a promising therapeutic option.[55] Existing dedicated devices are implanted in orthotopic or heterotopic positions, such as bioprostheses in the superior and inferior vena cava. The NAVIGATE (NaviGate Cardiac Structures, CA, USA) is a self-expanding bioprosthesis for an orthotopic replacement that consists of three xenogeneic pericardial leaflets seated in a tapered nitinol stent with atrial winglets and ventricular graspers for anchoring the tricuspid annulus and leaflets without protruding into adjacent chambers. Yet, only short case series have been published.[56,57]

Transfemoral transcatheter tricuspid valve replacement with the 28-F EVOQUE system (Edwards Lifesciences, Irvine, California) has been reported by Fam NP et al with promising results in terms of echocardiographic and clinical benefits.[58]

Other devices have been tested, but they are yet to be used in clinical setting. Hence, although nowadays the clinical implementation of transcatheter tricuspid valve replacement remains at its early stages, it has an interesting potential.

CONTROVERSIES

The timing of treatment of severe FTR is still debated. The emerging paradigm is that an earlier, safer, and effective transcatheter correction may provide the most beneficial results. However, this appealing hypothesis needs to be confirmed in appropriately sized prospective randomized trials. **Fig. 2** attempts a possible decision-making algorithm based on our personal clinical experience and available data.

Besides the timing of the intervention, the choice of the most appropriate transcatheter therapeutic option in the single patient also remains challenging. This also happens because transcatheter tricuspid valve interventions pose several anatomic and technical challenges. For instance, the thinner leaflets and the larger coaptation gaps make leaflet approximation more difficult to achieve than on the left side. It is possible that the use of the PASCAL, the new iteration of the MitraClip XTR system, by featuring extended arms, and the dedicated TriClip system, may facilitate grasping.[46] In the case of more advanced stages of FTR, the use of combined procedures (eg, sequential annuloplasty and edge-to-edge repair) may lead to better results. Every center aiming at determining eligibility for annuloplasty, caval stent/valve implantation, and valve replacement has to be familiar with advanced imaging, including multidetector computed tomography and 3D transesophageal echocardiography.

FUTURE DIRECTIONS: MITRAL AND TRICUSPID VALVES PERCUTANEOUS REPAIR

In patients with advanced HFrEF and severe FMR undergoing transcatheter mitral valve repair, there is an urgent need for long-term survival data and development of proper selection criteria to avoid futility. New information is available from MITRA-FR and COAPT Trials. Nevertheless, whether the knowledge derived from analyzing the differences and similarities of these 2 trials can help in decision making, in the real world, is unclear. Hence, further prospective studies and large registries are needed to help patient selection. We hope the RESHAPE-HF2 (Clinical Evaluation of the Safety and Effectiveness of the MitraClip System in the Treatment of Clinically Significant Functional Mitral Regurgitation 2; NCT02444338) and the MATTERHORN (Multicenter, Randomized, Controlled Study to Assess Mitral Valve Reconstruction for Advanced Insufficiency of Functional or Ischemic Origin; NCT02371512) trials might provide additional information to predict positive clinical outcomes after transcatheter mitral repair in HFrEF patients.

Moving to the heterogeneity of the pathophysiological phenotypes, we should not forget that besides leaflet restriction, the mechanisms of FMR are numerous and interconnected. Hence, the

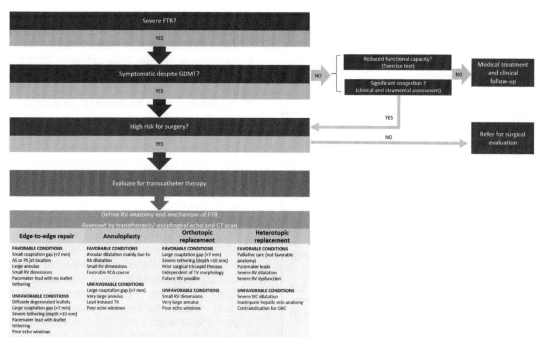

Fig. 2. Decision algorithm for transcatheter tricuspid valve interventions. AS, anteroseptal; CT, computed tomography; IVC, inferior vena cava; OAC, oral anticoagulation; PS, posteroseptal; RCA, right coronary artery; TV, tricuspid valve; ViV, valve-in-valve.

correction of one single mechanism might result in the improvement or the worsening of another. For instance, FMR reduction may favor reverse LV remodeling and revert annular dilatation. However, correcting a valvular lesion to address a ventricular problem could represent an only partial therapeutic approach. Based on this concept, transcatheter edge-to-edge repair, indirect and direct mitral valve annuloplasty, chordal replacement should altogether represent complementary options. However, solid data on which to base the combined use of transcatheter techniques are still missing.

Similar to FMR, patients with severe FTR represent a complex and heterogeneous population, and identifying the optimal transcatheter technique and the timing of treatment is crucial. Although the initial clinical experience with devices derived by mitral transcatheter techniques has been promising, it is still to be determined the patient who could benefit the most from these treatments. In the current experimental phase, most of the patients receiving FTR treatment have advanced HF and several comorbidities. In these cases, the percutaneous treatment is performed for "compassionate" use, or for excessive surgical risk. Therefore, the potential of transcatheter techniques to address FTR at an earlier stage has to be explored.

Development of new imaging techniques and validation of the existing ones is required for a more accurate and reproducible grading of TR severity, as well as for the anatomic screening.

Moreover, given the complexity of mitral and tricuspid valve disease and the increasingly large armamentarium to treat them, a multidisciplinary discussion remains the main guarantor that every patient is treated with the optimal therapeutic strategy.

Given the financial stakes of percutaneous valve intervention, industry has been heavily investing in the development of technologies. Hence, it is likely that new transcatheter solutions will become mainstream within the next years. The cost and cost-effectiveness of these strategies will need to be carefully weighted.

SUMMARY

Over the last years, numerous transcatheter techniques have been developed aiming at providing new therapeutic opportunities for patients affected by HFrEF. The number of patients treated is increasing over time and indications are expanding.

A rigorous patient selection, the availability of safe and effective devices, and a meticulous research approach are all essential to direct these developments to the satisfaction of patients' unmet clinical needs.

Transcatheter mitral and tricuspid valve therapies are establishing as a new cornerstone of the therapy of stage C-D HFrEF.

CLINICS CARE POINTS

- In heart failure with reduced ejection fraction, the advent of transcatheter therapies to address secondary (functional) mitral and tricuspid regurgitation offers new and previously unimaginable therapeutic opportunities.

- Nowadays, MitraClip is becoming an established therapy for severe functional mitral regurgitation when not associated with end-stage left ventricular dysfunction.

- Edge-to-edge tricuspid repair is the most developed transcatheter option currently available for functional tricuspid regurgitation.

- Transcatheter annuloplasty and valve replacement for functional atrioventricular regurgitations are still under investigation.

- The future appears bright for transcatheter mitral and tricuspid therapies, albeit their definitive place in routine clinical practice and in therapeutic algorithms is yet to be refined.

DISCLOSURE

The authors have nothing to disclose.

REFERENCES

1. Goel SS, Bajaj N, Aggarwal B, et al. Prevalence and outcomes of unoperated patients with severe symptomatic mitral regurgitation and heart failure: comprehensive analysis to determine the potential role of MitraClip for this unmet need. J Am Coll Cardiol 2014;63:185–6.
2. Goliasch G, Bartko PE, Pavo N, et al. Refining the prognostic impact of functional mitral regurgitation in chronic heart failure. Eur Heart J 2018;39:39–46.
3. Badano LP, Muraru D, Enriquez-Sarano M. Assessment of functional tricuspid regurgitation. Eur Heart J 2013;34:1875–85.
4. Topilsky Y, Nkomo VT, Vatury O, et al. Clinical outcome of isolated tricuspid regurgitation. JACC Cardiovasc Imaging 2014;7:1185–94.
5. Otto CM, Nishimura RA, Bonow RO, et al. 2020 ACC/AHA Guideline for the management of patients with valvular heart disease: a report of the American College of Cardiology/American Heart Association Joint Committee on clinical practice guidelines. J Am Coll Cardiol 2020;17:S0735–1097.
6. Baumgartner H, Falk V, Bax JJ, et al. 2017 ESC/EACTS Guidelines for the management of valvular heart disease. Eur Heart J 2017;38:2739–91.
7. Ponikowski P, Voors AA, Anker SD, et al. 2016 ESC Guidelines for the diagnosis and treatment of acute and chronic heart failure: The Task Force for the diagnosis and treatment of acute and chronic heart failure of the European Society of Cardiology (ESC) Developed with the special contribution of the Heart Failure Association (HFA) of the ESC. Eur Heart J 2016;18:891–975.
8. Yancy CW, Jessup M, Bozkurt B, et al. 2017 ACC/AHA/HFSA Focused Update of the 2013 ACCF/AHA Guideline for the Management of Heart Failure: A Report of the American College of Cardiology/American Heart Association Task Force on Clinical Practice Guidelines and the Heart Failure Society of America. Circulation 2017;136:e137–61.
9. Coats AJS, Anker SD, Baumbach A, et al. The management of secondary mitral regurgitation in patients with heart failure: a joint position statement from the Heart Failure Association (HFA), European Association of Cardiovascular Imaging (EACVI), European Heart Rhythm Association (EHRA), and European Association of Percutaneous Cardiovascular Interventions (EAPCI) of the ESC. Eur Heart J 2021;42:1254–69.
10. Bursi F, Barbieri A, Grigioni F, et al. Prognostic implications of functional mitral regurgitation according to the severity of the underlying chronic heart failure: a long- term outcome study. Eur J Heart Fail 2010;12:382–8.
11. Cioffi G, Tarantini L, De Feo S, et al. Functional mitral regurgitation predicts 1-year mortality in elderly patients with systolic chronic heart failure. Eur J Heart Fail 2005;7:1112–7.
12. Patel JB, Borgeson DD, Barnes ME, et al. Mitral regurgitation in patients with advanced systolic heart failure. J Card Fail 2004;10:285–91.
13. Grigioni F, Enriquez-Sarano M, Zehr KJ, et al. Ischemic mitral regurgitation: long-term outcome and prognostic implications with quantitative Doppler assessment. Circulation 2001;103:1759–64.
14. Rossi A, Dini FL, Faggiano P, et al. Independent prognostic value of functional mitral regurgitation in patients with heart failure. A quantitative analysis of 1256 patients with ischaemic and non-ischaemic dilated cardiomyopathy. Heart 2011;97:1675–80.
15. Trichon BH, Felker GM, Shaw LK, et al. Relation of frequency and severity of mitral regurgitation to survival among patients with left ventricular systolic dysfunction and heart failure. Am J Cardiol 2003;91:538–43.

16. Onishi T, Onishi T, Marek JJ, et al. Mechanistic features associated with improvement in mitral regurgitation after cardiac resynchronization therapy and their relation to long-term patient outcome. Circulation 2013;6:685–93.

17. Mirabel M, Iung B, Baron G, et al. What are the characteristics of patients with severe, symptomatic, mitral regurgitation who are denied surgery? Eur Heart J 2007;28:1358–65.

18. Maisano F, Torracca L, Oppizzi M, et al. The edge-to-edge technique: a simplified method to correct mitral insufficiency. Eur J Cardiothorac Surg 1998; 13:240–6.

19. Feldman T, Foster E, Glower DD, et al. Percutaneous repair or surgery for mitral regurgitation. N Engl J Med 2011;364:1395–406.

20. Tamburino C, Ussia GP, Maisano F, et al. Percutaneous mitral valve repair with the MitraClip system: acute results from a real world setting. Eur Heart J 2010;31:1382–9.

21. Franzen O, van der Heyden J, Baldus S, et al. Mitra-Clip therapy in patients with end-stage systolic heart failure. Eur J Heart Fail 2011;13:569–76.

22. Maisano F, Franzen O, Baldus S, et al. Percutaneous mitral valve interventions in the real world: early and 1-year results from the ACCESS-EU, a prospective, multicenter, nonrandomized post-approval study of the MitraClip therapy in Europe. J Am Coll Cardiol 2013;62:1052–61.

23. Schafer U, Maisano F, Butter C, et al. Impact of Preprocedural Left Ventricular Ejection Fraction on 1-Year Outcomes After MitraClip Implantation (from the ACCESS-EU Phase I, a prospective, Multicenter, Nonrandomized Postapproval Study of the MitraClip Therapy in Europe). Am J Cardiol 2016;118:873–80.

24. Stone GW, Lindenfeld JA, Abraham WT, et al. Transcatheter mitral-valve repair in patients with heart failure. N Engl J Med 2018;379:2307–18.

25. Obadia JF, Messika-Zeitoun D, Leurent G, et al. for the MITRA-FR Investigators. Percutaneous repair or medical treatment for secondary mitral regurgitation. N Engl J Med 2018;379:2297–306.

26. Chiarito M, Pagnesi M, Martino E, et al. Outcome after percutaneous edge-to-edge mitral repair for functional and degenerative mitral regurgitation: a systematic review and meta-analysis. Heart 2018; 104:306–12.

27. Grasso C, Capodanno D, Scandura S, et al. One- and twelve-month safety and efficacy outcomes of patients undergoing edge-to-edge percutaneous mitral valve repair (from the GRASP Registry). Am J Cardiol 2013;111:1482–7.

28. Buzzatti N, Maisano F, Latib A, et al. Comparison of outcomes of percutaneous MitraClip versus surgical repair or replacement for degenerative mitral regurgitation in octogenarians. Am J Cardiol 2015;115: 487–92.

29. Iung B, Armoiry X, Vahanian A, et al. Percutaneous repair or medical treatment for secondary mitral regurgitation: outcomes at 2 years. Eur J Heart Fail 2019;21:1619–27.

30. Sorajja P, Moat N, Badhwar V, et al. Initial Feasibility Study of a New Transcatheter Mitral Prosthesis: The First 100 Patients. J Am Coll Cardiol 2019;73:1250–60.

31. Grayburn PA, Sannino A, Packer M. Proportionate and disproportionate functional mitral regurgitation: a new conceptual framework that reconciles the results of the MITRA-FR and COAPT trials. JACC Cardiovasc Imaging 2019;12:353–62.

32. Arsalan M, Walther T, Smith RL, et al. Tricuspid regurgitation diagnosis and treatment. Eur Heart J 2017;38:634-38.

33. Yoganathan A, Khan SNM, Khan H, et al. Tricuspid valve diseases: Interventions on the forgotten heart valve. J Card Surg 2021;36:219–28.

34. Nath J, Foster E, Heidenreich PA. Impact of tricuspid regurgitation on long-term survival. J Am Coll Cardiol 2004;43:405–9.

35. Harjola VP, Mebazaa A, Čelutkienė J, et al. Contemporary management of acute right ventricular failure: a statement from the Heart Failure Association and the Working Group on Pulmonary Circulation and Right Ventricular Function of the European Society of Cardiology: contemporary management of acute RV failure. Eur J Heart Fail 2016;18:226-4.

36. Konstam MA, Kiernan MS, Bernstein D, et al. Evaluation and management of right-sided heart failure: a scientific statement from the American Heart Association. Circulation 2018;137:e578–622.

37. Overtchouk P, Piazza N, Granada J, et al. Advances in transcatheter mitral and tricuspid therapies. BMC Cardiovasc Disord 2020;20:1.

38. Giannini F, Colombo A. Percutaneous treatment of tricuspid valve in refractory right heart failure. Eur Heart J Suppl 2019;21(Suppl B):B43–7.

39. Braun D, Nabauer M, Orban M, et al. One-year results of transcatheter treatment of severe tricuspid regurgitation using the edge-to-edge repair technique. EuroIntervention 2018;14:e413–5.

40. Nickenig G, Kowalski M, Hausleiter J, et al. Transcatheter treatment of severe tricuspid regurgitation with the edge-to-edge mitraclip technique. Circulation 2017;135:1802–14.

41. Taramasso M, Alessandrini H, Latib A, et al. Outcomes after current transcatheter tricuspid valve intervention: mid-term results from the international trivalve registry. JACC Cardiovasc Interv 2019;12: 155–65.

42. Nickenig G, Weber M, Lurz P, et al. Transcatheter edge-to-edge repair for reduction of tricuspid regurgitation: 6-month outcomes of the TRILUMINATE single arm study. Lancet 2019;394:2002–11.

43. Orban M, Braun D, Deseive S, et al. Transcatheter edge-to-edge repair for tricuspid regurgitation is

associated with right ventricular reverse remodeling in patients with right-sided heart failure. JACC Cardiovasc Imaging 2019;12:559–60.

44. Rommel KP, Besler C, Noack T, et al. Physiological and clinical consequences of right ventricular volume overload reduction after transcatheter treatment for tricuspid regurgitation. JACC Cardiovasc Interv 2019;12:1423–34.

45. Karam N, Braun D, Mehr M, et al. Impact of transcatheter tricuspid valve repair for severe tricuspid regurgitation on kidney and liver function. JACC Cardiovasc Interv 2019;12:1413–20.

46. Fam NP, Ho EC, Zahrani M, et al. Transcatheter Tricuspid Valve Repair With the PASCAL System. JACC Cardiovasc Interv 2018;11:407–8.

47. Sugiura A, Vogelhuber J, Öztürk C, et al. PASCAL versus MitraClip-XTR edge-to-edge device for the treatment of tricuspid regurgitation: a propensity-matched analysis. Clin Res Cardiol 2021;110:451–9.

48. Perlman G, Praz F, Puri R, et al. Transcatheter Tricuspid Valve Repair With a New Transcatheter Coaptation System for the Treatment of Severe Tricuspid Regurgitation: 1-Year Clinical and Echocardiographic Results. JACC Cardiovasc Interv 2017;10:1994–2003.

49. Hahn RT, Meduri CU, Davidson CJ, et al. Early Feasibility Study of a Transcatheter Tricuspid Valve Annuloplasty: SCOUT Trial 30-Day Results. J Am Coll Cardiol 2017;69:1795–806.

50. Taramasso M, Maisano F. Transcatheter interventions for tricuspid regurgitation: TriCinch (4Tech). EuroIntervention 2016;12:Y110–2.

51. Gheorghe L, Swaans M, Denti P, et al. Transcatheter Tricuspid Valve Repair With a Novel Cinching System. JACC Cardiovasc Interv 2018;11:e199–201.

52. Latib A, Agricola E, Pozzoli A, et al. First-in-man implantation of a tricuspid annular remodeling device for functional tricuspid regurgitation. JACC Cardiovasc Interv 2015;8:e211–4.

53. Nickenig G, Weber M, Schueler R, et al. 6-Month Outcomes of Tricuspid Valve Reconstruction for Patients With Severe Tricuspid Regurgitation. J Am Coll Cardiol 2019;73:1905–15.

54. Nickenig G, Weber M, Schüler R, et al. Tricuspid valve repair with the Cardioband system: two-year outcomes of the multicentre, prospective TRI-REPAIR study. EuroIntervention. 2021;16:e1264–71.

55. Taramasso M, Benfari G, van der Bijl P, et al. Transcatheter versus medical treatment of symptomatic severe tricuspid regurgitation. J Am Coll Cardiol 2019;74:2998–3008.

56. Hahn RT, George I, Kodali SK, et al. Early single-site experience with transcatheter tricuspid valve replacement. JACC Cardiovasc Imaging 2019;12:416–29.

57. Navia JL, Kapadia S, Elgharably H, et al. First-in-Human Implantations of the NaviGate Bioprosthesis in a Severely Dilated Tricuspid Annulus and in a Failed Tricuspid Annuloplasty Ring. Circ Cardiovasc Interv 2017;10:e0058401.

58. Fam NP, Ong G, Deva DP, et al. Transfemoral Transcatheter Tricuspid Valve Replacement. JACC Cardiovasc Interv 2020;13:e93–4.

Left Ventricular Assist Device
Indication, Timing, and Management

Maria Frigerio, MD*

KEYWORDS

- Advanced heart failure • Mechanical circulatory support • Ventricular assist device
- Heart transplant • Heart replacement • LVAD • Right ventricular failure

KEY POINTS

- Long-term therapy with a continuous flow left ventricular (LV) assist device (CF-LVAD) should be considered in patients with advanced to refractory heart failure, with pure/predominant LV systolic dysfunction.
- Despite steady improvement of postoperative results over the years, with 1- and 2-year estimated survival currently exceeding 80% and 70%, respectively, it seems that LVAD is still considered almost only for patients with truly end-stage HF: most of them are inotrope-dependent, and many are in critical conditions.
- Main barriers to the expansion of the use of LVAD in ambulatory patients with advanced heart failure are (1) perceived burden of responsibilities related to self-care; (2) limited availability of expert care outside of the implanting hospitals; (3) persistent risk for device-related complications and hospitalizations during long-term follow-up; (4) lower probability of being transplanted in patients implanted with bridge-to-transplant strategy, especially in comparison with candidates supported with temporary circulatory assist devices.

INTRODUCTION

Mechanically assisted circulation has been conceived about 70 years ago for ensuring organ perfusion after cardiac arrest for open-heart surgery. A few decades later, heart transplantation (HTx) became feasible, thus providing an opportunity for extended survival to patients with end-stage heart failure (HF). Meanwhile, the progresses of cardiac surgery and biomedical engineering resulted in the development and use of several devices for short-term or durable, partial or complete replacement of cardiac function (**Table 1**). Intracorporeal (vs external) pumps, and reduction in size and weight of pump controllers and of rechargeable batteries, represent major technological improvements that allowed patients' mobilization and discharge on mechanical circulatory support

(MCS), opening the way to long-term therapy.[1] An important milestone is represented by a randomized clinical trial that demonstrated the superiority of a left ventricular assist device (LVAD) over medical therapy in inotrope-dependent patients with advanced HF, who were deemed unsuitable for HTx.[2] From 2001 to now, the expected 1-year survival of implanted patients increased from about 50% with a pulsatile-flow device[2] to more than 80% with most recent continuous-flow pumps.[3,4] Although total artificial heart (TAH) or biventricular support and pulsatile flow appear conceptually closer to native heart physiology, so far the best clinical results in terms of survival, freedom from hospitalizations for device-related complications, and quality of life have been obtained with continuous-flow devices supporting only the left ventricle (CF-LVAD).[5] This paper summarizes

2nd Section of Cardiology, Heart Failure and Transplant Unit, DeGasperis CardioCenter, Niguarda Great Metropolitan Hospital, Milan, Italy
* Cardiologia 2-Insufficienza Cardiaca e Trapianto - DeGasperis CardioCenter, Grande Ospedale Metropolitano Niguarda, Piazza Ospedale Maggiore 3, 20162 Milano, Italy.
E-mail address: maria.frigerio@ospedaleniguarda.it

Heart Failure Clin 17 (2021) 619–634
https://doi.org/10.1016/j.hfc.2021.05.007
1551-7136/21/© 2021 Elsevier Inc. All rights reserved.

Table 1
Mechanical circulatory support: common terms and abbreviations

Setting/Terms	Abbreviation	Notes/Details
Concept		
Heart Replacement, (−)/Therapy	HR, HRT	Refers to durable therapies such as HTx, long-term VAD, TAH
Mechanical Circulatory Support, (−)/Device	MCS, MCSD	Refers to any circulatory support device, irrespective of durability position, etc.
Device type		
Artificial heart, total/(−)	TAH	Of course, it is intended only as a durable device, and preferentially if not exclusively as BTT
Ventricular assist device	VAD	It refers to a variety of surgically or percutaneously implanted devices, may vary widely in terms of performance invasiveness and predicted/observed complications
Left ventricular/(−) Right ventricular/(−) Biventricular/(−)	LVAD RVAD BVAD	
Duration/durability		
Temporary	t-MCS, (−)/D	• For short-term use (d to wk)
Long-term, durable	//	• Intended for use of several mo/y (ideally permanent)
Place of the pump		Referring to the pump only
Intracorporeal		• aka "implantable," other components may be external
Paracorporeal		
Type of flow		
Pulsatile	PF-	• Generally synchronized with cardiac rhythm, automatic shift to fixed HR in case of arrest, low flow
Continuous	CF-	• May be artificially augmented every some cardiac cycles to imitate pulsatility
Axial		eg, Incor Berlin Heart, HeartMate II
Centrifugal		eg, Heartware HVAD, HeartMate3
Intention to treat		
Bridge to transplant	• BTT	• pt is on the HTx waiting list
Bridge to candidacy	• BTC	• pt has contraindications or risk factors for HTx, that are expected to resolve/improve with MCS
Bridge to recovery	• BTR	• pt is expected to improve to allow weaning (usually short-term MCS)
Bridge to decision	• BTD	• Probability of recovery and pt suitability for HRT unknown
Destination therapy	• DT	• pt deemed unsuitable for HTX (long-term MCS, usually LVAD)

contemporary evidences and basic knowledges regarding their use as a long-term therapy. Updated reviews on other device-based options for chronic, advanced HF, and temporary MCS in cardiogenic shock can be found elsewhere.[6–8]

INDICATIONS

HF is defined as a clinical syndrome that derives from the inability of the heart to maintain an adequate cardiac output—or to do so without an increase of filling pressures. Shifting the blood from the left ventricle (LV) to the aorta, LVADs are highly effective in correcting the hemodynamic abnormalities in patients with pure or predominant LV dysfunction. In the late stages of the disease, patients may develop RV dysfunction with peripheral and/or visceral congestion, nevertheless, many of them improve after LVAD implant. On the contrary, those with primary, severe, or frankly predominant RV dysfunction are not good candidates for LVAD therapy.[9] Patients with recurrent ventricular tachyarrhythmias, with multiple ICD interventions as main symptoms, should be considered with caution. In fact, CF-LVAD may not be adequate to support circulation and avoid syncope during sustained, high-rate ventricular tachycardia (VT) or ventricular fibrillation (VF), and surgical trauma plus reparative changes after apical cannulation may indeed facilitate arrhythmias.[9]

With these limitations, LVAD implant remains the only option—besides HTx—for patients with severe, irreversible LV dysfunction, and refractory/recurrent symptoms and signs of congestion and/or hypoperfusion despite optimal therapy.[9,10] These patients are typically represented by those requiring continuous i.v. inotropes and/or vasopressors, corresponding to profile 3 (or, more broadly, 2–4) according to the definitions proposed by the Intermacs consortium (**Table 2**).[11] The Intermacs classification is mainly descriptive and is based on symptoms and therapies rather than on objective parameters; however, it correlates with outcomes either with or without surgery.[12,13] Short-term MCS is initially preferred in patients with overt cardiogenic shock (Intermacs profile 1), then weaning or transition to long-term support (or, when reasonable and feasible, to emergency HTx) should be evaluated.[14] The risk-benefit trade-off of LVAD implant versus a wait-and-see strategy on medical therapy in patients with advanced but less severe disease (Intermacs profiles 4–5 and higher) has not been established clearly.[15] The advantages on HF-related symptoms and survival must be weighed against the risks for device-related complications, especially strokes, infections, and pump thrombosis. The HeartMate3 centrifugal pump appears to be associated with a relatively low rate of severe neurological complications and gastrointestinal bleeding, according to the results of a randomized clinical trial and in observational registries[3,12,16] (**Tables 3** and **4**).

Traditionally, the scope of LVAD has been defined in relation to HTx, with most of the patients being labeled as "bridge to transplant" (BTT) when listed for HTx or "Destination therapy" (DT) when deemed unsuitable for HTx (see **Table 1**). However, these categories merely reflect the initial "intention to treat." Donor availability and allocation policy may facilitate or, conversely, delay the access to HTx in implanted patients.[5,9,10,12,17,18] As waiting time on support lengthens, BTT and DT patients are similarly exposed to long-term device-related complications, and the evolution or the appearance of comorbidities commonly observed with aging. Most of the available knowledge on post-LVAD outcomes derive from the US experience, as collected and described in the Intermacs Registry. Given the proportion of BTT patients (~45%) and the rate of events within 2 years (including HTx, 26% of the entire cohort) in this Registry until 2018, postoperative outcomes and events beyond 2 years are reported from a limited number of patients.[12] Country-, center-, and patient-specific considerations must be taken into account when evaluating LVAD indication and timing.

PREOPERATIVE EVALUATION

Evaluating patients for a possible indication for LVAD implantation is similar to the screening process for HTx candidacy.[19,20] The essential points are:

- *Estimation of prognosis on medical therapy*: as for HTx listing, multiparametric scores may be applied to ambulatory patients (Intermacs ≥4). The ISHLT guidelines for HTx candidacy[19] suggest the Heart Failure Survival Score (HFSS)[21] or the Seattle Heart Failure Model (SHFM),[22] but the latter may be overoptimistic, and the 2 scores may provide very different estimates of the risk for the same patient. The Metabolic Exercise Cardiac Kidney Index (MECKI) multiparametric score appears more accurate.[23,24]
- *Psychosocial evaluation*: living with an LVAD impacts on self-image, and requires to take responsibilities for long-term management. The availability of a caregiver and the organization of local care should be discussed and planned in advance. Patients with acute onset of refractory HF may be unprepared for psychological implications of long-term LVAD, and could require additional postoperative support and education.
- *Characterization of heart disease*: cardiac imaging and hemodynamics are helpful for defining specific aspects that may require special attention and/or consideration for additional, concomitant procedures.
  - *Right ventricular function.* This is perhaps the most critical point of patient evaluation for LVAD implant. Many preoperative variables, alone or in combination, have been identified as related to the occurrence of postoperative RVF (**Table 5**) nevertheless the accuracy of any predictive index or score is limited because of (1) lack of uniform criteria for defining RVF (high right atrial pressure, prolonged need for inotropes, RVAD implant, refractory congestion, hypotension, and death may be

Table 2
Intermacs classification for advanced heart failure

Class - Profile	Description[11]	Intermacs[12] 2014–16 N = 8049	Intermacs[12] 2017–18 N = 4967	Euromacs[16] 2006–17 N = 2689
1. Crash and burn	Rapid evolution to cardiogenic shock	14.3%	17.1%	11%
2. Sliding on inotropes	Worsening symptoms and/or end-organ dysfunction—needs escalation of drugs	34.7%	35.7%	32%
3. Dependent stability	Stable on inotropes, but deteriorating at weaning attempts	37.1%	35.4%	26%
4. Resting symptoms	Minimal/no physical activity, confined in bed, requires assistance	11.9%	10.0%	27%
5. Housebound	Exertion intolerant. Some physical activity, may be able to dress and wash him or herself, unable to walk out.	1.5%	1.2%	
6. Walking wounded	Exertion limited. May walk for ~ 1 block, but shows worsening symptoms when lying in bed, or worsening end-organ dysfunction	0.4%	0.4%	
7. Advanced NYHA III	Severe but stable functional limitation	0.2%	0%,2%	
Modifiers:				
TCS	Temporary Circulatory support (applies to Intermacs 1–3)			
A:	Arrhythmias (repetitive/storms)			
FF:	Frequent flyer			

The table reports the description of Intermacs profiles and their distribution across patients included in large US and European Registries.

considered), (2) slow accumulation of data (ie, low number of patients per center/per year, (3) doubts on reliability of parameters obtained in patients receiving different types of LVAD, (4) heterogenicity of entry patient characteristics, background therapy, propensity for use of inotropes, and/or for implantation of a temporary RVAD.[25–27] A recently published score that has been derived from about 2000 patients and validated in about 900 patients, implanted with a CF-LVAD from 2006 to 2017 and enrolled in the EUROMACS Registry, is interesting for several reasons: (1) it combines echocardiographic, hemodynamic, clinical, and laboratory variables; (2) it can be calculated with a quantitative (equation with individual coefficients) or semiquantitative approach (adding predefined points); and has been designed to re-evaluate the patient immediately after LVAD implant.[26] However, less than 4% of the cases had received the most recently approved device (HM3). Secondary tricuspid valve regurgitation often accompanies RV dysfunction in patients with advanced CHF. The role of its correction at the time of LVAD implant has not been fully elucidated.[28]

○ *Aortic insufficiency.* Aortic insufficiency may compromise the expected hemodynamic benefit of CF-LVAD, even when it is mild. With continuous flow, aortic regurgitation is not counteracted by the synchronized changes of preload and afterload that normally occur during each cardiac cycle, and increases LV preload. Moreover, lack of pulsatility appears to increase the regurgitant flow over time by "fixing" aortic valve cusps. Thus, correction of aortic valve

Table 3
Outcomes with axial flow CF-LVAD or full-magnetic levitated centrifugal CF-LVAD- Results of the MOMENTUM-3 randomized trial

	FML Centrifugal	Axial	RR (95%CI)	P
Number	516	512		
Primary end-point: survival free from disabling stroke and need of pump exchange at 2 y	397%, 77% (73.1–80.5)	332%, 65% (60.5–69.0)	0.84 (0.78–0.91)	<0.001
Withdrew	5	10		
Pump exchange/removal	14%, 2.7% (1.5–4.5)	73%, 14.3% (11.4–17.6)	0.19 (0.11–0.33)	
Disabling stroke	20%, 3.9% (2.4–5.9)	30%, 5.9% (4.0–17.6)	0.66 (0.38–1.15)	
Death	80%, 15.5% (12.5–18.9)	67%, 13.1% (10.3–16.3)	1.18 (0.88–1.60)	

Abbreviations: axial refers to HeartMate II LVAD; FML, full-magnetic levitation, refers to HeartMate 3.
Data from Mehra MR, Uriel N, Naka Y, et al. A fully magnetically levitated left ventricular assist device-final report. N Engl J Med. 2019;380:1618-1627.

Table 4
Survival and freedom from major complications with different models of CF-LVAD, according to Intermacs Registry

CF-LVAD Type	Axial	HL Centrifugal	FML Centrifugal
Number	6938	4786	1292
At-risk at 1 y[a]	4771	2539	551
At-risk at 2 y[a]	3268	1065	20
Survival,			
1-y, %	82	81	87
2-y, %	72	72	84
Freedom from CVA,			
1-y, %	88	84	93
2-y %	82	78	93
Freedom from major infection,			
1-y, %	60	57	67
2-y %	49	45	59
Freedom from RVF,			
1-y, %	71	62	66
2-y %	66	56	63
Freedom from GI bleeding,			
1-y, %	75	80	88
2-y %	67	74	85

Abbreviations: CF-LVAD, continuous-flow left ventricular assist device; axial refers mainly to HeartMate II device; CVA, cerebrovascular accident; FML, full-magnetic levitation, refers to HeartMate 3; GI, gastrointestinal; HL, hybrid levitation, refers mainly to HeartWare HVAD; RVF, right ventricular failure.
P<.0001 for all comparisons.
[a] Number at-risk refers to Survival only.
Data from Teuteberg JJ, Cleveland JC, Cowger J, et al. The Society of Thoracic Surgeons Intermacs 2019 Annual Report: The changing landscape of devices and indications. Ann Thoracic surgery 2020;109:649-660.

Table 5
Risk factors for Right Ventricular failure after LVAD implant

Domain	Parameters
Demography	Female gender
Clinical	Body size, small High-dose/multiple inotropes Renal replacement therapy Ventilator IABP
Biochemistry and biomarkers	WBC count, high INR, Bilirubin, high MELD Score
Echocardiography	Moderate to severe preoperative RVD[a] Tricuspid regurgitation, severe RV/LV diameter ratio, high RV free wall longitudinal strain, low TAPSE, low
Hemodynamics	CVP, RAP/PCWP ratio, high RVSWI[b], low

Abbreviations: CVP, central venous pressure; IABP, intra-aortic balloon pump; INR, international normalized ratio; MELD, modified end-stage liver disease score; PCWP, pulmonary capillary wedge pressure; RAP, right atrial pressure; RVD, right ventricular dysfunction; RVSWI, right ventricular stroke work index; TAPSE, tricuspid annular plane systolic excursion; WBC, white blood cell.

A selection of the most relevant preoperative parameters that have been found to be independently associated with the postoperative occurrence of RV failure after contemporary CF-LVAD implants are listed.

[a] The presence of preoperative severe RVD (qualitatively assessed) is not surprisingly one of the strongest predictors of postoperative RVF – it would be interesting to find predictors when baseline RVF is not overtly compromised.

[b] RVSWI: RV Stroke volume index X (mean pulmonary artery pressure − CVP) X 0.0136, g/m^2.

regurgitation with a conservative procedure or a biological prosthesis at the time of LVAD implant appears advisable.[29]

o *Mitral insufficiency.* Mitral valve (MV) insufficiency secondary to LV dysfunction is common, and functional regurgitation is expected to be markedly reduced by LVAD implant alone. Controversial data are reported on the impact of moderate to severe preoperative mitral regurgitation on postimplant outcomes, and on the risks and benefits of concomitant MV repair or replacement.[30,31] As elegantly explained by Grayburn and colleagues,[32] functional and anatomic components may coexist in secondary MV insufficiency: it is possible that the latter are responsible for "disproportionate" mitral insufficiency, which could benefit from correction at the time of LVAD implantation.

o *Coronary artery disease.* Coronary artery anatomy is generally known before LVAD implant. No general recommendations are available regarding associated revascularization procedures.

• *Comorbidities:* The proportion of patients undergoing LVAD implant with DT indication is growing, and it is quite obvious that some comorbidities may be present in patients with advanced or refractory HF, often of 60 years of age or older, that are considered for LVAD while HTx candidacy has been denied. Several comorbidities are known to influence the outcome after LVAD implant; however, they do not automatically represent definite contraindications.

o *Multisystem organ failure (MOF).* Acute, severe, worsening MOF unresponsive to advanced support, chronic severe chronic renal insufficiency, liver cirrhosis, and lung disease (severe obstructive pulmonary disease, or pulmonary fibrosis, eg, due to job-related exposure or to amiodarone therapy) are associated with poor outcomes, high risk, and marginal improvement of quality of life, and may contraindicate LVAD implant.

o *Cerebrovascular* and severe *peripheral vessel disease* should be considered with caution, for the risk of stroke and of altered systemic vasoreactivity after LVAD implant.

○ *Cancer.* Delaying HTx candidacy is advisable early after successful cancer therapy, and LVAD may be the preferred option in hemodynamically unstable patients. Chemotherapy-associated cardiomyopathy often compromises both ventricles, and severe LV dysfunction may present with little or no dilation—that is not the ideal pathophysiological profile for LVAD.[33] LVAD implant should be considered with caution in patients with active cancer, due to the overall burden of the 2 conditions, and the risks for thrombosis and infection often associated with cancer and related therapy.

○ *Gastrointestinal (GI) bleeding.* Preimplant screening for conditions associated with actual or potential bleeding is advisable because of indefinite need for postoperative anticoagulation and antiplatelet therapy. Moreover, CF-LVAD portends a risk for a peculiar form of GI bleeding (see complications).

• *General conditions*: Besides evaluating the presence and severity of definite diseases, other health-related aspects should be assessed.

○ *BMI and nutritional status.* Severe obesity and, on the other side, poor nutrition and cachexia are associated with a higher probability of postimplant complications and deaths.[20]

○ *Physical functioning.* Prolonged confinement in bed, catecholamine treatment, poor nutrition, all concur in further reducing mobility and muscular mass in refractory HF patients.

○ *"Frailty"* is a holistic concept that has been introduced in geriatric medicine. It encompasses physical and psychological conditions, cognitive status, and disability, and is inversely related to the capability to survive the exposure to stressors. It appears reasonable that frailty could be related to outcome in LVAD recipients, especially in the elderlies and/or in patients with a long history of severe disease. However, some components of "frailty" are probably reversible, and may be favorably influenced by LVAD.[34,35]

PERIOPERATIVE MANAGEMENT

Perioperative management of LVAD recipients requires specific competences and skills that cannot be covered within a few paragraphs.

• *Preoperatively*, the following points should be addressed:

○ *Screening for infections.* Besides surveillance for nosocomial infections and planning for perioperative antimicrobial prophylaxis as per local practices, nasal swab for Staphylococcus colonization (and, in case, treatment with mupirocin ointment) are recommended, since Staph. species are among the most frequent bacteria implicated in device-related postoperative infections. Since 2020, nasopharyngeal swab for excluding SARS-CoV 2 infection is required for patients undergoing any major surgery.

○ *Hemodynamic optimization.* When possible, it is suggested to resolve lung congestion and end-organ dysfunction before the operation, with the help of drug therapy and/or IABP (or t-MCSD in most critical patients).

○ *"Prehabilitation."* This term indicates a comprehensive strategy for optimization of nutritional status, respiratory and muscular function before the operation, with the scope to reduce the duration of mechanically assisted ventilation, overall and ICU length of stay, and the risk for infections.[36] Considering the specific requirements of LVAD patients, part of the educational program for self-care and caring for the device could be anticipated in the preoperative phase, to reduce postoperative stress by increasing self-confidence.

• *Planned strategies for RV failure*: although RVF remains a serious threat for postimplant survival, it seems that its anticipation -and, in case, timely institution of temporary RV support before overt insufficiency has deployed its effects on multisystem organ function may favor subsequent successful weaning.[37]

• *Early postoperative management*: during the operation and in the first days thereafter, LVAD recipients require special attention from specialized personnel.[38] Crucial points are summarized here.

○ *Hemodynamic profile.* After LVAD implant, hemodynamic and clinical improvement depends largely on the interaction between the patient and the device. Immediate reduction of PCWP is generally observed. Cardiac output is the result of the combination of pump power (that correlates to pump output), residual LV function, adaptation of the RV to increased preload, volume status, and peripheral resistances. Initial setting of pump power in the low range, judicious use of inotropes, vasodilators, or inodilators to increase biventricular contractility and reduce LV afterload, and maintenance of euvolemia may reduce the risk of early RV failure. Normal/low PCWP (<12 mm Hg), reduction of pulmonary artery pressure, limited increase of right atrial (or central venous) pressure (ideally ≤10 mm Hg), adequate mean arterial pressure (ideally ~60–70 mm Hg) while reducing inotropes and increasing pump power indicate the adaptation of the RV to the new condition. Volume status should be regulated to avoid overload and, at the opposite, the so-called "suction" phenomenon, that is, the collapse of LV walls that occurs when it is too empty, which paradoxically causes a drop of cardiac output and an increase of PCWP. The higher the value of pump power, the lower the contribution of LV contraction to cardiac output: ultimately, the aortic valve remains always closed, which may predispose to thrombosis, reduced coronary flow, and valve insufficiency. In contemporary CF-LVAD, self-regulatory algorithms aimed to prevent and/or anticipate suction, and to reduce pump output periodically, for short periods, to facilitate the opening of the aortic valve every 4 to 8 cardiac cycles, may be activated.

○ *Anticoagulation and antiplatelet therapy.* CF-LVAD requires permanent anticoagulation, initially with i.v. heparin and then with vitamin K antagonists (warfarin, acenocoumarin), with INR target range of 2 to 2.5–3. The association with antiplatelet therapy is recommended by the manufacturers of most devices. Dosing, transition, and association of anticoagulant and antiplatelet agents must take into account time from surgery, bleeding, presence or absence of bowel motility, and concomitant therapies. Besides standard laboratory parameters to monitor anticoagulants, thromboelastography, and other specific tests may help in guiding therapy.

○ *Prevention of driveline-related infections.* The supply of energy to intracorporeal VADs is guaranteed by room electricity or by rechargeable batteries that are connected to the central unit that is called controller. The controller is connected to the pump by a plastic-coated, flexible cable, which enters the skin close to the right iliac spine. This permanent skin discontinuation is said to represent the "Achille's heel" of commercially available LVADs, because it may be the first site of an infection that from the surface goes deeper, causing abscesses sepsis and mediastinitis.[39] Initially, superficial colonization is generally caused by common skin-hosted bacteria, which are sensitive to most antibiotics, but drug-resistant agents may emerge over time. Infections may increase thrombogenicity, and antimicrobials may interfere with warfarin, thus increasing the risk for pump thrombosis, bleeding, and stroke. Accurate skin cleaning and disinfection before entering the operating room and tight fixing of the cable to the skin before exit are other important steps. Stable adhesion of reparative tissue to the cable is fundamental to limit driveline-mediated infection, and the cable should be fixed to avoid direct trauma and tearing of the exit site in case of inadvertent traction of its distal portion. Sterile dressing of the exit site should be carefully performed by trained personnel. Silver nitrate–based appliances may help in preventing infections.[40] The ideal frequency and modality of planned dressing have not been established, and protocols vary among centers. Some techniques and instructions for taking care of the driveline exit site are provided by manufacturers, single centers, and individuals, and are available on the web as manuals, handouts, or tutorials.

○ *Psychological support and education for the patients and their caregivers.* LVAD is a highly demanding therapy for the patient and the family. Formal training can be partially self-administered and improves confidence and skills.[41] Ability and self-confidence in performing basic tasks (**Table 6**) must be assessed before discharge.

○ *Criteria for discharge*: after LVAD implant, patients may be discharged when they are clinically stable (ie, they are fully mobilized without signs of decompensation, indexes of anticoagulation are within the expected range, there are no major/unexpected or unexplained abnormalities of laboratory parameters), have learned the basic principles and practical maneuvers for device maintenance, are comfortable with pharmacologic therapy and lifestyle, and/or may receive the help they need from family members, caregivers, proximity health care professionals, or home-based services. Cardiac rehabilitation facilities may help in the transition from hospital to home.

LONG-TERM MANAGEMENT AND COMPLICATIONS

• *Organization of follow-up:* After discharge, LVAD recipients should be followed

Table 6
Basic knowledge and skills required by LVAD recipients/caregivers before discharge

Self-maintenance, general	Emergency phone number(s) Daily weight Daily temperature Drug schedule
Planned activities	Exercise plan Dietary plan INR check How to get anticoagulant dosing Follow-up plan
Device maintenance	Battery changing and charging Battery check of level of charge Switch from battery to room energy supply Change the controller How to store and protect home monitor and spare parts How to wear the device How to avoid trauma How to avoid watering How to avoid cable damage
Driveline and exit site care	Exit site check, cleansing, and dressing Positioning and securing the cable
Device knowledge, other	Basic parameters and alarms Dos and donts in case of alarms

indefinitely. Follow-up protocols may vary according to local organization of health care and resources, but should be directed by health care professionals with sufficient knowledge and experience for understanding patient-device interaction, and for taking care of both. Appointments at predefined time intervals should be planned. One-stop service (patient visit, EKG, check of the device, blood testing, visual examination of the driveline exit site, echocardiography, and other diagnostic tests as needed, at the same place on the same day) is preferable over multiple, separated appointments. Patients who are on the HTx waiting list should undergo periodic right heart catheterization to exclude pulmonary hypertension (PH). There should be room for on-demand, supplementary controls, and there should be a 24/7 service for phone consultation. Exchange of information between the experts' team and proximity physicians or specialists is advisable. Remote

control/telemedicine services could be of help, especially when expert personnel is not available close to the patient.[42] Expanding the competencies for long-term surveillance and care of LVAD recipients beyond the implanting centers could facilitate their everyday life.

- Maintenance therapy:
  - *Heart failure therapy:* after LVAD implant, most of the patients do not show a significant improvement of LV function, although volume reduction is frequently observed as a result of unloading. Very few patients recover to the point that LVAD can be safely removed.[12] The role of standard CHF therapy, which is targeted to neurohormonal activation, has not been fully elucidated; however, its maintenance may be recommended based on observational data.[43,44] In general, LVAD recipients do not require high-dose diuretics (if any), which may provoke hypotension and suction. Very few or

no data are available regarding the use of sacubitril/valsartan and of newer, recently approved drugs for CHF, in LVAD patients. The data on the effects and usefulness of cardiac resynchronization therapy after LVAD implant are controversial.[45,46]

  o *Blood pressure control:* in patients with CF-LVAD, measuring arterial blood pressure (BP) is often impossible with standard equipments, and oscillometers or standard sphygmomanometer plus vascular Doppler ultrasound of radial artery may be used. Although systolic BP is obviously attenuated and postural hypotension may represent a problem, especially in the early postoperative days, hypertension may persist, appear or reappear after LVAD implant, and represents a risk factor for the occurrence of hemorrhagic stroke when MAP is >90 mm Hg.[4,47] Moreover, hypertension increases LV afterload, and may worsen aortic insufficiency. Keeping BP under control may be a good reason for prescribing neurohormonal inhibitors, with target MAP values of 70 to 80 mm Hg.[48]

  o *Anticoagulation and antiplatelet therapy:* see "Early postoperative management."

- *LVAD-related complications:* the occurrence of complications typically related to the presence of the device remains an important obstacle to the expansion of LVAD implants among ambulatory HF patients. Complications may cause death or permanent disability, often require hospitalizations, and worsen self-perceived quality of life. Complications may prompt higher priority on the waiting list for HTx, or removal from the list for deterioration. The incidence of LVAD-related complications in contemporary patients is summarized in **Table 4**.

  o *Stroke.* Stroke is among the most feared complications in LVAD recipients. The distinction between ischemic versus hemorrhagic, and disabling versus nondisabling strokes may lead to different estimates of the burden of this complication.[47] Age, obesity, atrial fibrillation, and lack of aspirin use appear to be related to the risk for ischemic stroke, whereas high BP and INR greater than 3 to that of hemorrhagic stroke.[47–49]

  o *Pump thrombosis and other causes of malfunction.* The incidence of LVAD thrombosis could be underreported, because the diagnosis may be elusive. Hemolysis and reduced pump output are the effects and key findings of pump thrombosis.[50,51] Minor changes of various indexes of pump function should be considered with much attention because they may anticipate overt thrombosis and device failure. It must be remembered that these alterations may vary according to the site of thrombosis (inflow, rotor, outflow) and the type of device.[51,52] Moreover, in the case of pump thrombosis, the LVAD controller may paradoxically generate "high output" signals, because increased energy consumption is required to maintain blood flow despite the presence of thrombus, and energy consumption is the main parameter entering the algorithm for calculating pump flow. Imaging techniques are not always of help. Echocardiography may identify thrombosis either morphologically and/or from flow changes, but it does not always allow to explore conduits and chambers clearly and completely.[53] Contrast-enhanced CT scan may identify the position and extent of the thrombus, but artifacts and the "noise" generated by artificial materials make interpretation of CT scan a difficult task. Several protocols for thrombolysis have been reported, with variable rates of success, but the most radical and effective treatment for LVAD thrombosis is pump exchange.[54,55] Aggressive antiplatelet therapy is then suggested with the aim to prevent recurrences. Pump malfunction may recognize other causes, for example, damages to the driveline, to the connection between the sources of energy and the controller, or to failure of the controller itself that may derive from direct trauma. In the author's experience, the few episodes of LVAD malfunction due to inappropriate behavior occurred with active, well-adapted, perhaps over-confident patients. Unexplained pump failures are very exceptional.

  o *Infections.* Infections of the tissue surrounding artificial materials that are part of a prosthesis or of a therapeutic device are not uncommon, and, as observed with prosthetic valves, intracardiac leads, and pockets of pacemakers, they are not limited to the first postoperative days or months. The risk for LVAD-related infections is initially high, then lowers, and increases again as follow-up lengthens.[12] **Table 7** summarizes the terminology for characterizing postimplant infections that have been proposed by the International Society for Heart and Lung Transplantation, to increase

Table 7
Terminology for describing LVAD-related infections according to the International Society for Heart and Lung Transplantation

Term	Explanation	Note
Infection		
Non-VAD infection	Infection unrelated to VAD	eg, urinary tract infection
VAD-related,	Device related, generic	eg, mediastinitis
VAD-specific	Typical and peculiar of VAD	Driveline related or unrelated
VAD-Specific		
Proven Probable Possible		• Needs microbiology data • Noninvasive clinical data may be sufficient
Driveline-related		
Superficial	Limited to layers outside fascia and muscle	
Deep	Infection beyond the fascia	

Data from Bhama JK, Bamsal U, Winger DG, et al. Clinical experience with temporary right ventricular mechanical circulatory support. J Thorac Cardiovasc Surg 2018;156:1885-1891.

consistency in reporting and facilitate comparative analysis.[39] Although infections with systemic symptoms and signs require aggressive treatment, a watchful wait-and-see strategy may be considered in patients with persistent/recurrent superficial colonization of the entry site by multisensitive microbial agents, to avoid selection of resistant lines. Clear signs of deepening of the infection are high fever, tenderness, and pain of the area surrounding the driveline, purulent secretion, leukocytosis and increased C-reactive protein and procalcitonin, but should be suspected also in case of minor symptoms and signs like low-grade fever and nonspecific fatigue or malaise. Local swabs, blood cultures, and imaging (soft tissue ultrasound imaging, radiography, CT scan, and, less frequently, scintigraphy with labeled leukocytes or positron-emission tomography [PET] with 5-fluorodesoxyglucose [FDG]) would help for diagnosis and evaluation of LVAD-related infections.[53] In HTx candidates, deep/systemic device-related infections may represent a criterion for increasing their priority or, at the opposite, for withdrawal (temporarily or definitely) from the waiting list. A significant impact of LVAD-related infections on post-transplant survival has not been demonstrated in large multicenter cohorts, but at least morbidity and length of stay are higher in this setting. Local treatment (debridement of necrotic/infected tissue, and application of vacuum therapy to help granulation and repair) are used for subcutaneous infection. In recent years, externalization and, after healing, repositioning of the cable or exchange of the entire device have been reported.[39]

○ *Gastrointestinal (GI) bleeding.* Besides requiring anticoagulation and antiplatelet therapy, CF-LVADs are associated with increased intraluminal pressure in the GI tract, low pulse pressure, and shear stress, leading to arteriovenous malformations, angiodysplasia, and acquired von Willebrand syndrome.[56] An unique complication of CF-LVAD implant is recurrent, obstinate bleeding from gastric and/or small bowel mucosa, that is associated with diffuse, multiple bleeding areas in the absence of focal, deep lesions as observed in typical peptic ulcer disease.[56] Although rarely lethal, it may cause profound anemia, and has a relevant impact on quality of life and hospitalizations. Octreotide is often used for empirical treatment.[57] Older age, ischemic heart disease, prior history of GI bleeding, preoperative and postoperative indexes of right ventricular failure, and renal insufficiency have been recognized as risk factors for GI bleeding.[58]

• Other complications
○ *Recurrent HF.* Except in case of pump thrombosis, other mechanical failures, or major intravascular volume changes, hemodynamics should remain quite stable in LVAD recipients over time. Nevertheless, recurrence of HF is not uncommon in the

long term. Patients with aortic insufficiency who remain symptomatic with aggressive afterload reduction could be considered for surgical or percutaneous treatment.[59] Late recurrent/worsening RV failure is another common cause. Irreversible PH contraindicates HTx but not LVAD implant, and in many of these patients, PH declines over time. When it persists, with the so-called "discoupling" between diastolic PAP and mean PCWP (gradient $\geq$ 5 mm Hg)[60] or when suboptimal LV unloading masks latent RV failure, the probability of the development of HF during follow-up is higher.[61] Suboptimal setting of the device or increased afterload due to poor BP control may also lead to late HF. Drugs that reduce contractility and/or increase fluid retention (eg, some anti-arrhythmia agents, calcium receptor blockers, or vasodilators such as doxazosin) may facilitate late HF. Although the contribution to cardiac output of residual LV function is generally marginal, its complete loss associated with permanent closure of the aortic valve may favor aortic root thrombosis and inadequate coronary perfusion. Atrial fibrillation, especially with high ventricular rate, may also precipitate HF, due to latent RV dysfunction and altered patient-device equilibrium.

o *Ventricular arrhythmias.* Sustained, high-rate VT may be better tolerated by LVAD-supported than by nonsupported HF patients, and with VF, loss of consciousness may be delayed. However, the hemodynamic performance of CF-LVAD is inferior with respect to that of older pulsatile devices, and repetitive ventricular arrhythmias can represent a relevant problem. On the other side, the role of ICD for primary prevention of sudden death is questionable.[46,62]

LEFT VENTRICULAR ASSIST DEVICES, TRANSPLANTATION, AND END-OF-LIFE CONSIDERATIONS IN REFRACTORY HEART FAILURE PATIENTS

Despite the improvement in postoperative results over the years, LVAD is still perceived as a demanding and somewhat "difficult" therapy. In the United States, Intermacs profiles 1 and 2 account for more than 50% of recently implanted patients, reflecting expanded use of tMCS and persistent reluctance toward LVAD use in ambulatory HF patients.[63] Moreover, after changing donor heart allocation rules in favor of patients on temporary MCS, the proportion of HTx in patients awaiting with an LVAD diminished, as did the number and the proportion of LVAD implanted with BTT indication.[64] The impact of these changes on post-transplant and, more importantly, overall survival, is still unknown. However, without any priority for noncomplicated LVAD patients, being implanted with BTT indication means in fact to delay HTx.[17] Thus, the declared goal of LVAD therapy is not achieved, and patient expectations are not satisfied, with a negative impact on their quality of life irrespective of device-related complications.[65] It is not surprising that listed patients would prefer HTx over LVAD implant, given that their doctors would do the same.[66] Earlier referral of patients with advanced HF to tertiary care centers is recommended,[9,67] but if HTx is scarcely available and LVAD is anyway delayed also in patients with DT indication, the majority of both HTx and LVAD implants will be performed in high urgency or emergency conditions, with suboptimal expected postoperative survival—which could imply lower reliance, interest, funding, and overall efforts in this field. With increasing availability of less invasive devices for tMCS, the pathways leading to heart replacement should be redesigned, putting immediate individual patients' needs and preferences in a midterm to long-term perspective, within a broad and realistic picture.

Patients with chronic refractory HF, and even more those with acutely worsening low-output state and shock, may not get full information about expected outcomes, lifestyle, responsibilities, and risk for complications with LVAD or alternative options—and may not able to foresee how they fit with their own expectations and values.[68] Patients and caregivers may be disoriented, frustrated, and overwhelmed in case of severe postimplant complications. Nevertheless, so far, the issue of withdrawing long-term LVAD therapy has probably been more a matter of bioethics than a request arising from patients or their representatives. In theory, LVAD should be interrupted upon patient's request—as any other therapy.[69] Bioethicists are interested in technicalities such as alarms shutdown, but seem to disregard that having an inactivated LVAD is a worse condition than simply not having it at all, because of free bidirectional flow along the conduits. This may be one of the reasons that make some doctors see LVAD stopping as a form of physician-assisted suicide if not euthanasia.[70]

Waiting for fully implantable LVADs, that could markedly increase patients' acceptance, it is important to make the most for improving patients and caregivers' skills and self-confidence, and for providing expert help and care physically close to patients, at least regarding standard maintenance.

Telemedicine services could facilitate contacts and support from referral centers to patients, caregivers, and local health care personnel.

CLINICS CARE POINTS

Evaluation for LVAD implant.

Before the operation, and according to patient's conditions, history, and risk factors, the following examinations and visits may be advisable.

- Assessment of severity of disease and estimate of prognosis without LVAD (consider actual data and trends)

  ○ Medical history, including therapy optimization and adherence

  ○ Prior/actual hospitalizations, use of inotropes, unplanned need for i.v. diuretics

  ○ NYHA functional class and Intermacs level

  ○ Cardiopulmonary exercise test

  ○ Kidney and liver function

  ○ Sodium (low), natriuretic peptide levels (high)

  ○ Multiparametric prognostic scores (see text)

- Consider if patient could improve with additional/alternative therapies/procedures (be aware of additional risks with multiple cardiac surgeries)

  ○ Medical therapy optimization/upgrade (on the other side, intolerance/need to reduce doses of ACE-inhibitors, angiotensin-receptor blockers, or beta-blockers—and/or need to increase/combine diuretics is unfavorable)

  ○ Wide QRS, left bundle branch morphology: cardiac resynchronization

  ○ Atrial fibrillation: ablation procedures

  ○ Ischemic etiology, angina, viable myocardium, contractile reserve: revascularization (surgical/percutaneous)

  ○ Severe MV regurgitation: surgical or percutaneous correction

- Suitability for LVAD, with good probability of improvement

  ○ Pure/predominant left ventricular dysfunction, dilated/hypokinetic model

  ○ No severe right ventricular dilation/dysfunction (see text—anticipate the need for temporary RV support)

  ○ No mechanical prosthetic valves (or plan exchange with biological prosthesis)

  ○ No aortic insufficiency (or plan correction)

  ○ Life-threatening arrhythmias, if any, in the setting of decompensated HF (see text).

- Assess the presence and severity of comorbidities that could increase the risk for death or complications, and/or reduce the overall perceived benefit

  ○ Cerebrovascular disease: Doppler ultrasound, cerebral CT scan

  ○ Gastrointestinal bleeding: endoscopy, virtual endoscopy by CT scan, video camera

  ○ Infections: routine monitoring of hospitalized patients as per local practices, SARS-CoV2 swab, nasal swab for Staph. spp, dental x-ray

  ○ Consider routine chest x-ray and upper abdomen echo for liver, gallbladder, spleen, kidneys evaluation

  ○ Lung status and function. Spirometry, consider CT scan

  ○ Cancer: as per gender age risk factor.

  ○ Peripheral vessels disease: pulse evaluation, consider doppler ultrasound

- Psychosocial status and patient preferences

  ○ Awareness and knowledge of disease, adherence to therapy and lifestyle

  ○ Health-related quality of life, expectations and values

  ○ Presence and role of family and relatives

  ○ Specific/perceived barriers and problems (eg, distance, language, etc.)

DISCLOSURE

The author declares that during the past 3 years, she has had an indirect financial relationship with the following companies: Abbott (support to the hospital for educational events); Novartis (invited speaker—support to the hospital for educational events); and Amgen (participation to a sponsored research protocol).

REFERENCES

1. Stewart GC, Mehra MR. A history of devices as an alternative to heart transplantation. Heart Fail Clin 2014;10(1 Suppl):S1–12.

2. Rose EA, Gelijns AC, Moskowitz AJ, et al. Long-term mechanical left ventricular assistance for end-stage heart failure. N Engl J Med 2001;345:1435–43.

3. Mehra MR, Uriel N, Naka Y, et al. A fully magnetically levitated left ventricular assist device-final report. N Engl J Med 2019;380:1618–27.

4. Milano CA, Rogers JG, Tatooles AJ, et al. HVAD: the ENDURANCE Supplemental Trial. JACC Heart Fail 2018;6:792–802.

5. Kirklin JK, Pagani FD, Kormos RL, et al. Eighth annual INTERMACS report: special focus on framing the impact of adverse events. J Heart Lung Transplant 2017;36:1080–6.

6. Melton N, Soleimani B, Dowling R. Current role of the Total Artificial Heart in the management of advanced heart failure. Curr Cardiol Rep 2019;21:142.

7. Shehab S, Hayward CS. Choosing between Left Ventricular Assist Devices and Biventricular Assist Devices. Card Fail Rev 2019;5:19–23.

8. Seliem A, Hall SA. The new era of cardiogenic shock: progress in mechanical circulatory support. Curr Heart Fail Rep 2020;17:325–32.

9. Crespo-Leiro MG, Metra M, Lund LH, et al. Advanced heart failure: a position statement of the Heart Failure Association of the European Society of Cardiology. Eur J Heart Fail 2018;20:1505–35.

10. Ammirati E, Oliva F, Cannata A, et al. Current indications for heart transplantation and left ventricular assist device: a practical point of view. Eur J Intern Med 2014;25:422–9.

11. Stevenson LW, Pagani FD, Young JB, et al. INTERMACS profiles of advanced heart failure: the current picture. J Heart Lung Transplant 2009;28:535–41.

12. Teuteberg JJ, Cleveland JC, Cowger J, et al. The Society of Thoracic Surgeons Intermacs 2019 Annual Report: The changing landscape of devices and indications. Ann Thorac Surg 2020;109:649–60.

13. Kittleson MM, Shah P, Lala A, et al. INTERMACS profiles and outcomes of ambulatory advanced heart failure patients: A report from the REVIVAL Registry. J Heart Lung Transplant 2020;39:16–26.

14. Saeed D, Potapov E, Loforte A, et al. Transition from temporary to durable circulatory support systems. J Am Coll Cardiol 2020;76:2956–64.

15. Shah KB, Starling RC, Rogers JG, et al. Left ventricular assist devices versus medical management in ambulatory heart failure patients: An analysis of INTERMACS Profiles 4 and 5 to 7 from the ROADMAP study. J Heart Lung Transplant 2018;37:706–14.

16. Akin S, Soliman O, de By TMMH, et al. on behalf of the EUROMACS investigators. Causes and predictors of early mortality in patients treated with left ventricular assist device implantation in the European Registry of Mechanical Circulatory Support. Intensive Care Med 2020;46:1349–60.

17. Ammirati E, Brambatti M, Braun OÖ, et al. Outcome of patients on heart transplant list treated with a continuous-flow left ventricular assist device: Insights from the TRans-Atlantic registry on VAd and TrAnsplant (TRAViATA). Int J Cardiol 2020;324:122–30.

18. Cantrelle C, Legeai C, Latouche A, et al. Access to heart transplantation: a proper analysis of the competing risks of death and transplantation is required to optimize graft allocation. Transplant Direct 2017;3:e198. https://doi.org/10.1097/TXD.0000000000000711.

19. Mehra MR, Canter CE, Hannan MM, et al. The 2016 International Society for Heart and Lung Transplantation listing criteria for heart transplantation: a 10-year update. J Heart Lung Transplant 2016;35:1–23.

20. Frigerio M, Cipriani M, Oliva F, et al. Preoperative assessment and clinical optimization. In: Montalto A, Loforte A, Musumeci F, et al, editors. Mechanical circulatory support for end-stage heart failure- A practical manual. Cham, Switzerland: Springer; 2017. p. 59–74.

21. Koelling TM, Joseph S, Aaronson KD. Heart Failure Survival Score continues to predict clinical outcomes in patients with heart failure receiving beta-blockers. J Heart Lung Transplant 2004;23:1414–22.

22. Levy WC, Mozaffarian D, Linker DT, et al. The Seattle Heart Failure Model: prediction of survival in heart failure. Circulation 2006;113:1424–33.

23. Agostoni P, Corrà U, Cattadori G, et al. Metabolic exercise test data combined with cardiac and kidney indexes, the MECKI score: a multiparametric approach to heart failure prognosis. Int J Cardiol 2013;167:2710–8.

24. Agostoni P, Paolillo S, Mapelli M, et al. Multiparametric prognostic scores in chronic heart failure with reduced ejection fraction: a long-term comparison. Eur J Heart Fail 2017. https://doi.org/10.1002/ejhf.989.

25. Bellavia D, Iacovoni A, Scardulla C, et al. Prediction of right ventricular failure after ventricular assist device implant: systematic review and meta-analysis of observational studies. Eur J Heart Fail 2017;19:926–46.

26. Soliman OII, Akin S, Muslem R, et al. Derivation and validation of a novel right-sided heart failure model after implantation of continuous flow Left Ventricular Assist Devices: The EUROMACS (European Registry for Patients with Mechanical Circulatory Support) Right-Sided Heart Failure Risk Score. Circulation 2018;137:891–906.

27. Ruiz-Cano MJ, Morshuis M, Koster A, et al. Risk factors of early right ventricular failure in patients undergoing LVAD implantation with intermediate Intermacs profile for advanced heart failure. J Card Surg 2020;35:1832–9.

28. Veen KM, Muslem R, Soliman OI, et al. Left ventricular assist device implantation with and without concomitant tricuspid valve surgery: a systematic review and meta-analysis. Eur J Cardiothorac Surg 2018;54:644-651.

29. Truby LK, Garan AR, Givens RC, et al. Aortic insufficiency during contemporary Left Ventricular Assist Device support - Analysis of the INTERMACS Registry. JACC Heart Fail 2018;6:951–60.

30. Stulak JM, Tchantchaleishvili V, Haglund NA, et al. Uncorrected pre-operative mitral valve regurgitation is not associated with adverse outcomes after continuous-flow left ventricular assist device implantation. J Heart Lung Transplant 2015;34:718–23.

31. Kassis H, Cherukuri K, Agarwal R, et al. Significance of residual mitral regurgitation after continuous flow left ventricular assist device implantation. JACC Heart Fail 2017;5:81–8.

32. Grayburn PA, Sannino A, Packer M. Proportionate and disproportionate functional mitral regurgitation: a new conceptual framework that reconciles the results of the MITRA-FR and COAPT trials. JACC Cardiovasc Imaging 2019;12:353–62.

33. Galand V, Flécher E, Chabanne C, et al. Outcome of Left Ventricular Assist Device Implantation in Patients With Uncommon Etiology Cardiomyopathy. Am J Cardiol 2020;125:1421–8.

34. Tse G, Gong M, Wong SH, et al. Frailty and clinical outcomes in advanced heart failure patients undergoing Left Ventricular assist device implantation: a systematic review and meta-analysis. J Am Med Dir Assoc 2018;19:255–61.

35. Maurer MS, Horn E, Reyentovich A, et al. Can a Left Ventricular Assist Device in advanced systolic heart failure improve or reverse the frailty phenotype? J Am Geriatr Soc 2017;65:2383–90.

36. McCann M, Stamp N, Ngui A, et al. Cardiac Prehabilitation. J Cardiothorac Vasc Anesth 2019;33:2255–65.

37. Bhama JK, Bamsal U, Winger DG, et al. Clinical experience with temporary right ventricular mechanical circulatory support. J Thorac Cardiovasc Surg 2018;156:1885–91.

38. Nepomuceno RG, Goldraich LA, De S, et al. Critical care management of the acute postimplant LVAD patient. Can J Cardiol 2020;36:313–6.

39. Kusne S, Mooney M, Danziger-Isakov L, et al. An ISHLT consensus document for prevention and management strategies for mechanical circulatory support infection. J Heart Lung Transplant 2017;36:1137–53.

40. Cagliostro B, Levin AP, Fried J, et al. Continuous-flow left ventricular assist devices and usefulness of a standardized strategy to reduce driveline infections. J Heart Lung Transplant 2016;35:108–14.

41. Barsuk JH, Wilcox JE, Cohen ER, et al. Simulation-based mastery learning improves patient and caregiver ventricular assist device self-care skills. A randomized pilot trial. Circ Cardiovasc Qual Outcomes 2019;12:e005794.

42. Ben Gal TB, Avraham BB, Abu-Hazira M, et al. The consequences of the COVID-19 pandemic for self-care in patients supported with a left ventricular assist device. Eur J Heart Fail 2020;22:933–6.

43. Yousefzai R, Brambatti M, Tran HA, et al. Benefits of neurohormonal therapy in patients with continuous-flow Left Ventricular Assist Devices. ASAIO J 2020;66:409–14.

44. McCullough M, Caraballo C, Ravindra NG, et al. Neurohormonal blockade and clinical outcomes in patients with heart failure supported by Left Ventricular Assist Devices. JAMA Cardiol 2020;5:175–82.

45. Roukoz H, Bhan A, Ravichandran A, et al. Continued versus suspended Cardiac Resynchronization Therapy after Left Ventricular Assist Device implantation. Sci Rep 2020;10:2573.

46. Cikes M, Jakus N, Claggett B, et al. Cardiac implantable electronic devices with a defibrillator component and all-cause mortality in left ventricular assist device carriers: results from the PCHF-VAD registry. Eur J Heart Fail 2019;21:1129–41.

47. Acharya D, Loyaga-Rendon R, Morgan CJ, et al. INTERMACS Analysis of stroke during support with continuous-flow Left Ventricular Assist Devices. Risk factors and outcomes. JACC Heart Fail 2017;5:703–11.

48. Bennett MK, Adatya S. Blood pressure management in mechanical circulatory support. J Thorac Surg 2015;12:2125–8.

49. Inamullah O, Chiang YP, Bishawi M, et al. Characteristics of strokes associated with centrifugal flow left ventricular assist devices. Sci Rep 2021;11:1645.

50. Byrati EY, Rame EJ. Diagnosis and management of LVAD thrombosis. Curr Treat Options Cardiovasc Med 2015;17:361.

51. Long B, Robertson J, Koyfman A, et al. Left ventricular assist devices and their complications: A review for emergency clinicians. Am J Emerg Med 2019;37:1562–70.

52. Consolo F, Esposti F, Gustar A, et al. Log files analysis and evaluation of circadian patterns for the early diagnosis of pump thrombosis with a centrifugal continuous-flow left ventricular assist device. J Heart Lung Transplant 2019;38:1077–86.

53. Almarzooq ZI, Varshney AS, Vaduganathan M, et al. Expanding the Scope of multimodality imaging in durable Mechanical Circulatory Support. J Am Coll Cardiol Imaging 2020;13:1069–81.

54. Seese L, Hickey G, Keebler M, et al. Limited efficacy of thrombolytics for pump thrombosis in durable Left Ventricular Assist Devices. Ann Thorac Surg 2020;110:2047–54.

55. Koda Y, Kitahara H, Kalantari S, et al. Surgical device exchange provides improved clinical outcomes compared to medical therapy in treating continuous-flow left ventricular assist device thrombosis. Artif Organs 2020;44:367–74.

56. Carlson LA, Maynes EJ, Choi JH, et al. Characteristics and outcomes of gastrointestinal bleeding in patients with continuous-flow left ventricular assist devices: A systematic review. Artif Organs 2020;44:1150–61.

57. Molina TL, Krisl JC, Donahue KR, et al. Gastrointestinal bleeding in Left Ventricular Assist Device:

Octreotide and other treatment modalities. ASAIO J 2018;64:433–9.

58. Yin MY, Ruckel S, Kfoury AG. Novel model to predict gastrointestinal bleeding during Left Ventricular Assist Device Support. The Utah Bleeding Risk Score. Circ Heart Fail 2018;11:e005267.

59. Goodwin ML, Bobba CM, Mokadam NA, et al. Continuous-Flow Left Ventricular Assist Devices and the aortic valve: interactions, issues, and surgical therapy. Curr Heart Fail Rep 2020;17:97–105.

60. Imamura T, Narang N, Kim G, et al. Decoupling between diastolic Pulmonary Artery and Pulmonary Capillary Wedge Pressures is associated with Right Ventricular Dysfunction and hemocompatibility-related adverse events in patients with Left Ventricular Assist Devices. J Am Heart Assoc 2020;9:e01480.

61. Tang PC, Haft JW, Romano MA, et al. Right ventricular function and residual mitral regurgitation after left ventricular assist device implantation determines the incidence of right heart failure. J Thorac Cardiovasc Surg 2020;159:897–905.

62. Clerkin KJ, Topkara VK, Demmer RT, et al. Implantable Cardioverter-Defibrillators in patients with a Continuous-Flow Left Ventricular Assist Device. An Analysis of the INTERMACS Registry. JACC Heart Fail 2017;5:916–26.

63. Molina EJ, Shah P, Kiernan MS, et al. The Society of Thoracic Surgeons Intermacs 2020 Annual Report. Ann Thorac Surg 2021;111:778–92.

64. Jawitz OK, Fudim M, Raman V, et al. Reassessing recipient mortality under the new heart allocation system. An updated UNOS Registry analysis. JACC Heart Fail 2020;8:548–56.

65. Voltolini A, Salvato G, Frigerio M, et al. Psychological outcomes of left ventricular assist device long term treatment: a 2-year follow-up study. Artif Organs 2020;44:67–71.

66. Mullan CW, Sen S, Ahmad T, et al. Left Ventricular Assist Devices versus heart transplantation for end-stage heart failure is a misleading equivalency. JACC Heart Fail 2021;9:290–2.

67. Thorvaldsen T, Lund LH. Focusing on referral rather than selection for advanced heart failure therapies. Card Fail Rev 2019;5:24–6.

68. Chuzi S, Hale S, Arnold J, et al. Pre-ventricular assist device palliative care consultation: a qualitative analysis. J Pain Symptom Manag 2019;57:100–7.

69. Thompson JH, Moser D. Experiences with end-of-life care with a left Ventricular assist device: an integrative review. Heart Lung 2020;49:451–7.

70. Pak ES, Jones CA, Mather PJ. Ethical challenges in care of patients on mechanical circulatory support at end-of-life. Curr Heart Fail Rep 2020;17:153–60.

Listing Criteria for Heart Transplant
Role of Cardiopulmonary Exercise Test and of Prognostic Scores

Andrea Segreti, MD[a],*, Giuseppe Verolino, MD[a],
Simone Pasquale Crispino, MD[a], Piergiuseppe Agostoni, MD, PhD[b,c]

KEYWORDS

• Advanced heart failure • Heart transplant • Cardiopulmonary exercise test • Prognostic scores

KEY POINTS

• Heart transplant (HT) is considered the standard of care for carefully selected patients with advanced heart failure.
• The cardiopulmonary exercise test is the accepted gold-standard technique for evaluating heart failure patients who are candidates for an HT.
• Considerations should be given to revising the existing listing criteria for an HT.
• Prognostic scores outperform individual markers in terms of discrimination and calibration.
• MECKI (Metabolic Exercise test data combined with Cardiac and Kidney Indexes) score demonstrates a higher discriminative capacity for HT listing compared with other prognostic scores.

INTRODUCTION

Heart failure (HF) is a clinical syndrome characterized by a reduced cardiac output or elevated intracardiac pressures at rest or during stress.[1] Its prevalence is approximately 1% to 2% of the adult population in developed countries, rising to at least 10% among people older than 70 years.[1] Several pharmacologic treatments currently available improve symptoms, functional capacity, and quality of life, reducing hospitalizations and associated mortality.[1] Unfortunately, a subset of patients with chronic HF develop persistent structural cardiac abnormalities and severe resting symptoms despite optimal conventional treatment. This condition is indicated as advanced HF (AdHF) and may require the application of long-term mechanical circulatory support (MCS) devices or a heart transplant (HT).[2]

HEART TRANSPLANT

On Dec. 3, 1967, Dr Christiaan Barnard in Cape Town, South Africa, performed the first human HT using a cadaveric donor.[3] Subsequently, recipient and donor selection developments and management of infectious complications and medical immunosuppression were significantly advanced, resulting in fewer complications and improved post-HT survival and quality of life.[2]

HT is now considered the standard of care for the management of carefully selected patients with AdHF presenting with limiting severe symptoms despite optimal conventional treatment, evidence of a poor prognosis, and no remaining treatment options.[2] HT significantly increases survival, exercise capacity, quality of life, and return to work compared with conventional treatment,

[a] Unit of Cardiovascular Science, Campus Bio-Medico University of Rome, Rome, Italy; [b] Centro Cardiologico Monzino, IRCCS, Milan, Italy; [c] Department of Clinical Sciences and Community Health, University of Milan, Milan, Italy
* Corresponding author. Unit of Cardiovascular Science, Campus Bio-Medico University of Rome, Via Álvaro del Portillo 200, Rome 00128, Italy.
E-mail address: a.segreti@unicampus.it

Heart Failure Clin 17 (2021) 635–646
https://doi.org/10.1016/j.hfc.2021.05.008
1551-7136/21/© 2021 Elsevier Inc. All rights reserved.

provided that careful selection criteria are applied and no contraindications are present.[1,2,4]

Although HT has become the gold-standard therapy for such patients, challenges continue to exist, and the patient evaluation before listing for HT involves various considerations.[2,4] Indeed, the number of patients with AdHF is growing, whereas the number of donor organs remains constant, representing a limiting factor.[4,5] Clinicians should confirm the diagnosis of refractory HF and ensure no other treatable etiologies or alternative explanations for advanced symptoms. Secondly, HT candidates' selection involves prognostic variables to identify patients with a high mortality risk without HT who also have a good expected survival after HT. Lastly, physicians should detect those comorbidities that may negatively affect perioperative and post-HT outcomes.[2]

Diagnostic tests like the cardiopulmonary exercise test (CPET),[6] right heart catheterization,[7] and prognostic scores[8] are valuable tools in the pre-HT evaluation.[2]

PROGNOSTIC STRATIFICATION

Various criteria are available to identify patients with HF requiring HT. Initially, selection criteria were almost universally represented by resting hemodynamic data and subjective measures of symptoms and perceived activity levels like the New York Heart Association (NYHA) scale, which grades 4 functional classes from less to more severe.[9] Such a subjective assessment of functional capacity can easily be obtained but is frequently inaccurate despite its usefulness, because it can change depending on the patient and physician's interpretation.[9] A more detailed ranking system for patients with severe HF is the Interagency Registry for Mechanically Assisted Circulatory Support (INTERMACS) classification, which above class 3 recognizes symptoms as the predominant issue.[1] Furthermore, measurements of cardiac function at rest, both invasive and noninvasive, are poorly predictive of patients' symptoms, exercise capacity, prognosis, or need for HT.[9]

The exercise test makes a variety of contributions to the understanding of functional impairment in HF.[10] Indeed, stratification of HF patients based on exercise capacity can effectively identify patients with poor prognoses and an HT indication. Consequently, the 2016 International Society of Heart and Lung Transplantation (ISHLT) guidelines place the CPET and the risk assessment scores at the forefront of the listing process for HT.[4]

It is not possible to perform a CPET in patients in INTERMACS classes 1 to 3, in the presence of uncontrolled arrhythmias, and in patients unable to exercise because of comorbidities or extreme frailty.[11] However, in most patients in INTERMACS classes 4 to 7, a symptom-limited maximal CPET can be performed, provided that clinicians select an exercise protocol adapted to the patient's functional capacity or use an ergometer that allows minimizing the orthopedic limitations.[11]

CARDIOPULMONARY EXERCISE TEST

The determinants of exercise limitation in AdHF include reduced cardiac output response, impaired pulmonary oxygen exchange, anemia reducing oxygen carrying capacity, abnormal blood flow distribution, and muscle dysfunction with reduced oxygen diffusion and extraction.[12–14]

A simple test to assess exercise capacity like the 6-minute walking test (6MWT), although helpful in broader populations for identifying patients with evident clinical compromise, is not accurate for functional capacity assessment in patients with AdHF.[2] Instead, CPET is the accepted gold-standard technique for a precise and objective noninvasive evaluation of the mechanisms limiting exercise capacity,[14] in grading disease severity, and the identification of patients with potential indications for HT or long-term MCS.[6] CPET is the most comprehensive whole-body test technique that reflects organ-specific maladaptive responses to exercise and allows a holistic evaluation of exercise performance, particularly relevant in chronic HF patients.[6,10]

Several variables obtained from the CPET have shown to carry strong prognostic power, independently and in multivariate models, justifying their routine use to assess HT candidates' risk.[15] CPET was introduced into the HF clinic in the 1980s and was rapidly adopted in clinical practice by HT centers to guide listing for HT following a landmark publication by Mancini and colleagues[16] in 1991 that documented the prognostic power of peak volume of oxygen consumption (pVO$_2$) in patients eligible for HT. In this pioneering study, 116 ambulatory patients affected by HF with reduced ejection fraction (HFrEF) were stratified based on pVO$_2$ values into 3 groups: pVO$_2$ ≤14 mL/kg/min and suitable for HT; pVO$_2$ ≤14 mL/kg/min but with contraindications to HT; and pVO$_2$>14 mL/kg/min. One-year survival rate was 48%, 47%, and 94%, respectively. Of note, patients with a pVO$_2$ ≤10 mL/kg/min had a significantly lower predicted survival.[16]

These study results led to the general recommendation that HT should be considered in HFrEF patients with a pVO_2 $\leq$14 mL/kg/min, and in contrast, HT could be safely deferred in those with a pVO_2>14 mL/kg/min.[16]

TREATMENT EFFECTS

After the cornerstone study of Mancini and colleagues,[16] advances in medical therapy and CPET interpretation have occurred. Because currently used therapies can improve HFrEF patients' survival, considerations should be given to revising the existing listing criteria.[1,17]

Indeed, the traditional threshold point of 14 mL/kg/min to refer patients to HT was based on data accumulated before the advent of β-blocker therapy in routine clinical management. Despite the marginal effects of β-blockers on pVO_2,[18] survival rates are significantly increased in patients with HF who receive β-blockers, and a low pVO_2 may be an even more powerful predictor of mortality in patients receiving β-blocker therapy than in those treated without them.[19] Accordingly, reconsideration of Mancini and colleagues's[16] proposed cutoff was performed in the β-blocker era to reassess indications for HT. For this purpose, several studies[20,21] found that patients taking β-blockers had a significant reduction of long-term risk of death or HT than those not taking β-blockers. To guide listing for HT, a pVO_2 value of $\leq$12 mL/kg/min was identified for patients taking β-blockers, while pVO_2 $\leq$14 mL/kg/min was confirmed in patients not taking β-blocker.[20,21] Of note, β-blockers use imparted a better outcome until pVO_2 values became very low (eg, $\leq$10 mL/kg/min), when survival rates were equally low.[18] Consistent with this concept, Cattadori and colleagues[20] performed a long-term prognostic evaluation by pVO_2 in ambulatory HF patients using the Metabolic Exercise test data combined with Cardiac and Kidney Indexes (MECKI) score database.[22] In 715 ambulatory patients with HF and severe exercise intolerance, as defined by pVO_2 criteria for HT, the survival rate was better in patients who received β-blockers than those who did not for a given pVO_2 class, except for patients with the lowest pVO_2 (ie, <8 mL/min/kg). These data confirm that pVO_2 maintains prognostic value independent of the presence of β-blocker therapy. Also, HF patients with severe exercise limitation and intolerant of β-blockers showed a worse prognosis than HT patients regardless of pVO_2, and these patients should be considered a higher risk population.[20]

In addition to these landmark studies, a continuing wealth of evidence has fortified the prognostic strength of pVO_2, so much so that the 2016 ISHLT listing criteria in the presence of a maximal CPET (ie, with a respiratory exchange ratio [RER] >1.05) recommend a pVO_2 $\leq$14 mL/kg/min in intolerant patients and a pVO_2 $\leq$12 mL/kg/min in patients receiving β-blocker therapy (**Table 1**).[4]

Also, implantable cardioverter defibrillators (ICDs) and cardiac resynchronization therapy (CRT) are now routinely prescribed for potential HT patients and have been demonstrated to improve primary clinical outcomes and improve survival in HFrEF patients.[1] In 46 patients with AdHF with significant dyssynchrony and who were candidates for HT, CRT delayed HT and improved NYHA class and exercise capacity (increase in pVO_2).[23] However, in the larger prospective substudy of the Comparison of Medical Therapy, Pacing and Defibrillation in Heart Failure (COMPANION) trial,[24] CRT did not increase pVO_2 at 6 months compared with optimal medical therapy, despite improved NYHA functional class and 6-MWT distance. Consistent with these data, the 10-year update of ISHLT guidelines published in 2016[4] maintained the pVO_2 cutoffs of previous guidelines despite the advent and broader application of CRT in HF[25] and the evidence that the prognostic value of pVO_2 has changed with time.[19]

PEAK VOLUME OF OXYGEN CONSUMPTION ADJUSTED VALUES

PVO_2 during exercise is influenced by the severity of HF but also by noncardiac factors as age, gender, body size, muscle mass, obesity, deconditioning, and type of exercise. Therefore, when considering a patient for HT, to enhance the predictive accuracy, one must consider interpreting predicted pVO_2 values, adjusted for these variables.[21]

Based on this assumption, Stelken and colleagues[26] retrospectively studied 181 chronic HF patients to compare the sensitivity of percentage achieved of the predicted pVO_2, considering age, gender, and weight, with the traditionally used absolute pVO_2 measured in milliliters per kilogram per minute. Multivariate analysis revealed that 50% predicted of the pVO_2 was the strongest predictor of cardiac events, superior to the cutoff value of pVO_2 of 14 mL/kg/min.[26]

Significantly, pVO_2 is traditionally corrected for total body weight and is reported in milliliters per kilogram per minute. However, adipose tissue is not aerobically active but can represent a significant portion of total body weight.[27] Therefore, normalization of pVO_2 for fat-free mass may be more accurate, as adjusting pVO_2 to total body weight may result in an underestimation of

Table 1
Valuable diagnostic tests in the precardiac transplant evaluation

Diagnostic Test	Parameters
CPET	If maximal (RER >1.05 and achievement of AT on optimal medical treatment): • $pVO_2 \leq 14$ mL/kg/min if on β-blockers (class I, level of evidence: B); • $pVO_2 \leq 12$ mL/kg/min if not on β-blockers (class I, level of evidence: B); • In <50 y and women, use percent of predicted $pVO_2 \leq 50\%$ in conjunction with pVO_2 (class IIa, level of evidence: B). If submaximal (RER <1.05): • V_E/VCO_2 slope >35 (class IIb, level of evidence: C). In obese (body mass index >30 kg/m^2) patients: • Lean body mass–adjusted pVO_2 <19 mL/kg/min (class IIb, level of evidence: B).
HF prognosis scores	Should be performed along with CPET to determine prognosis and guide listing for HT for ambulatory patients. An estimated 1-y survival as calculated by the SHFM of <80% or an HFSS in the high-/medium-risk range should be considered as reasonable cut points for listing (class IIb, level of evidence: C). MECKI score prognosis estimation.[a]
Right heart catheterization	Should be performed on all adult candidates in preparation for listing for HT and periodically until HT (class I, level of evidence: C). Should be performed at 3- to 6-month intervals in listed patients, especially in the presence of reversible pulmonary hypertension or worsening of HF symptoms (class I, level of evidence: C). A vasodilator challenge should be administered when the pulmonary artery systolic pressure is ≥50 mm Hg and either the transpulmonary pressure gradient is ≥15 or the pulmonary vascular resistance is >3 Wood units while maintaining an SBP >85 mm Hg) (class I, level of evidence: C).

Abbreviations: V_E/VCO_2 slope, minute ventilation (VE)/carbon dioxide production (VCO_2) slope.
[a] For MECKI, there is no validated cutoff yet; nevertheless, its performance to predict the right candidate to HT was superior to other scores.[62–64]
Adapted from Mehra MR, Canter CE, Hannan MM, et al. The 2016 International Society for Heart Lung Transplantation listing criteria for heart transplantation: A 10-year update. J Heart Lung Transplant 2016;35(1):1-23; with permission.

pVO_2.[14] In fact, Osman and colleagues[27] demonstrated that in patients with HFrEF, a value of pVO_2 lean (ie, corrected for lean body mass) <19 mL/kg/min, rather than the traditional cutpoint of 14 mL/kg/min, had a more comprehensive and accurate prognostic discriminator of major cardiac events (death or urgent HT).[27]

As a consequence, ISHLT guidelines state that in obese patients (ie, with a body mass index >30 kg/m^2), adjusting pVO_2 to lean body mass may be considered for timing HT and that a lean body mass-adjusted pVO_2 of <19 mL/kg/min can serve as an optimal threshold (see **Table 1**).[4]

VO_2 at the anaerobic threshold (AT) (VO_2AT) (ie, when anaerobic metabolism influence ventilation), has been considered as ancillary to pVO_2, and, originally, AT identification was considered needed for a reliable assessment of pVO_2.[21] Later,

only the presence of an RER greater than 1.0 was considered mandatory for pVO_2 assessment, although some authors discuss this statement.[21] In reality, AT is reached but not identifiable in a sizable percentage of severe HF patients, and this datum has a strong negative prognostic power.[28,29]

The AT has been proposed as a submaximal index of exercise capacity, independent of the patient's motivation.[21] In a prospective study in 223 ambulatory patients with HF prioritized for HT, Gitt and colleagues[30] compared the pVO_2 and the submaximal parameters to predict patients' survival rate. A VO_2AT of less than 11 mL/kg/min combined with a minute ventilation (V_E)/carbon dioxide production (VCO_2) slope (V_E/VCO_2 slope) of greater than 34 was a better indicator of risk associated with early cardiac death than pVO_2 alone.[30]

Notably, hemodynamic responses to exercise are greatly affected by gender, and a threshold value of 14 mL/kg/min may be inappropriate for women.[31] In HF patients who were candidates for HT, Elmariah and colleagues[32] observed that women compared with men had a lower pVO_2, reached the AT in a lower percentage, and had a lower peak RER, despite being younger. However, women had higher HT-free survival.[32] Similarly, another paper reported that the best way to assess the effects of gender on aerobic capacity is to use predicted pVO_2 ($ppVO_2$) that incorporates age, gender, height, and weight.[33] These data indicate that different thresholds for pVO_2 by gender may be necessary for timing HT. The traditional pVO_2 cutoff value for HT candidate selection might be disproportionate in women in whom, if adopted, might be referred to HT too soon. As a result, ISHLT guidelines state that in young patients (<50 years) and women, it is reasonable to consider using alternate standards in conjunction with pVO_2 to guide listing, including $ppVO_2$ of no more than 50% (see **Table 1**).[4]

Besides the aforementioned case of β-blockers, the concept that CPET must be performed when ongoing therapy, both pharmacologic and device-driven, has been optimized is absolutely relevant. Indeed, the prognostic power of pVO_2, V_E/VCO_2 slope, and other CPET parameters has been confirmed in different years, but the cut-point values have been modified.[19] The combined risk of cardiovascular death, urgent HT, and LVAD implantation progressively increases as pVO_2 decreases or the V_E/VCO_2 slope value increases, respectively.[19] The implementation of guidelines and the continuous update of pharmacologic and device-based HF treatment observed in the last years are likely to be the primary explanation for the improvement of HFrEF prognosis and observed increase and decrease, respectively, of the cut-point values of pVO_2 and V_E/VCO_2 slope over time (**Fig. 1**).[19]

Therefore, it is conceivable that the widespread use of any new treatment option will likely further improve survival and possibly risk cutoff values. Sacubitril-valsartan is recommended to further reduce the risk of hospitalization and death in patients with HFrEF.[1] This drug increases pVO_2 values and reduces V_E/VCO_2 slope.[34,35] Six months of sacubitril-valsartan treatment decreased the percentage of patients with pVO_2 ≤12 mL/min/kg from 37% to 11% and those with V_E/VCO_2 slope greater than 35 from 52.4% to 17.1%. These results are significant and underline the concepts that for proper HT assessment by CPET, patients had to be on optimal medical treatment, which nowadays includes, if tolerated,

sacubitril-valsartan.[35] Also, HF patients awaiting HT with an initial pVO_2 below the threshold for HT listing can be taken off from the active waiting list if pVO_2 significantly improves following a period of treatment optimization.[36] Accordingly, ISHLT 2016 guidelines recommend that listed patients in an outpatient, ambulatory, noninotropic therapy-dependent state should be continually evaluated for maximal pharmacologic and device therapy and must be re-evaluated at 3- to 6-month intervals with CPET and HF survival prognostic scores to assess their response to therapy. If they have improved significantly, they should be considered for delisting (see **Table 1**).[4]

BEYOND PEAK VOLUME OF OXYGEN CONSUMPTION

PVO_2 is the gold standard for evaluating exercise tolerance and is a fundamental part of a comprehensive HT evaluation.

Whereas pVO_2 values of less than 10 and greater than 18 mL/kg/min usually identify high- and low-risk patients, respectively, patients with an intermediate pVO_2 fall within a grey area of medium-risk, not amenable to further prognostic stratification based solely on pVO_2.[33] Moreover, Grigioni and colleagues[37] demonstrated that HF patient candidates for HT with only a pre-HT moderate impairment of pVO_2 are at a high risk of failing to improve exercise performance significantly after HT.[37] Therefore, particularly in this subgroup of patients, other prognostic parameters obtained by CPET, in addition to pVO_2, should be considered.

Nevertheless, maximal exercise effort is not always achieved during CPET. However, some variables with prognostic values obtained during submaximal CPET may help inform HT candidacy.[38] Indeed, an impressive and convincing body of published reports identifies ventilatory efficiency parameters like V_E/VCO_2 slope as a more powerful prognostic index than pVO_2 in HF patients, because they can be measured throughout the entire exercise duration and are independent of patient motivation.[39,40]

The rationale behind ventilation assessment is that HF patients exhibit excessive exercise-induced hyperventilation, proportional to the disease severity.[41] Consequently, the V_E/VCO_2 slope during exercise is steeper in patients with more severe disease.[41] This feature has several causes, including lung mechanics alterations, reduced lung diffusion, increased ventilatory need because of increased CO_2 production, enhanced dead space ventilation, and overactive reflexes from metaboreceptors, baroreceptors, and chemoreceptors.[41,42]

A

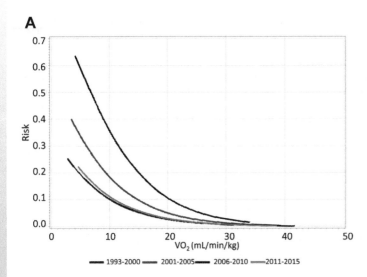

B

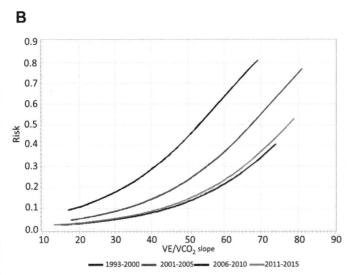

Fig. 1. The predicted 2-year cumulative risks of the composite event (cardiovascular mortality, urgent HT, or LVAD implantation), associated with VO$_2$ and VE/VCO$_2$ slope values within each time range. (*From* Paolillo S, Veglia F, Salvioni E, et al. Heart failure prognosis over time: how the prognostic role of oxygen consumption and ventilatory efficiency during exercise has changed in the last 20 years. *Eur J Heart Fail* 2019;21(2):208-217; with permission.)

Increased ventilation during exercise relative to metabolic rate has proved to be a valuable prognostic indicator in HF, being as good or better than pVO$_2$ alone, even in patients with obesity, on β-blockers, and with diastolic dysfunction.[43]

Arena and colleagues[40] developed a 4-level ventilatory classification of HF patients based on V$_E$/VCO$_2$ slope: I no more than 29; II 30.0 to 35.9; III: 36.0 to 44.9; and IV at least 45.0. A value of at least 45 indicates disease severity and portends a particularly high risk for adverse cardiovascular events. In fact, 2 years, survival free of death, HT or MCS implantation for classes I to IV was 97.2%, 85.2%, 72.3%, and 44.2%, respectively.[40]

Similarly, other studies found that the increase of V$_E$/VCO$_2$ slope was the most accurate predictor of cardiac death, urgent HT, or need for MCS,[39,44] and using V$_E$/VCO$_2$ slope as a criterion for HT selection could reclassify correctly 18.3% more patients than the classical pVO$_2$-based criteria.[39]

As a result of the previously reported studies, ISHLT guidelines recommend that in case of a submaximal effort (RER <1.05), the use of V$_E$/VCO$_2$ slope greater than 35 as a determinant in listing for HT may be considered (see **Table 1**).[4]

Another negative prognostic marker is the presence of exercise-induced periodic breathing

(EPB), identified as a regularly recurring waxing and waning of tidal volume caused by oscillations in the central respiratory drive.[45] There is compelling evidence that EPB is a robust independent prognosticator in HFrEF, because it is related to a higher risk of events.[45] Indeed, the authors of an interesting study[46] found that in a group of patients with AdHF under evaluation for HT, EPB was frequent (about 30%).[46] When EPB was present, it almost independently tripled the average risk of cardiac death.[46] In the same study, EPB was associated with lower $P_{ET}CO_2$ at rest and steeper V_E/VCO_2 slope during exercise (ie, excessive ventilatory response).[46] These findings are especially relevant in clinical practice, because the presence of this disorder does not depend on patients' maximal effort or achievement of a pVO_2.[46]

MULTIVARIATE APPROACH COMBINING CARDIOPULMONARY EXERCISE TEST VARIABLES

Besides gas exchange parameters, other exercise variables obtained by CPET have been investigated to stratify further chronic HF patients referred for HT. For example, failure to achieve during exercise systolic blood pressure (SBP) greater than 120 mm Hg, chronotropic incompetence, and slow heart rate recovery (HRR) in the first-minute after exercise represent negative prognostic markers.[6] A multivariate approach that combines CPET parameters further improves the ability to stratify patients and provides a more comprehensive insight into HF pathophysiology, compared with single variables.[6,8,30]

Myers and colleagues[47] produced a stratification score that integrates 5 CPET variables: V_E/VCO_2 slope (≥ 34), HRR (≤ 6 bpm), oxygen uptake efficiency slope (OUES) (≤ 1.4), $P_{ET}CO_2$ (<33 mm Hg), and pVO_2 (≤ 14 mL/kg/min). The score ranges were 0 to 5, 6 to 10, 11 to 15, and 16 to 20, with patients with a score greater than 15 having 3-year mortality of 12.2% and a relative risk greater than 9 for total events, whereas a score of less than 5 was associated with an annual mortality rate of 1.2%.[47] Similarly, the PROBE score[48] considers together pVO_2 (4 Wb's classification classes), V_E/VCO_2 slope (4 Arena's classification classes) and EPB (0 = no; 1 = yes).[48]

As a result, in HFrEF patients, a pVO_2 of no more than 12 if taking β-blockers or no more than 14 mL/kg/min if not taking β-blockers, a V_E/VCO_2 slope greater than 36, the presence of EPB, an OUES of no more than 1.4, VO_2AT lower than 9 mL/kg/min, reaching SBP less than 120 mm Hg, and an HRR less than 6 bpm, indicate a 1-year mortality rate of greater than 20%.[6]

SPECIFIC CONSIDERATIONS AND FUTURE APPLICATIONS OF CARDIOPULMONARY EXERCISE TEST FOR LISTING PATIENTS

Deserving of consideration are the frequent concomitant coexistence of HF and atrial fibrillation (AF)[1] and the question of whether HF patients with AF can be precisely stratified with the current CPET cutoffs for HT selection. Because the combination of HF and AF provides a worse prognosis, a timely referral for HT or MCS could be particularly important to reduce AF's negative prognostic effect in HF patients.[49] Agostoni and colleagues[50] demonstrated that an unidentifiable AT was observed in 27% of AF and 15% of SR patients with HF and was associated with impaired exercise performance. AF with respect to SR patients had a reduced exercise performance with lower pVO_2 and peak oxygen pulse and a trend toward higher V_E/VCO_2 slope values.[50] However, at AT, AF patients had higher VO_2 and heart rate (HR) with a lower oxygen pulse, likely related to the higher chronotropic response to exercise in AF patients.[50] This last observation raises uncertainties about using AT data to define the performance and prognosis of HF patients with AF.[50] In another study carried out in patients with HFrEF and possible indication for HT or MCS, AF patients had a higher incidence of cardiac death and HT and a lower exercise capacity.[49] Although AF carried a worse prognosis, the current pVO_2 cutoff for HT selection precisely stratified this group of high-risk patients, indicating that HF patients with AF and a CPET under the current pVO_2 cut-point for HT selection should be quickly referred for HT or MCS.[49] Of note, pVO_2 cutoff seems to have a higher positive predictive value than V_E/VCO_2 slope cutoff for the prediction of the primary outcome in HF patients with AF.[49]

Another important consideration is the possible utility of simultaneous CPET and cardiac output measures during exercise in listing patients for HT. Because both cardiac output response to exercise and pVO_2 are critical to define the severity of HF and provide valuable independent prognostic information, these variables should be used in combination for selecting HT candidates.[51,52] Cardiac output has a pivotal role in understanding the physiopathology of exercise limitation and evaluation of many interventions, such as the use of inotropic drugs, CRT, mitral percutaneous procedures, and MCS devices.[51] Indeed, after optimization of medical treatment, different hemodynamic responses to exercise in HF candidates for HT can be present, as an increased pVO_2 can be achieved by cardiac output improvement, increased extraction of peripheral oxygen, or both.[51] According to the Fick principle, concomitant VO_2 and cardiac output detection during exercise allow calculation of arteriovenous oxygen difference.[25] Plotting these 3 variables together permits one to discriminate exercise limitations caused by altered left ventricle pump function from those due to other causes, including muscle enzyme deficiency and deconditioning.[52] The ideal method for determining cardiac output during exercise should be noninvasive, with the inert gas rebreathing method with continuous analysis of respired gases being a reliable, safe, and inexpensive method.[52] As suggested by Yearly and colleagues,[25] concomitant CPET and noninvasive cardiac output measurement should identify the patient with favorable central remodeling and potential for further improvement, which may ultimately result in removal from the HT list. On the other hand, those patients with an increase of pVO_2 but an absence of appreciable change in cardiac output should remain on the HT list because of persisting severe cardiac dysfunction. Nevertheless, these patients deserve careful attention, because comprehension of their favorable remodeling of the periphery may provide another therapeutic option for HF patients not candidates for HT or MCS treatment.[25] Therefore, studies are required to evaluate the prognostic power of CPET and simultaneous noninvasive cardiac output measurement in stratifying patients for HT.

Another consideration is the presence of significant functional mitral regurgitation that negatively affects exercise capacity in patients with HFrEF who are potential candidates for HT or destination LVAD.[53] Percutaneous mitral valve repair has proven to improve overall cardiopulmonary performance in this population, including increased pVO_2, exercise time, AT, peak oxygen pulse, and workload.[53] However, the true impact of this treatment remains a grey zone.[54] Therefore, further trials are required to determine better the impact on actual cutoff recommendations of this treatment and if clinical improvement in patients with functional mitral regurgitation translates to better survival outcomes and safe deference of advanced HF therapies.[53]

Finally, different types of HF severity and prognosis biomarkers of HF have emerged and among these biomarkers, B-type natriuretic peptide is the most studied.[55] However, another noninvasive technique like analysis of volatile organic compounds in the breath has been proven to be effective in detecting and classifying many diseases, including chronic coronary syndromes[56] and HF.[57] For example, higher levels of exhaled breath acetone in patients with HF are associated with an increased risk of death or HT within 12 months.[55] This new noninvasive test might be a useful tool for timely detecting HF patients candidates to HT.

PROGNOSTIC SCORES

As previously reported, several single variables have been used in the prognostic stratification of HF. Because of the composite nature of HF syndrome, no single variable can account for all prognostic dimensions.[8] Thus, a multiparametric approach considering multivariable prognostic scores outperforms individual markers both in terms of discrimination and calibration.[2,38]

The last ISHLT guidelines show that besides functional criteria of HT suitability, derived from CPET, risk scores should be considered for better assessment of clinical background and consequently complete the understanding of risk level.[4] Different scores are available, and each one includes clinical, laboratory, therapeutic, and demographic elements within.

The first one is Heart Failure Severity Score (HFSS),[58] a prognosis index developed in 1997 in a population of 268 patients with AdHF. The HFSS stratifies the patient's risk using 7 parameters: resting HR, mean blood pressure, left ventricular ejection fraction (LVEF), serum sodium, presence or absence of ischemic heart disease, presence of intraventricular conduction delay (QRS $\geq$120 milliseconds), and pVO_2.[58] HFSS performance aims to improve risk stratification compared to the pVO_2 alone by dividing patients into 3 categories to define their prognosis. A score of at least 8.10 identifies a low-risk patient, whereas scores of 7.2 to 8.09 and no more than 7.19 indicate a medium and high risk, respectively. Patients in medium- and high-risk groups are most likely to die or require urgent HT in the following year (1-year survival of 72% and 43%, respectively); on the contrary, HT can be safely deferred in patients in the low-risk group (1-year survival 93%). Consequently, ISHLT guidelines explain that aside from CPET evaluation and pVO_2 value, subjects with high-medium risk derived from HFSS may be reasonable candidates for HT.[4]

Otherwise, among candidates for HT, estimating long-term prognosis is pivotal too; dealing with this issue, the Seattle Heart Failure Model (SHFM)[59] through a system including 20 parameters, proposed a long-term estimation of 1-, 3- and 5-year survival. SHFM included the impact of medical and device interventions that are not included in other score systems. The SHFM is based on age, gender, NYHA class, weight, LVEF, SBP, medications, a few laboratory values, and other clinical information. Furthermore, the model has incorporated newer HF therapies with a meaningful impact on survival, including ICDs and CRT. This system derived an accurate 1-year survival estimation; as stated by ISHLT guidelines, survival probability less than 80% defines a good candidate for listing.[4] Although an in-depth consideration of characteristics and intervention could provide a better definition of the clinical setting, a more complex system may be cumbersome and unpractical. Nonetheless, the prognosis prediction capacity of each score alone seems less efficient than both parameters' association.

SHFM and HFSS have roughly the same ability to predict 1- and 2-year adverse events, and a correlation between them is present.[60] Both these scores have better performance than NYHA class (parameter included in SHFM), although this last indicator keeps its role in prognosis definition.[60] According to some, these 2 scores might have their best capacity and utility in patients with medium risk, because this group represents the grey zone of HT suitability.[60]

The consideration of a broad spectrum of parameters allows obtaining the proper clinical judgment. Although it has a less relevant role, the Meta-Analysis Global Group in Chronic Heart Failure (MAGGIC) score[61] is another system derived from a large cohort of patients affected by HF with preserved or reduced ejection fraction, showing a good performance compared with SHFM.[62] However, the MAGGIC score has not been validated in the AdHF population, and for that reason, it may have a marginal role in HT indication.

The most recent prognostic score, MECKI score,[22] has shown a brilliant prognosis estimation performance and a good versatility. Agostoni and colleagues[22] developed the MECKI score to identify the risk of cardiovascular death and urgent HT from a cohort of 2715 patients with HFrEF. The score is composed of the following easy-to-obtain 6 continuous variables independently related to prognosis: 2 variables derived from the CPET (pVO_2 expressed as % predicted and V_E/VCO_2 slope), 3 variables from laboratory data (serum sodium, hemoglobin, and glomerular filtration rate obtained by the Modification of Diet in Renal Disease [GFR-MDRD] formula), and 1 variable from transthoracic echocardiography (LVEF).[22] An algorithm for the immediate calculation of the MECKI score, defining the risk of cardiovascular death and urgent HT at 2 years, is available online (https://www.cardiologicomonzino.it/it/mecki-score/). Of note, in the MECKI score analysis, the percentage of predicted pVO_2 was superior to the absolute value in determining prognosis.

Compared with other scores not validated in the HT population, the MECKI score combines easy utilization and high predictive power, allowed by a comprehensive internal and external validation cohort. Summing things up, this system predicts death for HF and a 2-year probability of urgent HT in patients who can perform at least a submaximal or symptoms-limited CPET.[22] Unlike other score systems, MECKI includes physiologic variability caused by demographic and gender differences within its parameters. The predicted percentage of pVO_2 is a derived index that considers age and resting HR; in the same way, the GFR-MDRD formula includes gender, age, and ethnicity. Indirectly, consideration of demographic characteristics allows better patient profiling. A comprehensive evaluation of the HF population with the MECKI score confirms its long-term prediction capacity and higher discriminative prognostic power compared with MAGGIC, HFSS, and SHFM scores.[63–65] Score systems undoubtedly represent a useful tool for HT candidate identification; however, according to the most recent revision of ISHLT guidelines, risk scores cannot be used alone but in association with physical evaluation.[4] A multiparametric approach may be the right way to follow, in consideration of patients' complexity and of the various disease presentation of AdHF (see **Table 1**).

SUMMARY

HT represents the gold-standard treatment for carefully selected patients with AdHF, but a shortage of donor organs limits its availability. Proper selection criteria and accurate prognostic determination are required to guarantee the patient's candidacy and allocate this scarce resource to the patients at the highest risk of cardiovascular events.

CPET and validated prognostic scores are objective methods that allow identification of candidates for HT. HT represents the gold-standard treatment for carefully selected patients with AdHF, but a shortage of donor organs limits its availability. Proper selection criteria and accurate prognostic determination are required to guarantee the patient's candidacy and allocate this scarce resource to the patients at the highest risk of cardiovascular events.

The progressive improvement of HF treatment strategies requires a continuous reevaluation of HT candidacy by a multivariate approach comprehensive of several indicators. Finally, more extensive utilization of CPET plus noninvasive measurements of cardiac output has the potential to become a valuable tool to better phenotype HFrEF patients and refine listing criteria for HT.

Clinics Care Points

- Patients with advanced heart failure candidates for a heart transplant (HT) should undergo maximal cardiopulmonary exercise testing (CPET).

- A maximal CPET should be performed on optimal medical treatment and is defined as one with a respiratory exchange ratio >1.05 and achievement of anaerobic threshold.

- When maximal CPET is performed, the pVO$_2$ cutpoint to consider for HT listing patients should be <14 ml/kg/min if on β-blockers or <12 ml/kg/min if not on β-blockers.

- In the case of submaximal CPET, a VE/VCO$_2$ slope value >35 could be considered for HT listing patients.

- As the value of pVO$_2$ can be influenced by many factors like age, gender, and lean-body, the pVO$_2$ value adjusted for these factors should improve the predictive accuracy.

- Multivariable prognostic scores obtained through different techniques support clinicians in the determinations of candidacy for HT.

- MECKI score has proven higher long-term prediction capacity and higher discriminative prognostic power than other prognostic scores.

REFERENCES

1. Ponikowski P, Voors AA, Anker SD, et al. 2016 ESC Guidelines for the diagnosis and treatment of acute and chronic heart failure: the task force for the diagnosis and treatment of acute and chronic heart failure of the European Society of Cardiology (ESC). Developed with the special contribution of the Heart Failure Association (HFA) of the ESC. Eur J Heart Fail 2016;18(8):891–975.

2. Crespo-Leiro MG, Metra M, Lund LH, et al. Advanced heart failure: a position statement of the Heart Failure Association of the European Society of Cardiology. Eur J Heart Fail 2018;20(11):1505–35.

3. Barnard CN. The operation. A human cardiac transplant: an interim report of a successful operation performed at Groote Schuur Hospital, Cape Town. S Afr Med J 1967;41(48):1271–4.

4. Mehra MR, Canter CE, Hannan MM, et al. The 2016 International Society for Heart Lung Transplantation listing criteria for heart transplantation: a 10-year update. J Heart Lung Transplant 2016;35(1):1–23.

5. Grigioni F, Potena L, Barbieri A, et al. Age and heart transplantation: results from a heart failure management unit. Clin Transplant 2008;22(2):150–5.

6. Malhotra R, Bakken K, D'Elia E, et al. Cardiopulmonary Exercise Testing in Heart Failure. JACC Heart Fail 2016;4(8):607–16.

7. Grigioni F, Potena L, Galie N, et al. Prognostic implications of serial assessments of pulmonary hypertension in severe chronic heart failure. J Heart Lung Transplant 2006;25(10):1241–6.

8. Mantegazza S, Badagliacca R, Nodari S. Management of heart failure in the new era: the role of scores. J Cardiovasc Med 2016;17(8):569–80.

9. Alraies MC, Eckman P. Adult heart transplant: indications and outcomes. J Thorac Dis 2014;6(8):1120–8.

10. Agostoni P, Dumitrescu D. How to perform and report a cardiopulmonary exercise test in patients with chronic heart failure. Int J Cardiol 2019;288:107–13.

11. Mendes M. Cardiopulmonary exercise test in the evaluation of heart transplant candidates with atrial fibrillation. Arq Bras Cardiol 2020;114(2):219–21.

12. Koike A, Wasserman K, Taniguchi K, et al. Critical capillary oxygen partial pressure and lactate threshold in patients with cardiovascular disease. J Am Coll Cardiol 1994;23(7):1644–50.

13. Del Torto A, Corrieri N, Vignati C, et al. Contribution of central and peripheral factors at peak exercise in heart failure patients with progressive severity of exercise limitation. Int J Cardiol 2017;248:252–6.

14. Del Buono MG, Arena R, Borlaug BA, et al. Exercise intolerance in patients with heart failure: JACC state-of-the-art review. J Am Coll Cardiol 2019;73(17):2209–25.

15. Guazzi M, Adams V, Conraads V, et al. EACPR/AHA scientific statement. Clinical recommendations for cardiopulmonary exercise testing data assessment in specific patient populations. Circulation 2012;126(18):2261–74.

16. Mancini DM, Eisen H, Kussmaul W, et al. Value of peak exercise oxygen consumption for optimal timing of cardiac transplantation in ambulatory patients with heart failure. Circulation 1991;83(3):778–86.

17. Barbieri A, Berti E, Marino M, et al. Comparative effectiveness of disease-modifying-drugs in elderly patients after incident hospitalization for heart failure. Int J Cardiol 2014;173(3):557–60.

18. O'Neill JO, Young JB, Pothier CE, et al. Peak oxygen consumption as a predictor of death in patients with heart failure receiving beta-blockers. Circulation 2005;111(18):2313–8.

19. Paolillo S, Veglia F, Salvioni E, et al. Heart failure prognosis over time: how the prognostic role of oxygen consumption and ventilatory efficiency during exercise has changed in the last 20 years. Eur J Heart Fail 2019;21(2):208–17.

20. Cattadori G, Agostoni P, Corra U, et al. Severe heart failure prognosis evaluation for transplant selection in the era of beta-blockers: role of peak oxygen consumption. Int J Cardiol 2013;168(5):5078–81.

21. Corra U, Mezzani A, Bosimini E, et al. Cardiopulmonary exercise testing and prognosis in chronic heart failure: a prognosticating algorithm for the individual patient. Chest 2004;126(3):942–50.

22. Agostoni P, Corra U, Cattadori G, et al. Metabolic exercise test data combined with cardiac and kidney indexes, the MECKI score: a multiparametric approach to heart failure prognosis. Int J Cardiol 2013;167(6):2710–8.

23. Vanderheyden M, Wellens F, Bartunek J, et al. Cardiac resynchronization therapy delays heart transplantation in patients with end-stage heart failure and mechanical dyssynchrony. J Heart Lung Transplant 2006;25(4):447–53.

24. De Marco T, Wolfel E, Feldman AM, et al. Impact of cardiac resynchronization therapy on exercise performance, functional capacity, and quality of life in systolic heart failure with QRS prolongation: COMPANION trial sub-study. J Card Fail 2008;14(1):9–18.

25. Yerly P, Hullin R. Cardiopulmonary exercise testing in advanced heart failure with reduced ejection fraction: time for in-depth analysis for central and peripheral contributors to peak VO2? Eur J Prev Cardiol 2019;26(15):1613–5.

26. Stelken AM, Younis LT, Jennison SH, et al. Prognostic value of cardiopulmonary exercise testing using percent achieved of predicted peak oxygen uptake for patients with ischemic and dilated cardiomyopathy. J Am Coll Cardiol 1996;27(2):345–52.

27. Osman AF, Mehra MR, Lavie CJ, et al. The incremental prognostic importance of body fat adjusted peak oxygen consumption in chronic heart failure. J Am Coll Cardiol 2000;36(7):2126–31.

28. Carriere C, Corra U, Piepoli M, et al. Anaerobic threshold and respiratory compensation point identification during cardiopulmonary exercise tests in chronic heart failure. Chest 2019;156(2):338–47.

29. Agostoni P, Corra U, Cattadori G, et al. Prognostic value of indeterminable anaerobic threshold in heart failure. Circ Heart Fail 2013;6(5):977–87.

30. Gitt AK, Wasserman K, Kilkowski C, et al. Exercise anaerobic threshold and ventilatory efficiency identify heart failure patients for high risk of early death. Circulation 2002;106(24):3079–84.

31. Franco V. Cardiopulmonary exercise test in chronic heart failure: beyond peak oxygen consumption. Curr Heart Fail Rep 2011;8(1):45–50.

32. Elmariah S, Goldberg LR, Allen MT, et al. Effects of gender on peak oxygen consumption and the timing of cardiac transplantation. J Am Coll Cardiol 2006;47(11):2237–42.

33. Corra U, Mezzani A, Giordano A, et al. Peak oxygen consumption and prognosis in heart failure: 14 mL/kg/min is not a "gender-neutral" reference. Int J Cardiol 2013;167(1):157–61.

34. Vitale G, Romano G, Di Franco A, et al. Early effects of sacubitril/valsartan on exercise tolerance in patients with heart failure with reduced ejection fraction. J Clin Med 2019;8(2):262.

35. Goncalves AV, Pereira-da-Silva T, Galrinho A, et al. Maximal oxygen uptake and ventilation improvement following sacubitril-valsartan therapy. Arq Bras Cardiol 2020;115(5):821–7.

36. Stevenson LW, Steimle AE, Fonarow G, et al. Improvement in exercise capacity of candidates awaiting heart transplantation. J Am Coll Cardiol 1995;25(1):163–70.

37. Grigioni F, Specchia S, Maietta P, et al. Changes in exercise capacity induced by heart transplantation: prognostic and therapeutic implications. Scand J Med Sci Sports. Aug 2011;21(4):519-25. doi:10.1111/j.1600-0838.2009.01065.x.

38. Paolillo S, Agostoni P. Prognostic role of cardiopulmonary exercise testing in clinical practice. Ann Am Thorac Soc 2017;14(Suppl 1):S53–8.

39. Ferreira AM, Tabet JY, Frankenstein L, et al. Ventilatory efficiency and the selection of patients for heart transplantation. Circ Heart Fail 2010;3(3):378–86.

40. Arena R, Myers J, Abella J, et al. Development of a ventilatory classification system in patients with heart failure. Circulation 2007;115(18):2410–7.

41. Agostoni P, Cattadori G, Bussotti M, et al. Cardiopulmonary interaction in heart failure. Pulm Pharmacol Ther 2007;20(2):130–4.

42. Segreti A, Grigioni F, Campodonico J, et al. Chemoreceptor hyperactivity in heart failure: Is lactate the culprit? Eur J Prev Cardiol 2020. 2047487320915548.

43. Sue DY. Excess ventilation during exercise and prognosis in chronic heart failure. Am J Respir Crit Care Med 2011;183(10):1302–10.

44. Pereira-da-Silva T, M Soares R, Papoila AL, et al. Optimizing risk stratification in heart failure and the selection of candidates for heart transplantation. Rev Port Cardiol 2018;37(2):129–37.

45. Agostoni P, Corra U, Emdin M. Periodic Breathing during Incremental Exercise. Ann Am Thorac Soc 2017;14(Suppl_1):S116–22.

46. Leite JJ, Mansur AJ, de Freitas HF, et al. Periodic breathing during incremental exercise predicts mortality in patients with chronic heart failure evaluated for cardiac transplantation. J Am Coll Cardiol 2003;41(12):2175–81.

47. Myers J, Oliveira R, Dewey F, et al. Validation of a cardiopulmonary exercise test score in heart failure. Circ Heart Fail 2013;6(2):211–8.

48. Guazzi M, Boracchi P, Arena R, et al. Development of a cardiopulmonary exercise prognostic score for optimizing risk stratification in heart failure: the (P)e(R)i(O)dic (B)reathing during (E)xercise (PROBE) study. J Card Fail 2010;16(10):799–805.

49. Goncalves AV, Pereira-da-Silva T, Soares R, et al. Prognostic prediction of cardiopulmonary exercise test parameters in heart failure patients with atrial fibrillation. Arq Bras Cardiol 2020;114(2):209–18.

50. Agostoni P, Emdin M, Corra U, et al. Permanent atrial fibrillation affects exercise capacity in chronic heart failure patients. Eur Heart J 2008;29(19):2367–72.

51. Vignati C, Cattadori G. Measuring Cardiac Output during Cardiopulmonary Exercise Testing. Ann Am Thorac Soc 2017;14(Suppl_1):S48–52.

52. Agostoni P, Cattadori G, Apostolo A, et al. Noninvasive measurement of cardiac output during exercise by inert gas rebreathing technique: a new tool for heart failure evaluation. J Am Coll Cardiol 2005; 46(9):1779–81.

53. Benito-Gonzalez T, Estevez-Loureiro R, Garrote-Coloma C, et al. MitraClip improves cardiopulmonary exercise test in patients with systolic heart failure and functional mitral regurgitation. ESC Heart Fail 2019;6(4):867–73.

54. Frigerio M, Fiocca L, Bedogni F, et al. [Grey zones on valvular heart disease: interventional cardiology versus cardiac surgery. Expert opinion]. G Ital Cardiol (Rome) 2020;21(2):111–8. Grey zones sulla cardiologia interventistica valvolare e cardiochirurgia a confronto. Opinioni degli esperti.

55. Marcondes-Braga FG, Batista GL, Gutz IG, et al. Impact of Exhaled Breath Acetone in the Prognosis of Patients with Heart Failure with Reduced Ejection Fraction (HFrEF). One Year of Clinical Follow-up. PLoS One 2016;11(12):e0168790.

56. Segreti A, Incalzi RA, Lombardi M, et al. Characterization of inflammatory profile by breath analysis in chronic coronary syndromes. J Cardiovasc Med (Hagerstown) 2020;21(9):675–81.

57. Marcondes-Braga FG, Batista GL, Bacal F, et al. Exhaled Breath Analysis in Heart Failure. Curr Heart Fail Rep 2016;13(4):166–71.

58. Aaronson KD, Schwartz JS, Chen TM, et al. Development and prospective validation of a clinical index to predict survival in ambulatory patients referred for cardiac transplant evaluation. Circulation 1997; 95(12):2660–7.

59. Levy WC, Mozaffarian D, Linker DT, et al. The Seattle Heart Failure Model: prediction of survival in heart failure. Circulation 2006;113(11):1424–33.

60. Goda A, Williams P, Mancini D, et al. Selecting patients for heart transplantation: comparison of the Heart Failure Survival Score (HFSS) and the Seattle Heart Failure Model (SHFM). J Heart Lung Transplant 2011;30(11):1236–43.

61. Pocock SJ, Ariti CA, McMurray JJ, et al. Predicting survival in heart failure: a risk score based on 39 372 patients from 30 studies. Eur Heart J 2013; 34(19):1404–13.

62. Canepa M, Fonseca C, Chioncel O, et al. Performance of prognostic risk scores in chronic heart failure patients enrolled in the European Society of Cardiology Heart Failure long-term registry. JACC Heart Fail 2018;6(6):452–62.

63. Freitas P, Aguiar C, Ferreira A, et al. Comparative analysis of four scores to stratify patients with heart failure and reduced ejection fraction. Am J Cardiol 2017;120(3):443–9.

64. Agostoni P, Paolillo S, Mapelli M, et al. Multiparametric prognostic scores in chronic heart failure with reduced ejection fraction: a long-term comparison. Eur J Heart Fail 2018;20(4):700–10.

65. Kouwert IJ, Bakker EA, Cramer MJ, et al. Comparison of MAGGIC and MECKI risk scores to predict mortality after cardiac rehabilitation among Dutch heart failure patients. Eur J Prev Cardiol 2020; 27(19):2126–30.

Right Heart Catheterization in Patients with Advanced Heart Failure
When to Perform? How to Interpret?

Michelle M. Kittleson, MD, PhD[a], Paola Prestinenzi, MD[b],
Luciano Potena, MD, PhD[b],*

KEYWORDS

• Right heart catheterization • Advanced heart failure • Cardiogenic shock

KEY POINTS

- Cardiogenic shock is a critical and deadly condition that requires accurate diagnosis, prompt and tailored therapeutic approach, careful monitoring of evolution, and response to initial therapy. In this setting, right heart catheterization (RHC) is a critical tool to diagnose shock subtype and monitor shock evolution, in particular the need for mechanical circulatory support. In acute heart failure (HF) with no clinical signs of shock, RHC may help to guide therapy and to uncover unusual mechanisms of HF and lack to therapy response (eg, constrictive/restrictive physiology).
- RHC is an essential component of the evaluation of patients for advanced HF therapies to both determine whether patients are limited enough to warrant consideration of heart transplant, justify the priority with which patients are listed, and to determine if there is pulmonary hypertension that may preclude or warrant optimization before heart transplantation.
- RHC is helpful to clarify the indication for durable mechanical circulatory support implantation. In particular, the RHC is used to evaluate right ventricular function before implantation and to optimize the level of pump support.
- Remote monitoring of pulmonary artery pressures with an implantable device reduces HF hospitalizations in patients with symptomatic HF regardless of ejection fraction.

INTRODUCTION

The first right heart catheterization (RHC) was performed by Werner Forssman, on himself, in 1929.[1] He inserted a cannula into his own antecubital vein through which he passed a catheter for 65 cm and then walked to the X-ray department, where a photograph was taken of the catheter in his right atrium. Although he went on to a career in urology, he was awarded the Nobel Prize for Medicine or Physiology in 1956 along with André Frédéric Cournand and Dickinson W. Richards "for their discoveries concerning heart catheterization and pathologic changes in the circulatory system."

Although Dr Forssman demonstrated the feasibility of this technique, it was not until 1970 that the procedure was refined for safe and routine clinical use. Jeremy Swan and William Ganz, through a combination of ingenuity, persistence, and serendipity,[2] pioneered the development of the pulmonary artery catheter (PAC) which could measure intracardiac pressures as well as cardiac output (CO)[3] and led to the development of the Forrester classification of heart failure (HF) based

[a] Department of Cardiology, Smidt Heart Institute, Cedars-Sinai, Los Angeles, CA, USA; [b] Heart Failure and Heart Transplant Program, IRCCS Policlinico di Sant'Orsola, Building 25 via Massarenti, 9, 40138 Bologna, Italy
* Corresponding author.
E-mail address: luciano.potena2@unibo.it

Heart Failure Clin 17 (2021) 647–660
https://doi.org/10.1016/j.hfc.2021.05.009
1551-7136/21/© 2021 Elsevier Inc. All rights reserved.

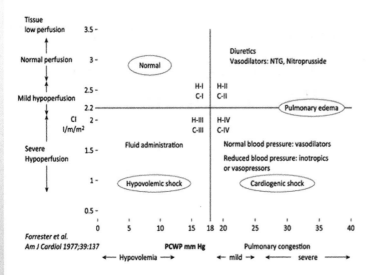

Fig. 1. Clinical classification of the mode of heart failure (Forrester classification). H I-IV refers to hemodynamic severity, with reference figures for CI and pulmonary capillary pressures shown on the vertical and horizontal axes, respectively. C I-IV refers to clinical severity. CI, cardiac index; NTG, nitroglycerin; PCWP, pulmonary capillary wedge pressure. (*From* Nieminen MS, Böhm M, Cowie MR, Drexler H, Filippatos GS, Jondeau G, et al. Executive summary of the guidelines on the diagnosis and treatment of acute heart failure: the Task Force on Acute Heart Failure of the European Society of Cardiology. Eur Heart J. 2005 Feb;26(4):384–416; with permission.)

on cardiac function, hemodynamic thresholds, and clinical presentation (**Fig. 1**).[4,5]

The current HF guidelines from both the American College of Cardiology (ACC)/American Heart Association (AHA),[6] as well as from the European Society of Cardiology (ESC),[7] offer recommended indications for RHC (**Table 1**). The ACC/AHA Guidelines recommend invasive hemodynamic monitoring with a PAC in patients who have respiratory distress or clinical evidence of impaired perfusion in whom the adequacy or excess of intracardiac filling pressures cannot be determined from clinical assessment. The ACC/AHA Guidelines note that invasive hemodynamic monitoring can be useful for carefully selected patients with acute HF who have persistent symptoms despite empirical adjustment of standard therapies and whose fluid status, perfusion, or systemic or pulmonary vascular resistance (PVR) is uncertain; whose systolic pressure remains low or is associated with symptoms, despite initial therapy; whose renal function is worsening with therapy; who require parenteral vasoactive agents; or who may need consideration for mechanical circulatory support (MCS) or transplantation. The ESC Guidelines are similar, also noting that RHC with a PAC should be considered in patients with probable pulmonary hypertension assessed by echocardiography to confirm pulmonary hypertension and its reversibility before the correction of valve/structural heart disease.

Thus, RHC is an established cornerstone of advanced HF management because a clear understanding of the patient's hemodynamic status offers insight into diagnosis, prognosis, and management. In this review, the authors will describe the role of RHC in the diagnosis and management

of shock, in the assessment of heart transplant candidacy, in the context of left ventricular assist devices, and also explore future directions of implantable monitoring devices for pulmonary artery (PA) and left atrial pressure monitoring.

RIGHT HEART CATHETERIZATION: BEST PRACTICES

RHC may be performed via central veins including the internal jugular, subclavian, femoral, or a large peripheral vein such as the brachial vein. Information obtained includes right atrial (RA) pressure, PA systolic and diastolic pressure, pulmonary capillary wedge pressure (PCWP), and CO via the Fick and thermodilution methods. Oxygen saturation of blood from the superior and inferior vena cava, RA, right ventricle (RV), and PA can also be obtained to assess for intracardiac shunts, although shunt interpretation is generally not performed as part of the assessment of advanced HF and beyond the scope of this review.

Best practices for RHC, including performing of the procedure and interpretation of the results, are summarized in **Table 2**. In addition to inspecting the waveform to determine current location of the catheter, operators should examine the pressure tracing quality looking carefully for signs of overdampening or underdampening; examples of the PA pressure tracings are shown in **Fig. 2**.

Methods to Estimate Cardiac Index and Its Interpretation

Cardiac index (CI; CO indexed to body surface area) can be measured by either the Fick method or thermodilution. The direct Fick method is the

Table 1
Guideline-directed indications for right heart catheterization

2013 American College of Cardiology/American Heart Association Guidelines[6]	2016 European Society of Cardiology Guidelines[7]
Class 1	
Invasive hemodynamic monitoring with a PAC should be performed to guide therapy in patients who have respiratory distress or clinical evidence of impaired perfusion in whom the adequacy or excess of intracardiac filling pressures cannot be determined from clinical assessment.	RHC with a PAC is recommended in patients with severe HF being evaluated for heart transplantation or mechanical circulatory support.
Class 2a	
Invasive hemodynamic monitoring can be useful for carefully selected patients with acute HF who have: • Persistent symptoms despite empirical adjustment of standard therapies and whose fluid status, perfusion, or systemic or pulmonary vascular resistance is uncertain; • Whose systolic pressure remains low, or is associated with symptoms, despite initial therapy; • Whose renal function is worsening with therapy; • Who require parenteral vasoactive agents; or • Who may need consideration for MCS or transplantation.	RHC with a PAC should be considered in patients with probable pulmonary hypertension assessed by echocardiography in order to confirm pulmonary hypertension and its reversibility before the correction of valve/structural heart disease
Class 2b	PAC may be considered in patients who, despite pharmacologic treatment, present refractory symptoms (particularly with hypotension and hypoperfusion) and may be considered to adjust therapy in patients with HF who remain severely symptomatic despite initial standard therapies and whose hemodynamic status is unclear
Class III: No benefit	
Routine use of invasive hemodynamic monitoring is not recommended in normotensive patients with acute decompensated HF and congestion with symptomatic response to diuretics and vasodilators.	

Class 1 denotes interventions that are indicated; Class 2a denotes interventions that may be useful; Class 2b denotes interventions that might be useful, and Class 3 denotes contraindications.

gold standard for determining CI but requires specialized equipment to directly measure oxygen consumption. Therefore, thermodilution and the indirect Fick methods are used more commonly. The indirect Fick method relies on estimated values for total body oxygen consumption, which is often inaccurate in patients with HF, pulmonary hypertension, and obesity.[8] Although thermodilution is perceived to be less accurate in the setting of tricuspid regurgitation and low CI, there is good correlation between thermodilution and direct Fick under these circumstances.[9] In contrast, an analysis of greater than 15,000 patients undergoing

RHC confirmed a poor correlation between thermodilution and indirect Fick methods ($r = 0.65$).[10] Thus, thermodilution is generally the preferred method of measuring CI with the exception of patients with intracardiac shunts. On the other hand, Fick method, relying on the measurement of mixed venous blood oxygen saturation (MvO2), may provide better reliability for continuous monitoring of estimated CI.

A decreased MvO2 is a sensitive marker of decreased CO because it reflects the balance between oxygen delivery and oxygen consumption. The MvO2 decreases in low-CO states

Table 2
Best practices for performing and interpreting the right heart catheterization

Preparation	1. Review patient characteristics and imaging to understand pretest probability of various diagnoses. Confirm hemodynamic findings fit the clinical scenario. 2. Operators should have an unobstructed view of hemodynamic monitors and real-time ECG.
Patient positioning	Supine position with legs flat; avoid recording while patient is talking, coughing, or under duress.
Sedation	Minimize systemic sedation when possible to avoid altered breathing patterns.
Leveling	Pressure transducer should be zeroed to atmospheric pressure at level of left atrium (halfway between the anterior sternum and table surface).
Tracing quality	Watch for signs of overdampening or underdampening (see **Fig. 2**). If underdampening is present, catheter ringing can be reduced by introducing a small amount of blood or contrast into the fluid filled catheter.
Respiratory cycle considerations	1. Pressure measurements should be recorded during spontaneous breathing without breath-hold maneuvers (due to concern for inadvertent Valsalva and preload alteration). 2. If Cheyne-Stokes breathing is present, operators should measure each pressure value during the same phase of the breath cycle. 3. End-expiratory measures are preferred for most situations.
PCWP measurement	1. Confirm complete PA occlusion with measurement of PCWP SaO_2 (should be >90–95% as reflective of post-capillary bed). 2. Report presence of large v waves suggestive of left heart disease and/or mitral regurgitation. 3. Mean PCWP throughout the cardiac cycle is accurate unless there are large v waves; in this situation, average the peak and trough of the a-wave of PCWP.
Cardiac output measurement	In the absence of intracardiac shunting, thermodilution is preferred over indirect Fick for estimation of cardiac output and associated hemodynamic calculation.

Abbreviations: ECG, electrocardiogram; LHD, left heart disease; SaO_2, mixed venous oxyhemoglobin saturation.
Adapted from Maron Bradley A., Kovacs Gabor, Vaidya Anjali, Bhatt Deepak L., Nishimura Rick A., Mak Susanna, et al. Cardiopulmonary Hemodynamics in Pulmonary Hypertension and Heart Failure. Journal of the American College of Cardiology. 2020 Dec 1;76(22):2671–81; with permission.

because of prolonged transit time of the blood in the peripheral vasculature and subsequent extraction of more O2. MvO2 of ≤50% suggest a critical PvO2 of 26 mm Hg—a level where tissue hypoxia likely present (a typical finding in pure cardiogenic shock [CS]). MvO2 of greater than 70% corresponds with high-flow states, and failure of peripheral tissues to extract oxygen and microcirculatory shunt that are present results in states of sepsis, hyperthyroidism, and severe liver disease and is a hallmark of pure distributive shock. Very high values of MvO2 (>90%) have been associated with worse outcomes.[11] MvO2 is therefore useful for diagnosing causes of shock and for trending values in individual patient. However, as a treatment target, normalizing MvO2 does not improve outcomes in critically ill patients.[12] MvO2 values however should be interpreted in light of hemoglobin concentration, ventilator parameters of the patient, and the body surface area. Anemia is associated with reduced MvO2, unless it leads to hyperdynamic circulatory state and then to high-output HF. MvO2 increases with increasing the Fio_2, and high levels of Fio_2 can increase the MvO2 to normal levels in low-output states. This is at least in part due to high arterial dissolved oxygen level and masks the tissue hypoxia. Therefore, Pao_2 should not be overlooked when assessing MvO2.[13]

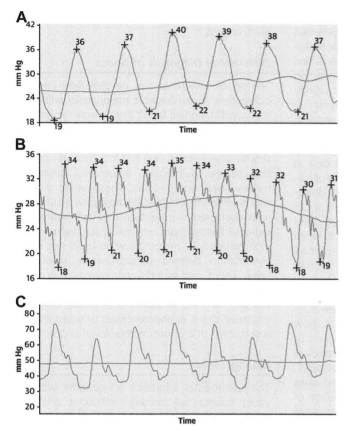

Fig. 2. Pulmonary artery pressure waveforms. (*A*) Overdampening. Note that the characteristic dicrotic notch is not seen. Overdampening occurs when air is introduced into the catheter or tubing and may result in reduction of the overall amplitude of the pressure tracing (mean pressure is usually not affected). This can be addressed by flushing the catheter or tubing. (*B*) Underdampening. Also called catheter ringing, this occurs when the frequency of the transmitted waveform (heart rate) approximates the natural resonance frequency of the transducer system. This falsely increases the amplitude of the waveform. Similar to overdampening, mean pressure is usually not affected. Ringing artifact may be reduced by introducing a small amount of a denser fluid, such as blood or contrast, into the catheter, with careful attention not to overdamp the signal. (*C*) Example of an optimal pulmonary artery pressure waveform with preserved dicrotic notch but minimal systolic and diastolic ringing artifact. (*From* Maron Bradley A., Kovacs Gabor, Vaidya Anjali, Bhatt Deepak L., Nishimura Rick A., Mak Susanna, et al. Cardiopulmonary Hemodynamics in Pulmonary Hypertension and Heart Failure. Journal of the American College of Cardiology. 2020 Dec 1;76(22):2671–81; with permission.)

Central venous oxygen saturation (ScvO2) is often used a surrogate for MvO2 because it is measured form any central venous catheter without the need for PAC. It contains only superior vena cava blood; hence, the normal values are lower than MvO2. It is not equivalent to nor does it predict the MvO2,[14–17] but the degree and direction of changes in ScvO2 do correlate with MvO2.[18]

Interpretation of the Pulmonary Capillary Wedge Pressure

In most situations, the PCWP should be recorded at end-expiration although without breath-hold maneuvers that can prompt Valsalva physiology. At end-expiration, intrathoracic pressure closely approximates zero and thus exerts minimal influence on intracardiac pressures. Because the mitral valve is open at end-diastole, left atrial pressure (and PCWP) should be equal to left ventricular end-diastolic pressure (LVEDP) in the absence of mitral stenosis. Because the c-wave (mitral valve closure) may be difficult to identify on the PCWP tracing, the peak and trough of the a-wave is averaged and correlates with the pre–c-wave value (**Fig. 3**). This value is the best estimate of LVEDP. However, mean PCWP, or PCWP averaged over

the cardiac cycle which encompasses the pressure waveform during both systole and diastole, generally approximates end-diastolic PCWP as an accurate estimation of LVEDP. However, the presence of large v waves (from mitral regurgitation or left heart disease) or atrial fibrillation often leads to a mean PCWP that is greater than the end-diastolic PCWP, and in this situation, the a-wave of the PCWP tracing should be measured. Finally, whenever the PCWP tracing morphology is atypical, the PCWP blood sample oxyhemoglobin saturation content should be analyzed. A truly wedged catheter will yield a mixed venous oxyhemoglobin saturation reflective of the postcapillary pulmonary bed, typically greater than 90% to 95%. Lower values should prompt repeat attempts to wedge, including alternate vascular areas or consideration of direct left ventrilicle measurement.[19]

CLINICAL APPLICATIONS OF RIGHT HEART CATHETERIZATION
Cardiogenic Shock

CS is a condition of low CO caused by impaired ventricular function and associated with signs of hypoperfusion, which may progress to multiorgan failure. In-hospital mortality for CS ranges between 40% and 60% and except for primary percutaneous coronary intervention for ST-elevation myocardial infarction, no therapeutic intervention has demonstrated efficacy in reducing mortality in CS.[20] In this context, appropriate and timely diagnosis for CS, and for the conditions preceding CS, is crucial to identify patients requiring specific approaches to support the circulation. Systemic hypotension and low CI are usually included in the definition, along with variable indicators of peripheral hypoperfusion.[21] However, a recent document providing a comprehensive definition of CS strata[22] supports the concept that low blood pressure is not always required to diagnose CS, while in the context of patients with chronic advanced HF who may slowly slide toward CS, it is challenging to assess hypoperfusion.

PAC monitoring facilitates triage and management of patients presenting with acute hemodynamic decompensation. Specifically, PACs allow operators to assess the relative contributions of right and left ventricular failure to guide medical therapy with vasoactive medications, inotropes, and MCS device(s) for CS.[23] PAC-derived data may significantly improve the understanding of the current hemodynamic conditions over what can be gained by physical examination only: Physicians predict CO in critically ill patients with only around 50% accuracy in the absence of direct hemodynamic data.[24–26] Despite the absence of randomized controlled trials of PACs in CS, registry analyses indicate that patients in CS with no PAC assessment had a higher in-hospital mortality than those with complete PAC assessment, indicating that knowledge of hemodynamic profiles may guide appropriate therapeutic interventions.[27–29]

Differential Diagnosis of Shock

The shock syndrome can be classified into four categories: 1) cardiogenic (myocardial infarction, myocarditis, and so forth); 2) hypovolemic (hemorrhage, dehydration, and so forth); 3) distributive (sepsis, systemic inflammatory response syndrome, anaphylaxis, and so forth); and 4) obstructive (acute pulmonary embolism, pulmonary hypertension, and so forth). The clinical presentation is often similar between the subtypes of shock with sustained hypotension and symptoms and signs of tissue hypoperfusion (cold clammy skin, high lactate >2.2 mmol/L, and so forth) and organ dysfunction (altered consciousness level, low urine output, and so forth), but each type is distinguished by a unique hemodynamic profile (**Table 3**). The PAC is essential in cases when the cause of shock is undetermined or when there is a suspicion of a mixed/multifactorial shock.

Management

The therapeutic approach to patients with CS varies substantially among institutions and clinicians. In general terms, the PAC in CS can be used to ensure that filling pressures are adequate, to guide changes in therapy and to assess the responses to treatment modifications (for example, to establish the relationship of filling pressures to the CO in the individual patient).

Pure cardiogenic shock

In cases of pure CS, the role of PAC could be limited to be used in patients who do not respond

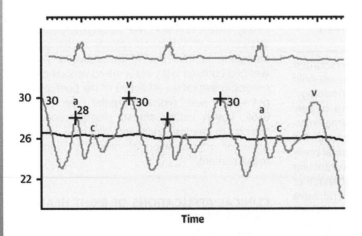

Fig. 3. Typical pulmonary capillary wedge pressure (PCWP) tracing. A-, c-, and v-waves as noted in red. End-diastole occurs just before the c-wave, and thus, pressure at this point correlates best with left ventricular end-diastolic pressure. When the c-wave is not well seen, averaging the peak and trough of the a-wave is recommended. In this example, the v-wave is normal amplitude. Mean PCWP (*black horizontal line*), which is an average pressure over the entire cardiac cycle, is essentially equal to end-diastolic PCWP. (*From* Maron Bradley A., Kovacs Gabor, Vaidya Anjali, Bhatt Deepak L., Nishimura Rick A., Mak Susanna, et al. Cardiopulmonary Hemodynamics in Pulmonary Hypertension and Heart Failure. Journal of the American College of Cardiology. 2020 Dec 1;76(22):2671–81; with permission.)

Table 3
Characteristics of shock subtypes

Type of Shock	PCWP	CO	SVR	MvO2 (%)
Hypovolemic	↓	← →, late↓	↑	>65 early <65 late
Distributive	← →,↓	↑ (usually)	↓	>65 (>90 worse outcomes)
Obstructive	← →,↓	← →, late↓	↑	>65
Cardiogenic	↑	↓	↑	<65
Mixed cardiogenic + distributive	Normal	Normal?	↓	Normal

to initial therapy. In general, patients with pure CS present as "cold and wet" (cool extremities and pulmonary congestion), and these features are reflected on PAC as reduced CI, increased systemic vascular resistance (SVR), and increased PCWP.

Mixed shock

An essential role of PAC for diagnosis and management is in cases of mixed type of shock that commonly affects patients with chronic HF when an inflammatory reaction triggers an acute admission. This type of shock where HF accompanied by systemic inflammatory response syndrome (mixed cardiogenic—distributive) is often underrecognized and undertreated without the PAC findings. Clinically, fever is not a consistent sign, and leukocytosis and elevation of inflammatory markers is not specific. Patients present as "wet and warm" which reflects a reduced CI, low-to-normal SVR, and an elevated PCWP. The patients with CS and inappropriately low SVR due to systemic inflammation that can progress to overt sepsis at baseline are at higher risk of mortality.[30]

RIGHT HEART CATHETERIZATION IN ACUTE HEART FAILURE

While in CS, the use of a PAC may provide some benefit for diagnosis and management, its routine use is not recommended in acute decompensation without shock based on a pivotal randomized trial which demonstrated potential harm of routine PAC monitoring in this setting.[31-33] These findings were confirmed by other registries, although there may have been confounding by indication, as sicker patients tend to receive PAC monitoring.[29] Nevertheless, in selected cases, PAC-derived hemodynamic profiles may have a relevant clinical utility.[34,35]

Diagnosis

The diagnosis of acutely decompensated HF can be often made with clinical, laboratory, and imaging data without the need for PAC. The use for diagnostic purpose should be limited only to cases when the diagnosis is uncertain (eg, restrictive cardiomyopathy vs constrictive pericarditis) and in selected cases of hemodynamically unstable patients with an unknown mechanism of deterioration.

In HF patients, it is important to differentiate patients with pre-existing heart disease with another illness that acts as a triggering factor for acute decompensation (eg, infection, acute renal failure, bleeding) from those without pre-existing heart disease who present with new-onset acute HF. Patients in the first group potentially could present more diagnostic uncertainties and may benefit from PAC to refine diagnosis and guide management at early stages.

Management

Initial treatment of acute heart failure is always targeted at achieving decongestion and maintenance of blood pressure without tissue hypoperfusion using diuretics and vasodilators. PAC can be considered in situations when direct information about volume status, intracardiac filling pressures, vascular resistance, and CO are clinically indeterminate, and for those refractory to initial therapy. These situations are becoming more frequent with increasing prevalence of comorbidities such as chronic kidney disease and pre-existing heart or pulmonary disease.

PAC-guided management should be considered in cases of

- No response to initial intravenous diuretics or a blunted response to diuretics in patients with significant renal dysfunction
- Worsening renal function when central hemodynamics are difficult to assess clinically
- Respiratory distress when central hemodynamics cannot be determined from clinical assessment (eg, to differentiate a "white lung" due to cardiogenic causes and noncardiogenic causes (ARDS) often difficult do differentiate on clinical and radiological criteria

- Right-sided congestion with uncertain central volume status
- Persistent hypotension and/or hypoperfusion despite increasing doses of parenteral vaso-active agents (the threshold and timing subject to clinical judgment and local protocols)

PAC in AHF management helps to identify early patients in the preshock phase and to classify the CS severity stages SCAI A-E.[22] In addition, it allows a full hemodynamic assessment for the timely initiation, choice, optimization, and escalation of MCS. The widespread availability of short-term percutaneous MCS devices has led to proposed management algorithms guided by PAC-derived invasive hemodynamic data in attempts to standardize patient care.[36,37]

AHF patients in whom diagnosis is made with clinical, laboratory, and imaging studies and their hospital course is uncomplicated with symptomatic response to diuretics and vasodilators do not need a PAC as a part of routine care.

RIGHT HEART CATHETERIZATION IN THE EVALUATION FOR ADVANCED HEART FAILURE THERAPIES
Indications

The 2016 Listing Criteria from the International Society of Heart and Lung Transplantation recommend that RHC should be performed on all adult heart transplant and durable MCS candidates.[38,39] The purpose of the RHC is two-fold: first, to evaluate the degree of decompensation as confirmation that evaluation for heart transplantation or durable MCS is warranted; and second, to assess the presence of potentially prohibitive pulmonary arterial hypertension, or of severe impairment of RV function.

Role of the Cardiac Index in Heart Transplant Evaluation

When elective RHC is performed in potential heart transplant candidates, the CI is a critical measurement to judge the degree of decompensation and, as described previously, guide administration of inotropic support if CS is present. In addition, the CI plays a major role in determining the heart transplant listing priority in the United Network of Organ Sharing allocation criteria in the United States. However, as CI may vary by the method used for measurement,[10] there is some evidence that the documentation of CI for the purposes of heart transplant listing may be influenced by the desire to justify a higher listing status and thus decrease wait time for a given heart transplant candidate.[40]

Role of the Pulmonary Artery Pressures in Heart Transplant Evaluation

Pulmonary hypertension from chronic elevation of LVEDP is a common complication of long-standing HF and, if unrecognized and untreated, can result in irreversible changes to the pulmonary vasculature.[41] Because a normal donor RV is unable to increase its external workload acutely to overcome elevated PVR, acute RV failure and CS may result early after transplant.[42] Elevated PVR remains a strong risk factor for RV failure and early postoperative mortality in the modern era.[43] Specifically, PA systolic pressure $\geq$60 mm Hg, PVR $\geq$5 Wood units, and transpulmonary gradient (mean PA pressure minus PCWP) $\geq$15–20 mm Hg are considered prohibitive for transplantation. The indications for and interpretation of the vasodilator challenge are shown in **Fig. 4**. If measures to reduce PA pressures, including diuretics, nitroprusside, milrinone, dobutamine, or inhaled nitric oxide, fail, temporary or durable MCS may be indicated for longer term unloading.[44,45]

RIGHT HEART CATHETERIZATION AND LEFT VENTRICULAR ASSIST DEVICES

RHC is crucial to confirm the clinical indication for LVAD which is determined by various parameters including low CO, reduced SvO2, and increased PCWP, despite optimized medical therapy. In particular, the RHC allows identification of the 3 major subtypes of cardiac decompensation to tailor appropriate therapies for each patients[46–51]: 1) LV-dominant (CVP<14, PCWP>18, CVP/PCWP<.86, pulmonary artery pulsatility index [PAPi]>1.5); 2) RV-dominant (CVP>14, PCWP<18, CVP/PCWP>.86, PAPi<1.5); or 3) biventricular (CVP>14, CVP/PCWP>.86, PAPi<1.5).

The classification scheme is relevant because LVAD efficacy relies on RV function for adequate preload, and post-LVAD right ventricular failure is a major cause of short- and long-term morbidity (longer ICU and hospital stay, hypotension with systemic hypoperfusion, renal failure, bleeding, recurrent hospitalizations) and mortality.[52–59] Clinically, RV function assessment in the setting of severe LV dysfunction is difficult. As expected, late clinical signs of advanced RV dysfunction such as severe tricuspid regurgitation, ascites, or increased bilirubin are risk factors for death after LVAD implantation.[58] Thus, LVAD support ideally should be implemented before significant RV failure develops. Therefore, the thorough preoperative characterization of RV function and predictors of RV function during LVAD support

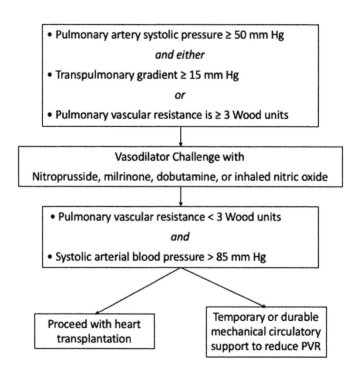

- Pulmonary artery systolic pressure ≥ 50 mm Hg

  and either

- Transpulmonary gradient ≥ 15 mm Hg

  or

- Pulmonary vascular resistance is ≥ 3 Wood units

↓

Vasodilator Challenge with
Nitroprusside, milrinone, dobutamine, or inhaled nitric oxide

↓

- Pulmonary vascular resistance < 3 Wood units

  and

- Systolic arterial blood pressure > 85 mm Hg

Proceed with heart transplantation   ←   Temporary or durable mechanical circulatory support to reduce PVR

Fig. 4. Management of pulmonary hypertension in a potential heart transplant candidate. If there is evidence of significant pulmonary hypertension, vasodilator challenge is indicated. If pharmacologic therapy fails, temporary or durable mechanical circulatory support may be required for left ventricular unloading.

for appropriate patient selection is of key importance in improving outcomes after LVAD.[60]

Invasive Assessment of Right Ventricle Systolic Function

There is no consensus on the RV function assessment before LVAD implantation. Several parameters and indices however have been shown to be predictive of RVF after LVAD implantation and are used in clinical practice.

Pulmonary vascular resistance

In some early studies, higher PVR was an independent predictor of RVF after LVAD implantation[56,61] because, theoretically, patients with higher PVR might be less likely to have an improvement in RV output/forward flow when the LV is decompressed, but its drawback as a parameter include the fact that it is inversely proportional to CO (calculated as [mPAP − PCWP]/CO x80); hence, it is significantly reduced by LVAD-induced increase in CO (if occurred). Of note, LVAD therapy can lead to reduction of PVR and restore candidacy for transplantation so elevated PVR may be itself an indication for LVAD.[45]

Right atrial pressure to pulmonary capillary wedge pressure ratio

Increased RAP to PCWP ratio was associated with worsening RV function, higher PVR, and an increased risk of adverse outcomes in HF

populations.[62,63] However, in the setting of pre-LVAD candidates, the evidence supporting this indicator as a risk factor for post-LVAD RF is inconsistent.[64,65]

Right ventricular stroke work index (RVSWI) calculated by the following formula, 0.0136 × stroke volume index × (mean PA pressure − RA pressure) with SVi calculated as CI by the Fick method divided by heart rate, reflects RV contractility. Low RVSWI predicts RVF after LVAD implantation,[66,67] but this indicator has potential drawbacks as it is derived from multiple measured parameters (prone to more error), is preload-dependent,[68] and has less predictive accuracy in patients implanted with continuous-flow versus pulsatile-flow LVADs (the former more commonly used).[67]

Both indices (RAP to PCWP ratio and RVSWI) depend largely on the RV preload and are influenced by the filling pressures, volume overload, and the presence of severe MR, which increases mean PCWP, so they need to be measured for predictive purpose on medically optimized patients (inotropes/vasodilators).

PAPi is defined as the ratio of PA pulse pressure to RA pressure and has recently emerged as an independent predictor of RVF after LVAD implantation. Notably, its predictive value exceeds that of traditional indices such as RAP:PCWP and RVSWI.[50,69] Its major strength is that it represents a pure right-sided hemodynamic effectiveness measure without the influence of the left heart. It predicts RVF better in patients who are on inotropes pre-LVAD implantation (partially because the commonly used inotropes unload the LV and lower PCWP and increase CI, all of which influence CVP/PCWP and RVSWi making them less predictive of RVF in that cohort).[51]

Pulmonary Artery Catheter After LVAD Implantation

Invasive hemodynamic assessment is particularly important in LVAD patients for whom device speed optimization may be dependent on measured CO. There is currently no gold standard for CO assessment after LVAD. A clinically relevant discrepancy in CO measurements between the indirect Fick CO versus termodilution method CO in LVAD patients with a bias of -0.72 L/min[70] has been shown, but it is not clear which method is superior. The reasons for this large discrepancy are uncertain, but as none of the methods measure CO directly, they are both prone to error. TD either overestimates CO in the setting of heat loss with low flow conditions, but this should not be present in LVAD-normalized CO or underestimates in the presence of TR. Continuous rather than pulsatile flow in LVAD patients could also contribute to the error in CO calculations. The changes in iFick CO underestimated CO compared with the flow reported from the outflow cannula, but the changes correlated well especially after closure of the aortic valve (AV).[71] The formulas of V_{O_2} estimation may not apply in LVAD populations and the gold standard of direct oxygen consumption measuring by calorimetry or could be more accurate but is difficult to achieve in day-to-day practice. Overall, more studies comparing different methods of CO evaluation (invasive and noninvasive) in LVAD population are needed, meanwhile the iFick method can be recommended over TD for measurements of CO in patients with LVADs.

Optimizing/Ramp Testing

LVAD therapy requires regular evaluation and optimization of hemodynamics with a standardized hemodynamic ramp protocol. Ramp testing is performed periodically for every LVAD patient (with the first one ideally more than 1 month after implantation in stable patients) and combines hemodynamic and echocardiographic parameters to optimize the performance of the device.

Various ramp testing protocols exist, but they all follow the same scheme: measurement at baseline LVAD speed the LV end-systolic dimension, LV end-diastolic dimension (interventricular septum position), the frequency of AV opening, and the degree of MR and AV regurgitation and PAC-derived filling pressures and CO (TD and Fick). After these measurements, the LVAD speed is modified (increased or decreased) by 100 rpm (HVAD) and 400 rpm (HMT III). The aforementioned echocardiographic and hemodynamic parameters are measured at each LVAD speed repeating all the echo and PAC measures. The ramp test is terminated when LV end-diastolic dimension is less than 3.0 cm or a significant suction event occurs. At the conclusion, LVAD speed is set targeting CVP less than 12 mm Hg and PCWP less than 18 mm Hg with the secondary goal of allowing intermittent AV opening and minimal MR.[72] LVAD patients in whom hemodynamics were optimized using a standardized protocol had significantly lower rate of hospital readmissions, primarily because of reduction of HF admissions.[73]

Beyond Right Heart Catheterization

Remote hemodynamic monitoring

In addition to invasive assessment of cardiac hemodynamics, there now exist sophisticated remote monitoring technologies that rely on implantable intracardiac devices to directly measure cardiac pressures. The two most widely studied wireless implantable hemodynamic monitors are a PA pressure monitor (CardioMEMS; CardioMEMS HF System, Abbott, Atlanta, GA), comprising a lead-less, battery-less pressure sensor percutaneously implanted in the PA, which remotely transmits PA pressure measurements, and a left atrial pressure transducer (HeartPOD device; HeartPOD, Savacor, Inc, from St Jude Medical, Inc, Minneapolis, Minnesota, USA) placed percutaneously via transseptal puncture within the interatrial septum with a communications module placed in a subcutaneous pocket.

To date, left atrial pressure transducers have not demonstrated clinical benefit. In LAPTOP-HF, patients transmitted left atrial pressure measurements and were instructed to adjust diuretic and vasodilator therapy based on a prespecified algorithm. While there was a reduction in HF hospitalizations in the intervention group, the study was terminated early by the data safety monitoring board because of several implant-related trans-septal complications, including cardiac perforations that required pericardiocentesis or surgical repair.[74]

In contrast, in the CHAMPION-HF trial, patients with symptomatic HF regardless of ejection fraction randomized to PA pressure monitoring versus usual care had a 37% reduction in HF hospitalizations over 15 months.[75] This benefit was noted in post-hoc analyses of patients with HF with both preserved[76] and reduced ejection fraction.[77] PA-pressing monitoring also reduces HF hospitalizations in routine clinical practice.[78–80] In one study, the mean rate of daily pressure transmission was 76%, suggesting that patient adherence to monitoring may be one component of its success.[80]

The CardioMEMS device is currently approved by the United States Food and Drug Administration to wirelessly monitor PA pressure and heart rate in New York Heart Association Class III patients who have been hospitalized for HF in the previous year. The Hemodynamic-GUIDED Management of HF (GUIDE-HF) trial (NCT03387813) is a prospective trial with a planned enrollment of 3600 patients with HF, regardless of ejection fraction, with either a history of an HF hospitalization in the preceding 12 months and/or an elevated N-terminal pro-b-type natriuretic peptide or b-type natriuretic peptide. GUIDE-HF will determine if the benefit of CardioMEMS-guided therapy extends to Class II and IV patients as well as those who have not been hospitalized within the past year; the projected completion date is April 2023.[81]

SUMMARY

The past few decades have resulted in remarkable advances in the use of RHC in the diagnosis and management of shock and advanced HF. Future advances will include refinement of the indications for use in patients with shock, HF with preserved ejection fraction, and pulmonary hypertension. Finally, the use of implantable hemodynamic monitors will allow the lessons learned from invasive RHC to be translated into outpatient clinical practice.

CLINICS CARE POINTS

- When patients have respiratory distress or clinical evidence of impaired perfusion and intracardiac filling pressures cannot be determined from clinical assessment, a pulmonary artery catheter (PAC) can be useful to diagnose the degree of cardiac decompensation.
- When interpreting the findings of right heart catheterization, examine the pressure-tracing quality for signs of overdampening or underdampening.
- Thermodilution is generally the preferred method of measuring cardiac index with the exception of patients with intracardiac shunts.

- Indirect Fick method based on mixed venous oxygen saturation may be preferred to continuously monitor cardiac output in intensive care unit setting.
- Monitoring of central venous pressure by a central line and assessment of lactate concentration and superior vena cava oxygen saturation provide an adequate surrogate for assessing cardiac output, filling pressure, and perfusion state when PAC is not available.
- A truly wedged catheter will yield a mixed venous oxyhemoglobin saturation reflective of the postcapillary pulmonary bed, typically greater than 90% to 95%. Lower values should prompt repeat attempts to wedge, including alternate vascular areas or consideration of direct LV measurement.
- Mean pulmonary wedge pressure should not exceed by more than 1 to 2 mm Hg diastolic pulmonary pressure unless the patient has significant pulmonary congestion or moderate to severe mitral regurgitation.
- Patients being evaluated for heart transplantation require right heart catheterization to assess the degree of decompensation which impacts the use of intravenous inotropic support and listing status and to assess for potentially prohibitive pulmonary hypertension.
- For patients with heart failure, a wireless implantable pulmonary artery sensor may allow better diuretic titration and reduce heart failure hospitalization.

DISCLOSURE

The authors have nothing to disclose.

REFERENCES

1. Thakkar AB, Desai SP. Swan, Ganz, and Their Catheter: Its Evolution Over the Past Half Century. Ann Intern Med 2018;169(9):636–42.
2. Forrester JS. A Tale of Serendipity, Ingenuity, and Chance: 50th Anniversary of Creation of the Swan-Ganz Catheter. J Am Coll Cardiol 2019;74(1):100–3.
3. Swan HJ, Ganz W, Forrester J, et al. Catheterization of the heart in man with use of a flow-directed balloon-tipped catheter. N Engl J Med 1970; 283(9):447–51.
4. Forrester JS, Diamond G, Chatterjee K, et al. Medical therapy of acute myocardial infarction by application of hemodynamic subsets (first of two parts). N Engl J Med 1976;295(24):1356–62.
5. Nohria A, Tsang SW, Fang JC, et al. Clinical assessment identifies hemodynamic profiles that predict

outcomes in patients admitted with heart failure. J Am Coll Cardiol 2003;41(10):1797–804.

6. Yancy CW, Jessup M, Bozkurt B, et al. 2013 ACCF/ AHA guideline for the management of heart failure: a report of the American College of Cardiology Foundation/American Heart Association Task Force on Practice Guidelines. J Am Coll Cardiol 2013; 62(16):e147–239.

7. Ponikowski P, Voors AA, Anker SD, et al. 2016 ESC Guidelines for the diagnosis and treatment of acute and chronic heart failure: The Task Force for the diagnosis and treatment of acute and chronic heart failure of the European Society of Cardiology (ESC) Developed with the special contribution of the Heart Failure Association (HFA) of the ESC. Eur Heart J 2016;37(27):2129–200.

8. Maron BA, Kovacs G, Vaidya A, et al. Cardiopulmonary Hemodynamics in Pulmonary Hypertension and Heart Failure. J Am Coll Cardiol 2020;76(22): 2671–81.

9. Hoeper MM, Maier R, Tongers J, et al. Determination of cardiac output by the Fick method, thermodilution, and acetylene rebreathing in pulmonary hypertension. Am J Respir Crit Care Med 1999;160(2): 535–41.

10. Opotowsky AR, Hess E, Maron BA, et al. Thermodilution vs Estimated Fick Cardiac Output Measurement in Clinical Practice: An Analysis of Mortality From the Veterans Affairs Clinical Assessment, Reporting, and Tracking (VA CART) Program and Vanderbilt University. JAMA Cardiol 2017;2(10): 1090–9.

11. Pope JV, Jones AE, Gaieski DF, et al. Multicenter study of central venous oxygen saturation (ScvO(2)) as a predictor of mortality in patients with sepsis. Ann Emerg Med 2010;55(1):40–6.e1.

12. Gattinoni L, Brazzi L, Pelosi P, et al. A trial of goal-oriented hemodynamic therapy in critically ill patients. SvO2 Collaborative Group. N Engl J Med 1995;333(16):1025–32.

13. Legrand M, Vallée F, Mateo J, et al. Influence of arterial dissolved oxygen level on venous oxygen saturation: don't forget the PaO2! Shock 2014;41(6): 510–3.

14. Dueck MH, Klimek M, Appenrodt S, et al. Trends but not individual values of central venous oxygen saturation agree with mixed venous oxygen saturation during varying hemodynamic conditions. Anesthesiology 2005;103(2):249–57.

15. Chawla LS, Zia H, Gutierrez G, et al. Lack of equivalence between central and mixed venous oxygen saturation. Chest 2004;126(6):1891–6.

16. Edwards JD, Mayall RM. Importance of the sampling site for measurement of mixed venous oxygen saturation in shock. Crit Care Med 1998;26(8):1356–60.

17. Martin C, Auffray JP, Badetti C, et al. Monitoring of central venous oxygen saturation versus mixed

venous oxygen saturation in critically ill patients. Intensive Care Med 1992;18(2):101–4.

18. Reinhart K, Kuhn H-J, Hartog C, et al. Continuous central venous and pulmonary artery oxygen saturation monitoring in the critically ill. Intensive Care Med 2004;30(8):1572–8.

19. Viray MC, Bonno EL, Gabrielle ND, et al. Role of Pulmonary Artery Wedge Pressure Saturation During Right Heart Catheterization: A Prospective Study. Circ Heart Fail 2020;13(11):e007981.

20. Hochman JS, Sleeper LA, Webb JG, et al. Early revascularization in acute myocardial infarction complicated by cardiogenic shock. SHOCK Investigators. Should We Emergently Revascularize Occluded Coronaries for Cardiogenic Shock. N Engl J Med 1999;341(9):625–34.

21. Tehrani BN, Truesdell AG, Psotka MA, et al. A Standardized and Comprehensive Approach to the Management of Cardiogenic Shock. JACC Heart Fail 2020;8(11):879–91.

22. Baran DA, Grines CL, Bailey S, et al. SCAI clinical expert consensus statement on the classification of cardiogenic shock. Catheter Cardiovasc Interv 2019;94(1):29–37.

23. Sionis A, Rivas-Lasarte M, Mebazaa A, et al. Current Use and Impact on 30-Day Mortality of Pulmonary Artery Catheter in Cardiogenic Shock Patients: Results From the CardShock Study. J Intensive Care Med 2020;35(12):1426–33.

24. Rali AS, Buechler T, Gotten BV, et al. Non-Invasive Cardiac Output Monitoring in Cardiogenic Shock: The NICOM Study. J Card Fail 2020; 26(2):160–5.

25. Eisenberg PR, Jaffe AS, Schuster DP. Clinical evaluation compared to pulmonary artery catheterization in the hemodynamic assessment of critically ill patients. Crit Care Med 1984;12(7):549–53.

26. Mimoz O, Rauss A, Rekik N, et al. Pulmonary artery catheterization in critically ill patients: a prospective analysis of outcome changes associated with catheter-prompted changes in therapy. Crit Care Med 1994;22(4):573–9.

27. Garan AR, Kanwar M, Thayer KL, et al. Complete Hemodynamic Profiling With Pulmonary Artery Catheters in Cardiogenic Shock Is Associated With Lower In-Hospital Mortality. JACC Heart Fail 2020; 8(11):903–13.

28. Chow J, Vadakken M, Whitlock R, et al. Pulmonary artery catheterization in cardiogenic shock: a systematic review and meta-analysis. Can J Cardiol 2020;36(10):S13–4.

29. Hernandez GA, Lemor A, Blumer V, et al. Trends in Utilization and Outcomes of Pulmonary Artery Catheterization in Heart Failure With and Without Cardiogenic Shock. J Card Fail 2019;25(5):364–71.

30. Kohsaka S, Menon V, Lowe AM, et al. Systemic inflammatory response syndrome after acute

myocardial infarction complicated by cardiogenic shock. Arch Intern Med 2005;165(14):1643–50.

31. Binanay C, Califf RM, Hasselblad V, et al. Evaluation study of congestive heart failure and pulmonary artery catheterization effectiveness: the ESCAPE trial. JAMA 2005;294(13):1625–33.

32. Richard C, Warszawski J, Anguel N, et al. Early use of the pulmonary artery catheter and outcomes in patients with shock and acute respiratory distress syndrome: a randomized controlled trial. JAMA 2003;290(20):2713–20.

33. Shah MR, Hasselblad V, Stevenson LW, et al. Impact of the pulmonary artery catheter in critically ill patients: meta-analysis of randomized clinical trials. JAMA 2005;294(13):1664–70.

34. Pandey A, Khera R, Kumar N, et al. Use of Pulmonary Artery Catheterization in US Patients With Heart Failure, 2001-2012. JAMA Intern Med 2016;176(1): 129–32.

35. Ikuta K, Wang Y, Robinson A, et al. National Trends in Use and Outcomes of Pulmonary Artery Catheters Among Medicare Beneficiaries, 1999-2013. JAMA Cardiol 2017 01;2(8):908–13.

36. Basir MB, Kapur NK, Patel K, et al. Improved Outcomes Associated with the use of Shock Protocols: Updates from the National Cardiogenic Shock Initiative. Catheter Cardiovasc Interv 2019;93(7): 1173–83.

37. Tehrani BN, Truesdell AG, Sherwood MW, et al. Standardized Team-Based Care for Cardiogenic Shock. J Am Coll Cardiol 2019;73(13):1659–69.

38. Mehra MR, Canter CE, Hannan MM, et al. The 2016 International Society for Heart Lung Transplantation listing criteria for heart transplantation: A 10-year update. J Heart Lung Transplant 2016;35(1): 1–23.

39. Feldman D, Pamboukian SV, Teuteberg JJ, et al. The 2013 International Society for Heart and Lung Transplantation Guidelines for mechanical circulatory support: executive summary. J Heart Lung Transplant 2013;32(2):157–87.

40. Parker WF, Chung K, Anderson AS, et al. Practice Changes at U.S. Transplant Centers After the New Adult Heart Allocation Policy. J Am Coll Cardiol 2020;75(23):2906–16.

41. Delgado JF, Conde E, Sánchez V, et al. Pulmonary vascular remodeling in pulmonary hypertension due to chronic heart failure. Eur J Heart Fail 2005; 7(6):1011–6.

42. Costard-Jäckle A, Fowler MB. Influence of preoperative pulmonary artery pressure on mortality after heart transplantation: testing of potential reversibility of pulmonary hypertension with nitroprusside is useful in defining a high risk group. J Am Coll Cardiol 1992;19(1):48–54.

43. Khush KK, Cherikh WS, Chambers DC, et al. The International Thoracic Organ Transplant Registry of the International Society for Heart and Lung Transplantation: Thirty-sixth adult heart transplantation report — 2019; focus theme: Donor and recipient size match. J Heart Lung Transplant 2019;38(10): 1056–66.

44. Tsukashita M, Takayama H, Takeda K, et al. Effect of pulmonary vascular resistance before left ventricular assist device implantation on short- and long-term post-transplant survival. J Thorac Cardiovasc Surg 2015;150(5):1352–60, 1361.e1-2.

45. Kutty RS, Parameshwar J, Lewis C, et al. Use of centrifugal left ventricular assist device as a bridge to candidacy in severe heart failure with secondary pulmonary hypertension. Eur J Cardiothorac Surg 2013;43(6):1237–42.

46. van Diepen S, Katz JN, Albert NM, et al. Contemporary Management of Cardiogenic Shock: A Scientific Statement From the American Heart Association. Circulation 2017;136(16):e232–68.

47. Kapur NK, Esposito ML, Bader Y, et al. Mechanical Circulatory Support Devices for Acute Right Ventricular Failure. Circulation 2017;136(3):314–26.

48. Lala A, Guo Y, Xu J, et al. Right Ventricular Dysfunction in Acute Myocardial Infarction Complicated by Cardiogenic Shock: A Hemodynamic Analysis of the Should We Emergently Revascularize Occluded Coronaries for Cardiogenic Shock (SHOCK) Trial and Registry. J Card Fail 2018;24(3):148–56.

49. Korabathina R, Heffernan KS, Paruchuri V, et al. The pulmonary artery pulsatility index identifies severe right ventricular dysfunction in acute inferior myocardial infarction. Catheter Cardiovasc Interv 2012; 80(4):593–600.

50. Morine KJ, Kiernan MS, Pham DT, et al. Pulmonary Artery Pulsatility Index Is Associated With Right Ventricular Failure After Left Ventricular Assist Device Surgery. J Card Fail 2016;22(2):110–6.

51. Kang G, Ha R, Banerjee D. Pulmonary artery pulsatility index predicts right ventricular failure after left ventricular assist device implantation. J Heart Lung Transplant 2016;35(1):67–73.

52. Kavarana MN, Pessin-Minsley MS, Urtecho J, et al. Right ventricular dysfunction and organ failure in left ventricular assist device recipients: a continuing problem. Ann Thorac Surg 2002;73(3):745–50.

53. Kormos RL, Teuteberg JJ, Pagani FD, et al. Right ventricular failure in patients with the HeartMate II continuous-flow left ventricular assist device: incidence, risk factors, and effect on outcomes. J Thorac Cardiovasc Surg 2010;139(5):1316–24.

54. Dang NC, Topkara VK, Mercando M, et al. Right heart failure after left ventricular assist device implantation in patients with chronic congestive heart failure. J Heart Lung Transplant 2006;25(1):1–6.

55. Morgan JA, John R, Lee BJ, et al. Is severe right ventricular failure in left ventricular assist device recipients a risk factor for unsuccessful bridging to

transplant and post-transplant mortality. Ann Thorac Surg 2004;77(3):859–63.

56. Drakos SG, Janicki L, Horne BD, et al. Risk factors predictive of right ventricular failure after left ventricular assist device implantation. Am J Cardiol 2010; 105(7):1030–5.

57. Baumwol J, Macdonald PS, Keogh AM, et al. Right heart failure and 'failure to thrive' after left ventricular assist device: clinical predictors and outcomes. J Heart Lung Transplant 2011;30(8):888–95.

58. Holman WL, Kormos RL, Naftel DC, et al. Predictors of death and transplant in patients with a mechanical circulatory support device: a multi-institutional study. J Heart Lung Transplant 2009;28(1):44–50.

59. Lietz K, Long JW, Kfoury AG, et al. Outcomes of left ventricular assist device implantation as destination therapy in the post-REMATCH era: implications for patient selection. Circulation 2007;116(5):497–505.

60. Hayek S, Sims DB, Markham DW, et al. Assessment of right ventricular function in left ventricular assist device candidates. Circ Cardiovasc Imaging 2014; 7(2):379–89.

61. Grant ADM, Smedira NG, Starling RC, et al. Independent and Incremental Role of Quantitative Right Ventricular Evaluation for the Prediction of Right Ventricular Failure After Left Ventricular Assist Device Implantation. J Am Coll Cardiol 2012;60(6):521–8.

62. Drazner MH, Velez-Martinez M, Ayers CR, et al. Relationship of right- to left-sided ventricular filling pressures in advanced heart failure: insights from the ESCAPE trial. Circ Heart Fail 2013;6(2):264–70.

63. Menachem JN, Felker GM, Patel CB. Right Atrial to Pulmonary Capillary Wedge Pressure Ratio Is Not Associated with Failure of Optimal Medical Management in the INTERMACS 4-5 Population. J Heart Lung Transplant 2013;32(4, Supplement):S22.

64. Cogswell Rebecca J, Masri S. Carolina. Abstract 18958: High Pre-Operative Right Atrial Pressure to Pulmonary Capillary Wedge Pressure Ratio is Not Associated With Right Ventricular Dysfunction After LVAD Implantation. Circulation 2013;128(suppl_22):A18958.

65. Bhat G, Ali A, Yost G, et al. Right Atrial to Pulmonary Capillary Wedge Pressure Ratio as Predictor for Postoperative Outcomes in Left Ventricular Assist Device Implantation. J Heart Lung Transplant 2017;36(4):S341.

66. Ochiai Y, McCarthy PM, Smedira NG, et al. Predictors of severe right ventricular failure after implantable left ventricular assist device insertion: analysis of 245 patients. Circulation 2002;106(12 Suppl 1):I198–202.

67. Bellavia D, Iacovoni A, Scardulla C, et al. Prediction of right ventricular failure after ventricular assist device implant: systematic review and meta-analysis of observational studies. Eur J Heart Fail 2017;19(7): 926–46.

68. Reed CE, Dorman BH, Spinale FG. Assessment of right ventricular contractile performance after pulmonary resection. Ann Thorac Surg 1993;56(3): 426–31. discussion 431-432.

69. Marshall D, Malick A, Truby L, et al. Pulmonary Artery Pulsatility Index (PAPi) is a Predictor of Right Ventricular Assist Device (RVAD) Use Following HeartMate 3 LVAD Implantation. J Heart Lung Transplant 2020;39(4, Supplement):S408.

70. Tehrani DM, Grinstein J, Kalantari S, et al. Cardiac Output Assessment in Patients Supported with Left Ventricular Assist Device: Discordance Between Thermodilution and Indirect Fick Cardiac Output Measurements. ASAIO J 2017;63(4):433–7.

71. Sayer G, Jeevanandam V, Ota T, et al. Invasive Hemodynamic Echocardiographic Ramp Test in the HeartAssist5 LVAD: Insights into Device Performance. ASAIO J 2017;63(2):e10.

72. Imamura T, Chung B, Nguyen A, et al. Clinical implications of hemodynamic assessment during left ventricular assist device therapy. J Cardiol 2018;71(4):352–8.

73. Imamura T, Jeevanandam V, Kim G, et al. Optimal Hemodynamics During Left Ventricular Assist Device Support Are Associated With Reduced Readmission Rates. Circ Heart Fail 2019;12(2):e005094.

74. Abraham WT, Adamson PB, Costanzo MR, et al. Hemodynamic Monitoring in Advanced Heart Failure: Results from the LAPTOP-HF Trial. J Card Fail 2016;22(11):940.

75. Abraham WT, Adamson PB, Bourge RC, et al. Wireless pulmonary artery haemodynamic monitoring in chronic heart failure: a randomised controlled trial. Lancet 2011;377(9766):658–66.

76. Adamson PB, Abraham WT, Bourge RC, et al. Wireless pulmonary artery pressure monitoring guides management to reduce decompensation in heart failure with preserved ejection fraction. Circ Heart Fail 2014;7(6):935–44.

77. Givertz MM, Stevenson LW, Costanzo MR, et al. Pulmonary Artery Pressure-Guided Management of Patients With Heart Failure and Reduced Ejection Fraction. J Am Coll Cardiol 2017;70(15):1875–86.

78. Heywood JT, Jermyn R, Shavelle D, et al. Impact of Practice-Based Management of Pulmonary Artery Pressures in 2000 Patients Implanted With the CardioMEMS Sensor. Circulation 2017;135(16):1509–17.

79. Desai AS, Bhimaraj A, Bharmi R, et al. Ambulatory Hemodynamic Monitoring Reduces Heart Failure Hospitalizations in 'Real-World' Clinical Practice. J Am Coll Cardiol 2017;69(19):2357–65.

80. Shavelle DM, Desai AS, Abraham WT, et al. Lower Rates of Heart Failure and All-Cause Hospitalizations During Pulmonary Artery Pressure-Guided Therapy for Ambulatory Heart Failure: One-Year Outcomes From the CardioMEMS Post-Approval Study. Circ Heart Fail 2020;13(8):e006863.

81. Lindenfeld J, Abraham WT, Maisel A, et al. Hemodynamic-GUIDEd management of Heart Failure (GUIDE-HF). Am Heart J 2019;214:18–27.

Advanced Heart Failure in Special Population
Cardiomyopathies and Myocarditis

Davide Stolfo, MD, Valentino Collini, MD, Gianfranco Sinagra, MD*

KEYWORDS

- Cardiomyopathies • Advanced heart failure • Genetic syndromes • Hypertrophic cardiomyopathy
- Restrictive cardiomyopathy • Arrhythmogenic ventricular dysplasia
- Left ventricular non-compaction cardiomyopathy • Myocarditis

KEY POINTS

- Cardiomyopathies are an important cause of heart failure (HF) especially in young populations.
- A timely recognition and treatment of patients at risk of progressive HF is important to avoid the development of advanced stage.
- Advanced stages of HF due to cardiomyopathies portend a poor prognosis and are the main cause of heart transplantation in young people.

DEFINITION OF CARDIOMYOPATHIES

The European Society of Cardiology (ESC) defines cardiomyopathy as "a myocardial disorder in which the heart muscle is structurally and functionally abnormal in the absence of coronary artery disease, hypertension, valvular disease, and congenital heart disease sufficient to explain the observed myocardial abnormality."[1]

Cardiomyopathies are frequently genetic and include a heterogeneous group of myocardial disorders that manifest with various structural and functional phenotypes: dilated cardiomyopathy, hypertrophic cardiomyopathy (HCM), restrictive cardiomyopathy (RCM), arrhythmogenic ventricular dysplasia, left ventricular noncompaction cardiomyopathy (LVNC). Severe systolic or diastolic dysfunction characterizes the advanced stages of HF and is among the main causes of transplantation in young populations.[2]

HYPERTROPHIC CARDIOMYOPATHY
Definition, Epidemiology, and Genetics

HCM is defined by an increase in myocardial wall thickness ($\geq$15 mm in adults, or $\geq$13 mm in adults with first-degree relatives with HCM) in one or more of the left ventricular (LV) wall segments not explained by abnormal loading conditions.[3] The estimated prevalence ranges from 1:200 to 1:500, and it is more common among young adults. HCM is the most common inherited heart disease and results from autosomal dominant sarcomere gene mutations in up to 60% of patients. Other etiologies that may mimic HCM (so-called phenocopy) include Fabry disease, glycogen and lysosomal storage diseases, and mitochondrial disorders with matrilinear transmission. Thin-filament gene mutations (TNNT2, TNNI3, TPM1, and ACTC) are associated with increased likelihood of advanced LV dysfunction and HF compared with thick-filament (MYH7 and MYBPC3) disease, whereas arrhythmic risk in both subsets is comparable.[4]

Patients with multiple genetic mutations in sarcomere proteins make up to 5% of the HCM population and are particularly susceptible to accelerated progression to end-stage disease.

Genetic testing is recommended in probands. If a proband with a positive test is identified, cascade screening (testing for the presence of the variant in family members) should be performed.

Cardiovascular Department, Azienda Sanitaria Universitaria Integrata, Trieste, Italy
* Corresponding author.
E-mail address: gianfranco.sinagra@asuits.sanita.fvg.it

Heart Failure Clin 17 (2021) 661–672
https://doi.org/10.1016/j.hfc.2021.05.010
1551-7136/21/© 2021 Elsevier Inc. All rights reserved.

Pathophysiology

In patients with HCM, HF symptoms have two distinct pathophysiologies:

1. HF can result from severe dynamic LV outflow tract (LVOT) obstruction. This form can be managed pharmacologically or with invasive therapies for septal reduction.
2. HF is caused by progressive and severe diastolic dysfunction or severe systolic dysfunction (defined by left ventricular ejection fraction (LVEF) <50%), subtended by extensive replacement fibrosis and chamber remodeling. This evolution is irreversible, tends to respond poorly to conventional pharmacologic treatment, and culminates in the rare (3%) but dramatic end-stage scenario.[5]

The manifestations of HCM in this advanced stage span between two extremes:

- Hypokinetic-restrictive form, characterized by a small and stiff LV with extreme diastolic dysfunction and mildly or more severe systolic impairment (**Fig. 1**).
- Hypokinetic-dilated form, characterized by volume increase and spherical remodeling of the LV. This variant may be indistinguishable from primary DCM, and the diagnosis of HCM relies either on prior documentation of asymmetrical LV hypertrophy or family history.

Several different mechanisms have been proposed to explain the evolution toward end-stage HCM, such as progressive cardiomyocyte energy depletion, microvascular ischemia, and replacement fibrosis, although its genesis remains largely unresolved.[6]

Advanced Heart Failure in Hypertrophic Cardiomyopathy

Classical symptoms are related to LVOT obstruction, mitral regurgitation, myocardial ischemia, diastolic dysfunction, abnormal vascular responses, and supraventricular or ventricular arrhythmias (VA). The most frequent symptoms are chest pain, shortness of breath, and palpitation. The prevalence of HF is reported to be 67%, and 17% of patients have New York Heart Association (NYHA) III–IV symptoms.[7] The progression to advanced HF occurs in 3% to 15% of individuals with an incidence ranging from 0.5% to 1.5% per year.[5]

Diagnosis

Multimodality imaging is essential to provide a comprehensive characterization. Accurate quantification of LV wall thickness, estimation of LV ejection fraction (EF), definition of LV apical aneurysm, mitral regurgitation, and extent of myocardial fibrosis are part of the HCM phenotype.

Overt dysfunction in echocardiography is characterized by severe functional LV deterioration and is generally associated with apparent regression of hypertrophy. Hypokinetic-dilated form is characterized by LV volume increase and spherical remodeling. In hypokinetic restrictive form, the distinctive feature is a small hypertrophic LV with severe diastolic dysfunction and mild systolic impairment.

Exercise echocardiography can be a valuable tool in the decision-making process aiding the differential diagnosis and unmasking LVOT gradient absent at rest that is associated to increased risk of symptoms onset at follow-up (3.2% vs 1.6% per year for nonobstructive patients).[8]

MRI is essential to complete the diagnostic workup and risk stratification process. Tissue characterization can help better define patients with upcoming end-stage evolution who frequently present widespread LV fibrosis. The progression of late gadolinium enhancement (LGE) or the identification of edema represents noninvasive markers of increased arrhythmic risk and is associated with mortality due to refractory HF.

Endomyocardial biopsy (EMB) may be considered when the results of other clinical assessments raise the suspicion of myocardial infiltration, active inflammation (ie, sarcoidosis), storage diseases, or phenocopies that cannot be confirmed by noninvasive strategies.

Management and Treatment

LVOT obstruction can generally be managed with medications (ie, beta-blockers, calcium-channel blockers, disopyramide) or, if refractory, with invasive surgical or percutaneous septal reduction therapies. The treatment of end-stage HCM resulting in severe HF lack of validated therapeutic alternatives.

Drug therapy

Current consensus and guidelines recommend the translation of conventional treatments for reduced EF HF to end-stage HCM. Thus, the sequential approach including antineurohormonal drugs and devices should be applied. EF below 50% is currently considered an indication to primary prevention Implantable Cardioverter Defibrillator (ICD) implantation, and cardiac resynchronization may be considered in patients with concomitant left-bundle branch block and wide QRS complex.[9]

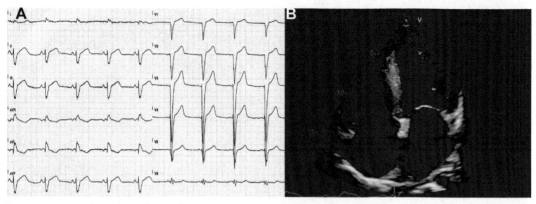

Fig. 1. A 53-year-old male with nonobstructive end-stage hypertrophic cardiomyopathy. (*A*) Left bundle-branch block with qs waves in right precordial leads and extreme fragmentation of QRS complex in V6. (*B*) Apical four-chamber view at transthoracic echocardiography. Note the diffuse concentric hypertrophy of the myocardium and the dilation of atrium and right ventricle.

However, adverse effects of drugs are not unusual in these patients: Hypotension occurs frequently with vasodilators, and diuretics often result in prerenal azotemia due to the steep LV pressure-volume relationship. Tolerability to medications with negative inotropic effect active against LVOT obstruction should be carefully reassessed.

Heart transplantation

Patients with advanced HF not otherwise amenable to other treatments should be considered for orthotopic heart transplantation (HT). Early inclusion on the HT waiting list should not be delayed in patients with younger age, family history, EF less than 50%, severe restrictive diastolic pattern, increased extension of LV fibrosis, elevated plasma levels of natriuretic peptides, or declining oxygen consumption rates.

The timeline of disease progression is generally rapid with a 4 to 14 years range from symptoms onset to end-stage HCM and a mean reported HT-free survival of 2.7 ± 2 years for patients with end-stage HCM.[5]

Left ventricular assist devices

Patients with HCM have traditionally been ineligible for LVAD support because of small LV cavities and relatively preserved EF. However, long-term mechanical supports have been reported in recent case series as a reasonable bridge to HT in selected patients with nonobstructive HCM and larger LV cavities (>46 mm). The reported 1-year survival on pump was 50%, with 31% of patients successfully transplanted and only 18% dead.[10]

Prognosis

End-stage HCM is associated with very high mortality (11% per year vs 1% per year in the overall HCM population), and HF morbidity and increased risk of sudden cardiac death.[5] Patients' perspectives after HF are instead reassuring, with 75% to 100% survival at 5 years and 61% to 94% survival at 10 years. Most recent data reported 8% mortality and 61% HT in the first year after inclusion on transplant list; after HF, 1-, 5-, and 10-year survival was 89%, 79%, and 66%, respectively.[11]

RESTRICTIVE CARDIOMYOPATHY
Definition, Etiology, and Genetics

RCM is rare (accounting for <5% of all cardiomyopathies) and caused by a heterogeneous group of diseases with a common physiology, predominating the impairment to the left or biventricular filling. The overall prognosis is generally poor.[12]

Idiopathic RCM is diagnosed in the absence of alternative causes such as infiltrative (ie, cardiac amyloidosis), storage diseases (ie, hemochromatosis), and inflammatory (ie, sarcoidosis). Isolated endomyocardial fibrosis and Löffler endocarditis (**Fig. 2**), that complicates systemic eosinophilic syndromes, are two nongenetic causes of RCM.

Genetic etiologies (such as mutations in troponin T-I, α-actin, and β-myosin heavy chain) with autosomal dominant pattern of transmission and complete penetrance have been demonstrated in 30% of all reported RCM and cause more severe presentations.[13]

Advanced Heart Failure in Restrictive Cardiomyopathy

RCM is a disorder resulting from the increased stiffness of the myocardium, which implicates the rising filling pressure within the ventricular chambers without a compensatory increase in volumes. Diastolic dysfunction progresses overtime and induces pulmonary and systemic

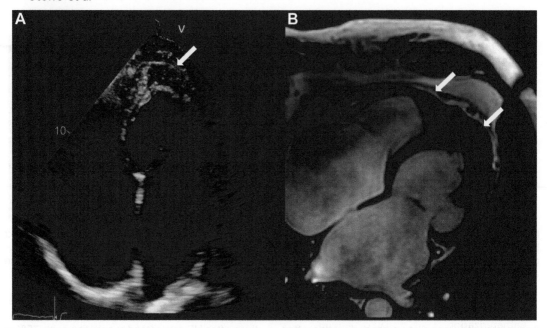

Fig. 2. A 61-year-old male with Churg-Strauss syndrome and Loeffler endocarditis. The restrictive physiology is attested by the massive enlargement of right and left atrium. (*A*) Apical four-chamber view at transthoracic echocardiography. (*B*) Cine cardiac magnetic resonance four-chamber view. Typical fibrous thickening of the endocardium leading to apical obliteration mimicking apical thrombus is present in both the ventricles (*white arrows*).

congestion. In the later stages, systolic LV dysfunction may arise.

The prevalence of HF in RCM is 83%, and 42% of patients present advanced functional class.[7] Dyspnea is the most frequent symptom (71%), followed by edema (46%), palpitation (33%), fatigue (32%), orthopnea, and chest pain.[14]

Electrocardiographic abnormalities are frequent but nonspecific. AF is frequent, particularly in the late stages (>50%).[14] Peripheral voltages are normal, pseudonecrosis may be present.

Diagnosis

The advanced stages of RCM are characterized by markedly increased left atrial volume, restrictive LV filling pattern, low septal and lateral e' velocities, and E/e' ratio ≥15. Wall thickness is usually normal. MRI aids the diagnostic characterization of the disease, including the definition of pericardial thickness that can support the alternative diagnosis of constrictive pericarditis. Interstitial fibrosis and myocyte hypertrophy are the most common findings at EMB. Differential diagnosis between RCM and constrictive pericarditis can be challenging and requires a multimodality approach (**Table 1**).

Management and Treatment

No therapy has proven to improve outcome in patients with RCM. Symptomatic therapy is the only option available, although poorly effective in the long term[15]:

- Diuretics are the mainstay of treatment to reduce volume overload. However, these patients rely on high filling pressures to maintain cardiac output, and excessive diuresis may result in tissue hypoperfusion.
- The use of β-blockers or calcium channel blockers should be carefully introduced because a fixed stroke volume requires a higher heart rate to maintain cardiac output.
- The use of ACE-inhibitors/angiotensin receptor blockers is extremely controversial, and hypotension occurs frequently with vasodilators.
- RCM patients are prone to digoxin toxicity.
- Anticoagulation may be helpful because of propensity for thrombus formation in large atria.

Heart transplantation

HT is considered for symptomatic RCM pediatric patients with reactive pulmonary hypertension[15] and in patients with refractory symptoms and end-stage HF.

Owing to lacking consensus on risk stratification, the International Society for Heart Lung Transplantation in 2016 provided a list of typical features associated with adverse outcome:

- Pulmonary congestion at diagnosis
- Angina or ischemic electrocardiogram (ECG) findings
- Male gender

Table 1
Differential diagnoses of RCM and constrictive pericarditis

	Restrictive Cardiomyopathy	Constrictive Pericarditis
History	Systemic disease	Previous diseases affecting the pericardium
Clinical signs	Regurgitant murmur, S3	Pericardial knock
X-ray chest	Cardiomegaly and pulmonary venous congestion	Calcified pericardium
Echocardiography	Wall thickening, sparkling myocardium E/A ratio >2, short DT, peak e′ <8 cm/s	Pericardial thickening, septal bounce, Respiratory variation in mitral inflow E peak velocity >25%, peak e′ >8 cm/s, annulus reversus
CT	Normal pericardium	Thickened/calcified pericardium
MRI	LGE with different patterns and distribution	Thickened pericardium
Catheterization hemodynamics	LVEDP – RVEDP $\geq$5 mm Hg RVSP $\geq$55 mm Hg RVEDP/RVSP $\leq$.33	LVEDP – RVEDP <5 mm Hg RVSP <55 mm Hg RVEDP/RVSP >.33
Biopsy	May reveal underlying cause	Normal myocardium

Abbreviation: DT, E-wave deceleration time; E/A, E-wave/A-wave; LVEDP, left ventricular end diastolic pressure; RCM, restrictive cardiomyopathy; RVEDP, right ventricular end diastolic pressure; RVSP, right ventricular systolic pressure.

- Reactive pulmonary hypertension
- Left atrial dimension greater than 60 mm
- Reduced LVEF
- Increased end-diastolic posterior wall thickness

Elevated pulmonary vascular resistance (PVR) (triggered by chronically elevated LV filling pressures) promotes fixed pulmonary hypertension that can contraindicate HT. Then periodic invasive hemodynamic assessment should be performed in patients considered for listing.

Left ventricular assist device

Patients with RCM are generally excluded from long-term mechanical circulatory support (MCS) because of the potential impairment to pump function caused by small cavities and restrictive physiology.[15] In a cohort of 94 patients, 1 year after LVAD implantation, 60.0%, 15.4%, and 24.6% are, respectively, alive on pump, transplanted, and dead.[10]

Prognosis

RCM has the poorest prognosis among the cardiomyopathies. Several studies have reported 50% of the mortality occurring within 2 years after diagnosis and 66% to 100% dying or being transplanted in the following years. The risk of death doubled with each increment in NYHA class, independently of other characteristics.[13] In a large cohort, the prevalence of HT due to RCM was 1.4%, and crude 1-, 5-, and 10-year overall survival after HT was 84%, 66%, and 45%. Most common causes of death within the first year were infection (34%) and multiple organ failure (17%).[16]

ARRHYTHMOGENIC VENTRICULAR CARDIOMYOPATHY
Definition, Prevalence, and Genetics

Arrhythmogenic ventricular cardiomyopathy (ACM) is a genetic heart muscle disease characterized by fibrofatty myocardial replacement, causing global and/or regional ventricular dysfunction and predisposing to potentially lethal scar-related VA. Originally described as a right ventricular (RV) disease, ACM is increasingly recognized as a biventricular entity, and the term arrhythmogenic right ventricular cardiomyopathy (ARVC) is reconsidered as a more comprehensive term: arrhythmogenic cardiomyopathy.[17]

ACM estimated prevalence ranges between 1 in 2000 and 1 in 5,000, and HF is reported in up to 20% of cases.[18]

Genetic transmission is more frequently autosomal dominant, and related mutations are identified in approximately 60% of index-patients.

Variants involve mainly desmosomal genes, including DSP, PKP2, DSG2, DSC2, and JUP. Earlier onset and worse prognosis have been reported in patients with multiple mutations (4%–6%).[19]

Pathophysiology and Clinical Presentation

Desmosome mutations causing cardiomyopathy relies on loss of adhesion between cardiac myocytes, which predisposes to the detachment of myocytes and progressive cellular loss that is replaced by fibrofatty tissue, macroscopically resulting in regional wall motion abnormalities and multiple aneurysms. The most frequent location is the so-called "triangle of dysplasia" (inflow, apex, and outflow tract of the RV). The LV is concomitantly involved in up to 75% of cases.[18]

Three phases are recognizable along the natural history:

- Early stage: Despite minimal or absent symptoms, the risk of sudden cardiac death is not negligible and promoted by exercise;
- Electrical phase: characterized by symptomatic arrhythmias, such as monomorphic ventricular tachycardia (VT);
- Progressive phase: leading to biventricular HF (**Fig. 3**) with fluid overload and symptoms of congestion. In this phase, scar-related re-entrant VT and ventricular fibrillation due to ongoing myocyte death and reactive inflammation are possible.

LV involvement was originally considered an end-stage complication of ARVC, occurring late, after the phase of right HF. However, emerging evidences suggest that the LV is part of the pathologic process in most patients since the earlier stages.[20]

Diagnosis

Classic criteria for diagnosis have been proposed in 2010 and are currently accepted for the definition of arrhythmogenic RV phenotype.[21] However, the emerging concept that ACM is a biventricular disease with a heterogeneous presentation questions the general applicability of such criteria. Thus, a wider approach to the disease is needed, with more comprehensive criteria.[17]

More frequently, ECG abnormalities are T-wave inversion in V1-V3, that can involve lateral and inferior leads in left-dominant or biventricular patterns. VT and ventricular ectopic beats with typical left-bundle branch morphology are frequent.

The most typical echocardiographic features are RV dilatation, akinetic-dyskinetic wall motion abnormalities, and myocardial aneurysms. RV or

biventricular systolic impairment characterizes the progression to HF.

MRI is the gold-standard imaging technique for diagnosis and phenotype characterization due to the optimal definition of RV size and function, the identification of regional wall motion abnormalities, and the tissue characterization that allows to identify early involvement of the LV. Subepicardial LGE indeed is a typical finding in ACM, particularly in carriers of DSP variants.[21,22]

Management and treatment

Advanced HF is rare (3.9% of ACM patients)[7] because screening programs and improved diagnostic strategies support early diagnosis. In patients with HF symptoms, the approach should follow current recommendations for Heart Failure with Reduced Ejection Fraction (HFrEF), with distinction in medical approach according to the predominant form of HF (right side vs left side).

ICD implantation has a class 1 recommendation in either patients with a history of cardiac arrest or sustained VT or in patients with severe RV or LV dysfunction (high-risk category with estimated event rate >10% per year).[18]

The use of MCS is usually warranted if patients are not responsive to drug therapy. However, the frequent biventricular or predominant RV failure is a potential contraindication to isolated left-side MCS.

The proportion of ACM patients with progressive HF that need to be considered for transplant listing is relatively small.[23]

Prognosis

Age at first symptom younger than 35 years appeared to be the only independent predictor of HT. In recent experiences, survival varies between 87% and 94% at 1 year, 81% and 91% at 5 years, and 77% and 81% at 10 years after HT.[23]

LEFT VENTRICULAR NONCOMPACTION CARDIOMYOPATHY
Definition, Epidemiology, and Natural History

LVNC is a rare condition characterized by prominent LV trabeculations, deep intertrabecular recesses communicating with the ventricular cavity, and a thin and compacted epicardial layer. Pathogenesis remains uncertain and is generally considered to result from the arrest of the normal process of trabecular growth early during embryonic development of myocardium.[24]

Reported prevalence is between 0.014% and 0.05% in the general population,[25] and as much

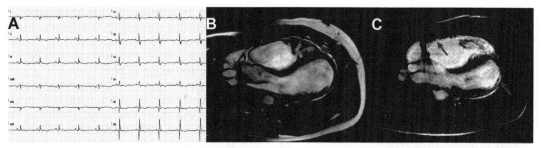

Fig. 3. A 46-year-old male with arrhythmogenic biventricular cardiomyopathy and end-stage heart failure listed for transplantation. (*A*) ECG shows high R wave in right precordial leads (right ventricle hypertrophy or posterior pseudonecrosis), lateral q waves (pseudonecrosis), and diffuse negative T waves. (*B*) Cine cardiac magnetic resonance four-chamber view showing the dilated right ventricle with apical akinesia and basal aneurysm, and the thinned akinetic lateral wall of the left ventricle. (*C*) At T1-weighted sequence, late gadolinium enhancement is present in the lateral-apical left ventricle (subepicardial distribution) and in the basal right ventricle (transmural distribution) (*red arrows*).

as 3% in adults presenting with HF. Genetic inheritance arises in at least 30%–50% of patients.

The disease can present throughout life with progressive LV systolic dysfunction and can lead to HF, which remains the most common presentation.[25] Gleva and colleagues evaluated 661 adults with LVNC: 2 of 3 having HF (30% in NYHA class III/IV) with a mean LVEF of 33%.[26] AF occurred in 21% of patients, 67% had nonsustained VT, and 30% had VT or prior cardiac arrest.[26]

Diagnosis

Diagnosis is based on multimodality imaging approach and can be challenging since different criteria have been proposed (**Box 1**) and lacking agreement between different imaging techniques is not rare.

Segments usually involved are midventricular (especially inferior and lateral ones) and apical, with evidence of direct blood flow from the ventricular cavity into deep intertrabecular recesses by color Doppler.

Management and Treatment

Management includes treatment of HF, arrhythmias, and thromboembolic events.

In patients with impaired LV function, long-term anticoagulation is mandatory because of a high risk of systemic thromboembolism.[33]

Validated criteria for the stratification of arrhythmic risk are lacking, and general indications for primary prevention ICD implantation match the current indications for the prevention of sudden cardiac death in HFrEF.

HT is the treatment of choice for patients with end-stage HF, and early listing should be considered in the same way as in patients with

nonischemic HFrEF. Destination or bridging strategies of long-term MCS are valid alternatives in patients ineligible for HT or with worsening hemodynamic status and long-time waiting list. The extensive trabeculations may predispose to thromboembolic events, pump thrombosis, and arrhythmias and, in some cases, challenge the management of MCS.[33]

Prognosis

Factors associated with poor outcome are larger LV dimensions, lower EF, the amount of delayed trabecular hyperenhancement, advanced NYHA class, AF, and wide QRS. The overall incidence of HF-related hospitalizations and HT are 3.53 and 2.17, respectively, per 100 person-years.[33]

MYOCARDITIS
Definition and Epidemiology

Myocarditis is defined as any inflammatory disease of the myocardium (**Box 2**). Pathogenesis is extremely heterogeneous, but viral infection is considered the most common.[34]

Males are more often affected (80%) than women, with the highest prevalence seen in children and young adults. The most frequent symptom at presentation is chest pain (prevalence >85%) followed by dyspnea. An associated immune disorder is frequent.[35] The estimated incidence among cases with unexplained HF is 10% to 17%.

Natural History

Progressive pathologic stages can be summarized into

Box 1
Diagnostic criteria for LVNC

Echocardiographic criteria:

- Prominent LV trabeculations, in the apical and midventricular areas of both the inferior and lateral walls.

- Epicardial surface to trabeculation trough divided by epicardial surface to trabeculation peak in end-diastole ≤0.5.[27]

- End-systolic ratio[28] or end-diastolic ratio[29] between noncompacted and compacted myocardium is greater than 2.

MRI criteria:

- Trabeculated left ventricular mass greater than 20% of the global ventricular mass at end-diastole.[30]

- Noncompacted/compacted myocardium greater than 2.3 at end diastole.[31]

- Trabeculated ventricular mass greater than 25% of the global ventricular mass, noncompacted mass greater than 15 g/m3.[32]

- Initial myocardial injury: dominated by the viral infection and replication, which causes the initial myocardial injury. In 40% to 60% of cases, complete spontaneous recovery or

---

Box 2
Causes of myocarditis

Infectious myocarditis:

- DNA viruses (ie, Parvovirus B19), RNA viruses (ie, coxsackieviruses)

- Bacterial (ie, *Staphylococcus*)

- Spirochaete Borrelia (Lyme disease)

- Protozoal (ie, *Trypanosoma cruzi*)

- Fungal (ie, *Aspergillus*)

- Parasitic (ie, *Trichinella spiralis*)

- Rickettsial (ie, *Coxiella burnetii*)

Immune-mediated myocarditis:

- Autoantigens (ie, infection-negative lymphocytic or giant cell; associated with autoimmune or immune-oriented disorders)

- Allergens (ie, vaccines or drugs)

- Alloantigens (ie, HT rejection)

Toxic myocarditis:

- Drugs (ie, chemotherapy)

- Physical agents (ie, radiation)

---

healing on a defect status is observed in 2 to 4 weeks, but about 25% will develop persistent cardiac dysfunction, and 12% to 25% may acutely deteriorate and either die or progress to end-stage DCM.[34]

- Autoimmune myocardial injury: Structural and functional damage of the myocardium activates the immune response, which can lead to severe extensive inflammation which can promote clinically evident HF (fulminant myocarditis [FM]).[35]

- Dilated cardiomyopathy: The immune response is eventually downregulated; however, myocardial inflammation can also persist. Persistent inflammation is characterized by an ongoing damage to the cardiomyocytes, and the loss of cardiac cells ultimately results in fibrosis and nonischemic HF. Before the introduction of etiologically targeted therapy, about 30% of cases progressed toward death or HT.[36]

Fulminant myocarditis

FM is more typical of some specific etiologies (giant-cell myocarditis and sarcoidosis) and is characterized by rapid onset of HF symptoms (in up to 80% of patients) that frequently follow more generic symptoms of viral infection (flu-like or gastrointestinal symptoms).[36] Classically, the disease rapidly deteriorates causing severe hemodynamic instability and, in some cases, is associated with life-threatening arrhythmias, requiring the rapid upgrade of support strategies. Increased markers of myocardial injury together with indicators of systemic inflammation are typical.[35,37]

Inflammatory cardiomyopathy

Inflammatory cardiomyopathy is defined as myocarditis associated with cardiac dysfunction and ventricular remodeling. Characterized by inflammatory cell infiltration into the myocardium and a high risk of deteriorating cardiac function, it is associated with a poor prognosis when complicated by LV dysfunction, HF, or arrhythmia.[38]

Diagnosis

Noninvasive testing

In the emergency setting, the diagnosis is mainly supported by clinical indicators. ECG abnormalities are constant but not specific. LV or biventricular dysfunction, nondilated LV, and pericardial effusion are the most frequent, but not specific, echocardiographic features. In unstable patients, MRI can be precluded, and straight endomyocardial biopsy (EBM) can be considered.[39]

In chronic myocarditis, echocardiography is useful to exclude other causes of HF and identify ventricular thrombi. RV dysfunction is an uncommon but important predictor of death or HT.

Cardiac magnetic resonance

MRI is the noninvasive reference standard for the diagnosis. It is based on the revised Lake Louise criteria (2018),[40] which target three aspects of myocardial inflammation:

- Myocardial hyperemia (early gadolinium enhancement in T1-weighted images)
- Interstitial edema (in T2-weighted fast spin echo fat suppression images).
- Myocardial fibrosis (LGE in T1-weighted sequences), which typically involves the subepicardial myocardial layer.

Endomyocardial biopsy

EBM remains the gold-standard technique for the diagnosis. However, the invasive nature of the procedure limits its applicability to selected cases. American guidelines recommend EBM in case of severe clinical presentation (recent HF or life-threatening arrhythmias).[41] The consensus from the European working group instead is more extensive in the application of EBM for the diagnostic confirmation.[34] However, EBM is crucial in the definition of the hystotype and in the identification of the viral genome in myocardial tissue to individualize the immunosuppressive treatment. Former gold-standard Dallas criteria for histologic diagnosis have been recently strengthened by the addition of immunohistochemistry and viral genome analysis that characterize the immune cell infiltrate and the specific pathogens.

Management and Treatment

Immunosuppressive treatment

Disease-specific therapy using immunomodulating strategies is extremely controversial, and there is a lack of agreement on the best strategy to adopt. In FM, immunosuppressive therapy with prednisone and azathioprine appears suitable for patients with EMB-proven active myocarditis that do not rapidly improve with conventional medical or invasive support strategies. Specific etiologies such as cardiac sarcoidosis, eosinophilic myocarditis, and giant-cell myocarditis have mandatory indications for first-line immunosuppression with steroids.

Inflammatory cardiomyopathy secondary to lymphocytic myocarditis can be considered for immunosuppressive treatment in cases with persisting LV dysfunction or recurrent VA despite optimization of medical treatment for HF but only in presence of convincing inflammatory infiltrates at EMB and in the absence of viral genome.[38]

Support therapies and antineurohormonal drugs

Remaining strategies have the target to support patients across the acute inflammatory phase to allow the recovery of myocardial function. Inotropes and vasopressors are indicated in case of presentation with cardiogenic shock or low cardiac output states.[39]

After the unstable phase, conventional antineurohormonal agents for the treatment of HF should be cautiously uptitrated in patients with persistent LV dysfunction. Implantation devices (ICD and Cardiac Resynchronization Therapy (CRT)) can be indicated after complete evidence-based therapy optimization, according to current international HFrEF guidelines.

Mechanical circulatory supports

FM may require short-term MCS in case of persistent severe hemodynamic instability or progressively declining status, despite uptitration of inotropes. Intra-aortic balloon pump and axial flow supporting devices (ie, Impella®; Danvers, Massachusetts) are indicated in patients with isolated or predominant LV failure, whereas venoarterial extracorporeal life support (ECMO) is preferred in case of biventricular myocarditis or if concomitant refractory respiratory failure is present.

Long-term MCS has to be considered when myocardial recovery does not occur despite maximization of treatments because it can allow the complete or partial recovery avoiding urgent HT.[42]

Heart transplantation

HT should be deferred in the acute phase as FM tends to spontaneous or treatment-promoted recovery, but urgent listing can be necessary in case of failing mechanical devices or if ventricular function does not improve despite prolonged support.

Inflammatory cardiomyopathy follows the course of DCM and may require the candidacy to HT for refractory HF in absence of recognizable inflammatory activity and despite full titration of HF medications. Increased risk of acute rejection and recurrency of inflammatory disease has been reported in former series.

In large US database, myocarditis accounts only for less than 1% of patients who receive HT, but these patients had higher acuity at listing and were frequently listed as status 1A (44%). Sixty-five percent of these patients received HT, 11% died while waiting, and 33% required MCS. One-, 5-, and 15-year survival of transplanted patients was 89%, 78%, and 56%, respectively.[43]

Prognosis

FM that survives the acute phase has been considered to have a benign prognosis because the rate of complete LV recovery is high. In particular, an improvement of LVEF greater than 20% or an LVEF greater than 50% at 6 months is associated with a favorable prognosis.[44]

Inflammatory cardiomyopathy complicated by LV dysfunction, HF, or arrhythmias is instead associated with a poorer prognosis, similar to other causes of nonischemic DCM.[38]

Ammirati and colleagues recently reported a 11% mortality/HT at 1 year in patients with complicated myocarditis at presentation (compared with 0% in those with uncomplicated myocarditis). Moreover, 4% of patients required L-VAD, and 15% VA-ECMO.[36]

SUMMARY

1. Definition of cardiomyopathies
2. HCM
3. Restrictive cardiomyopathy
4. Arrhythmogenic ventricular cardiomyopathy
5. Left ventricular noncompaction cardiomyopathy
6. Myocarditis

CLINICS CARE POINTS

- Advanced heart failure (HF) in cardiomyopathies is rare but is an important cause of HF, especially in young populations.
- Comprehensive understanding of the epidemiology, underlying mechanisms, natural course, and recent therapeutic advances can have a far-reaching impact on the management and prognosis.
- Regardless of the underlying etiology, end-stage HF in cardiomyopathies is a predictor of poor outcome.
- HT should be considered in patients who progress to advanced HF despite guideline-directed medical therapy because it can restore a high quality of life with excellent long-term survival nowadays.

DISCLOSURE

The authors have nothing to disclose.

REFERENCES

1. Elliott P, Andersson B, Arbustini E, et al. Classification of the cardiomyopathies: a position statement from the European Society Of Cardiology Working Group on Myocardial and Pericardial Diseases. Eur Heart J 2008;29:270–6.
2. Seferović PM, Polovina M, Bauersachs J, et al. Heart failure in cardiomyopathies: a position paper from the Heart Failure Association of the European Society of Cardiology. Eur J Heart Fail 2019;21(5):553–76.
3. Elliott PM, Anastasakis A, Borger MA, et al. ESC Guidelines on diagnosis and management of hypertrophic cardiomyopathy: The Task Force for the Diagnosis and Management of Hypertrophic Cardiomyopathy of the European Society of Cardiology (ESC). Eur Heart J 2014;35(39):2733–79.
4. Morita H, Rehm HL, Menesses A, et al. Shared genetic causes of cardiac hypertrophy in children and adults. N Engl J Med 2008;358:1899–908.
5. Harris KM, Spirito P, Maron MS, et al. Prevalence, clinical profile, and significance of left ventricular remodeling in the end-stage phase of hypertrophic cardiomyopathy. Circulation 2006;114:216–25.
6. Olivotto I, Cecchi F, Poggesi C, et al. Patterns of Disease Progression in Hypertrophic Cardiomyopathy. An Individualized Approach to Clinical Staging. Circ Heart Fail 2012;5:535–46.
7. Charron P, Elliott PM, Gimeno JR, et al. The cardiomyopathy registry of the EURObservational Research Programme of the European Society of Cardiology: baseline data and contemporary management of adult patients with cardiomyopathies. Eur Heart J 2018;39:1784–93.
8. Magri D, Re F, Limongelli G, et al. Heart failure progression in hypertrophic cardiomyopathy-possible insights from cardiopulmonary exercise testing. Circ J 2016;80:2204–11.
9. Ommen SR, Mital S, Burke M, et al. AHA/ACC guideline for the diagnosis and treatment of patients with hypertrophic cardiomyopathy. Circulation 2020;142(25):533–57.
10. Patel SR, Saeed O, Naftel D, et al. Outcomes of restrictive and hypertrophic cardiomyopathies after LVAD: an INTERMACS analysis. J Card Fail 2017;23:859–67.
11. DePasquale EC, Deng M, Ardehali A, et al. Outcomes of Heart Transplantation in Adults with Hypertrophic Cardiomyopathy (HCM): UNOS Registry Analysis. J Heart Lung Transplant 2016;35(4):S64.
12. William JM, Daniel PJ. Epidemiology of the inherited cardiomyopathies. Nat Rev Cardiol 2021;18(1):22–36.
13. Kaski JP, Syrris P, Burch M, et al. Idiopathic restrictive cardiomyopathy in children is caused by

mutations in cardiac sarcomere protein genes. Heart 2008;94:1478–84.

14. Ammash NM, Seward JB, Bailey KR, et al. Clinical profile and outcome of idiopathic restrictive cardiomyopathy. Circulation 2000;101:2490–6.

15. Muchtar E, Blauwet LA, Gertz MA. Restrictive cardiomyopathy: genetics, pathogenesis, clinical manifestations, diagnosis, and therapy. Circ Res 2017; 121:819–37.

16. DePasquale EC, Nasir K, Jacoby DL. Outcomes of adults with restrictive cardiomyopathy after heart transplantation. J Heart Lung Transplant 2012; 31(12):1269–75.

17. Corrado D, Marra M, Zorzi A, et al. Diagnosis of arrhythmogenic cardiomyopathy: The Padua criteria. International Journal of Cardiology. Int J Cardiol 2020;319:106–14.

18. Corrado D, Basso C, Judge DP. Arrhythmogenic Cardiomyopathy. Circ Res 2017;121(7):784–802.

19. Bhonsale A, Groeneweg JA, James CA, et al. Impact of genotype on clinical course in arrhythmogenic right ventricular dysplasia/cardiomyopathy-associated mutation carriers. Eur Heart J 2015;36: 847–55.

20. Bauce B, Basso C, Rampazzo A, et al. Clinical profile of four families with arrhythmogenic right ventricular cardiomyopathy caused by dominant desmoplakin mutations. Eur Heart J 2005;26: 1666–75.

21. Marcus FI, McKenna WJ, Sherrill D, et al. Diagnosis of arrhythmogenic right ventricular cardiomyopathy/dysplasia: Proposed Modification of the Task Force Criteria. Eur Heart J 2010;31(7):806–14.

22. Jeffrey AT, William JMK, Dominic JA, et al. 2019 HRS expert consensus statement on evaluation, risk stratification, and management of arrhythmogenic cardiomyopathy. Heart Rhythm 2019;16(11): e301–72.

23. Gilljam T, Haugaa KH, Jensen HK, et al. Heart transplantation in arrhythmogenic right ventricular cardiomyopathy - Experience from the Nordic ARVC Registry. Int J Cardiol 2018;250:201–6.

24. Ichida F. Left ventricular noncompaction. Circ J 2009;73:19–26.

25. Bartram U, Bauer J, Schranz D. Primary noncompaction of the ventricular myocardium from the morphogenetic standpoint. Pediatr Cardiol 2007; 28:325–32.

26. Gleva MJ, Wang Y, Curtis JP, et al. Complications Associated With Implantable Cardioverter Defibrillators in Adults With Congenital Heart Disease or Left Ventricular Noncompaction Cardiomyopathy. Am J Cardiol 2017;120:1891–8.

27. Chin TK, Perloff JK, Williams RG, et al. Isolated noncompaction of left ventricular myocardium. A study of eight cases. Circulation 1990;82:507–13.

28. Jenni R, Oechslin E, Schneider J, et al. Echocardiographic and pathoanatomical characteristics of isolated left ventricular non-compaction: a step towards classification as a distinct cardiomyopathy. Heart 2001;86:666–71.

29. Stollberger C, Gerecke B, Finsterer J, et al. Refinement of echocardiographic criteria for left ventricular noncompaction. Int J Cardiol 2013;165:463–7.

30. Jacquier A, Thuny F, Jop B. Measurement of trabeculated left ventricular mass using cardiac magnetic resonance imaging in the diagnosis of left ventricular non-compaction. Eur Heart J 2010;31:1098–104.

31. Petersen SE, Selvanayagam JB, Wiesmann F. Left ventricular non-compaction: insights from cardiovascular magnetic resonance imaging. J Am Coll Cardiol 2005;46:101–5.

32. Grothoff M, Pachowsky M, Hoffmann J. Value of cardiovascular MR in diagnosing left ventricular non-compaction cardiomyopathy and in discriminating between other cardiomyopathies. Eur Radiol 2012; 22:2699–709.

33. Nay A, Doimo S, Ricci F, et al. Prognostic Significance of Left Ventricular Noncompaction: Systematic Review and Meta-Analysis of Observational Studies. Circ Cardiovasc Imaging 2020;13(1):e009712.

34. Caforio AL, Pankuweit S, Arbustini E, et al. Current state of knowledge on aetiology, diagnosis, management, and therapy of myocarditis: a position statement of the European Society of Cardiology Working Group on Myocardial and Pericardial Diseases. Eur Heart J 2013;34:2636–48.

35. Ammirati E, Cipriani M, Moro C, et al. Clinical presentation and outcome in a contemporary cohort of patients with acute myocarditis: The Multicenter Lombardy Registry. Circulation 2018;138:1088–99.

36. Ammirati E, Veronese G, Cipriani M, et al. Acute and fulminant myocarditis: a pragmatic clinical approach to diagnosis and treatment. Curr Cardiol Rep 2018; 20:114.

37. Veronese G, Ammirati E, Cipriani M, et al. Fulminant myocarditis: characteristics, treatment, and outcomes. Anatol J Cardiol 2018;19:279–86.

38. Tschöpe C, Ammirati E, Bozkurt B, et al. Myocarditis and inflammatory cardiomyopathy: current evidence and future directions. Nat Rev Cardiol Nat Rev Cardiol 2020;1–25.

39. Sinagra G, Anzini M, Pereira NL, et al. Myocarditis in clinical practice. Mayo Clin Proc 2016;91:1256–66.

40. Ferreira VM, Schulz-Menger J, Holmvang G, et al. Cardiovascular magnetic resonance in nonischemic myocardial inflammation: expert recommendations. J Am Coll Cardiol 2018;72:3158–76.

41. Kociol RD, Cooper LT, Fang JC, et al. Recognition and Initial Management of Fulminant Myocarditis A Scientific Statement From the. Am Heart Assoc 2020;141:e69–92.

42. Tschöpe C, Van Linthout S, Klein O, et al. Mechanical unloading by fulminant myocarditis: LV-IMPELLA, ECMELLA, BI-PELLA and PROPELLA concepts. J Cardiovasc Transl Res 2019;12(2): 116–23.

43. ElAmm C, Al-Kindi SG, Oliveira GH. Characteristics and Outcomes of Patients With Myocarditis Listed for Heart Transplantation. Circ Heart Fail 2016;9: e003259.

44. Anzini M, Merlo M, Sabbadini G, et al. Long-term evolution and prognostic stratification of biopsy-proven active myocarditis. Circulation 2013; 128(22):2384–94.

Advanced Heart Failure in Special Population— Pediatric Age

Emanuele Monda, MD[a], Michele Lioncino, MD[a], Roberta Pacileo, MD[a],
Marta Rubino, MD[a], Annapaola Cirillo, MD[a], Adelaide Fusco, MD[a],
Augusto Esposito, MD[a], Federica Verrillo, MD[a], Francesco Di Fraia, MD[a],
Alfredo Mauriello, MD[a], Viviana Tessitore, MD[a], Martina Caiazza, MD[a],
Arturo Cesaro, MD[a], Paolo Calabrò, MD, PhD[a],
Maria Giovanna Russo, MD, PhD[a], Giuseppe Limongelli, MD, PhD, FESC[a,b,c,*]

KEYWORDS

• Heart failure • Children • Cardiac transplantation • Mechanical circulatory support

KEY POINTS

- The etiology of heart failure (HF) in pediatric population is heterogeneous with the main causes in Europe and USA represented by congenital heart diseases and cardiomyopathies.
- The diagnosis of HF in pediatric age is challenging and requires a multiparametric approach because of the lack of specific signs and symptoms.
- The treatment of chronic HF aims to improve decrease of pulmonary wedge pressure, increase in cardiac output, improve symptomatic status, and prevent disease progression.
- The role of pediatric mechanic circulatory support has been assessed as an alternative treatment in patients in whom heart transplant could not be performed.
- Heart transplantation is the gold standard for children with advanced HF.

INTRODUCTION

Heart failure (HF) is an important health care issue in children because of its considerable morbidity and mortality. It represents a complex syndrome in which a primary insult to the heart results in a cascade of secondary response, leading to cardiac and extracardiac involvement.[1] It is characterized by typical symptoms and signs caused by structural and/or functional cardiac abnormalities, resulting in reduced cardiac output and/or elevated intracardiac pressures.[2] Irrespective of the precise nature of the primary cause, the clinical evolution of HF shares common features, so the progression of this condition results in a predictable cascade of events. Although potentially reversible in the first phase, in the absence of specific treatment, it can result in advanced HF and ultimately death.[3] Advanced HF encompasses patients who remained symptomatic despite optimal medical treatment and includes patients who require special care, such as continuous inotropic therapy, mechanical circulatory support, or heart transplantation (HT).[4] This article discusses the epidemiology, causes, pathophysiology, clinical manifestation, medical treatment, device therapy, and HT in pediatric

[a] Inherited and Rare Cardiovascular Diseases Unit, Department of Translational Medical Sciences, University of Campania "Luigi Vanvitelli", Monaldi Hospital, Via Leonardo Bianchi 1, 80131, Naples, Italy; [b] Institute of Cardiovascular Sciences, University College of London and St. Bartholomew's Hospital, Grower Street, London WC1E 6DD, UK; [c] Low Prevalence and Complex Diseases of the Heart-ERN GUARD-Heart, Italy
* Corresponding author. Inherited and Rare Cardiovascular Diseases Unit, Department of Translational Medical Sciences, University of Campania "Luigi Vanvitelli", Monaldi Hospital, Via Leonardo Bianchi 1, 80131, Naples, Italy
E-mail address: limongelligiuseppe@libero.it

Heart Failure Clin 17 (2021) 673–683
https://doi.org/10.1016/j.hfc.2021.05.011
1551-7136/21/© 2021 Elsevier Inc. All rights reserved.

HF, with a particular emphasis on patients with advanced HF.

EPIDEMIOLOGY

The incidence of pediatric HF is difficult to define because of the different definition used for HF in the literature. Rossano and colleagues[5] reported the incidence of pediatric HF-related hospitalization in the United States as 11.000 to 14.000 children (≤18 years) annually, describing an overall hospital mortality of 7.4%. In their cohort, congenital heart diseases (CHDs) represent the most common cause of HF (60%–69%), followed by cardiomyopathies (CMPs) (13%), arrhythmias (12%–15%), and myocarditis (2%).

A recent systematic review investigated the epidemiology and the main cause of pediatric HF showing an incidence of 0.8 to 7.4/100.000.[6] Of interest, HF etiology varied across regions with lower respiratory tract infections and severe anemia predominating in lower income countries, and CHDs and CMPs in the higher income countries.

Different types of CHDs can lead to HF, ranging from simple lesions (eg, ventricular septal defects) to more complex disorders (eg, hypoplastic left heart syndrome), and account for the higher rate of HF admissions (55%–60%) in the first year of life.[5] Regarding CMPs, evidence shows that the proportion of HF was highest among patients with dilated cardiomyopathy (DCM), followed by those with restrictive and hypertrophy cardiomyopathy.[7,8]

The etiology of HF significantly affects the prognosis of pediatric patients. For example, Andrews and colleagues[9] described the incidence of the HF-related hospitalizations in pediatric patients with CMPs as about 1/100.000 patients younger than 16 years, and in their cohort, 34% died or underwent HT within the first year of hospital admission. Furthermore, HF patients are often hospitalized for prolonged period, with a significant impact in terms of cost and detriment to families.[10]

ETIOLOGY

The etiology of HF in pediatric population is heterogeneous, and the possible causes substantially differ from those found in the adult population (**Table 1**). With the disappearance of rheumatic fever, the main causes in Europe and USA are CHDs and CMPs.[6] There are no comprehensive data on the incidence and etiology of pediatric HF, nonetheless CHDs account for almost 82% of the cases of HF in infants[11]; it is calculated that slightly half of the HF cases are due to CHDs, although the incidence of HF in CHDs was estimated to be nearly 24%. In contrast, 65% to 80% of children with CMPs had HF, but these represent only a little proportion of total HF cases, thus reflecting the higher prevalence of CHD than CMP among pediatric population.[11] The etiologies may vary depending on the age of presentation.

At birth, HF can be caused by fetal CMPs or by extracardiac conditions (such as sepsis, hypoglycemia, or hypocalcemia). Fetal arrhythmias, and in particular re-entry or focal tachyarrhythmias, can manifest with severe HF already at birth, especially in case of prolonged duration of arrhythmic events during gestational age. In the first week of life, patients with critical duct-dependent CHDs, such left ventricular outflow tract obstructive lesions (eg, critical aortic stenosis in newborns) or systemic right ventricular systolic dysfunction

Table 1
Etiology of heart failure in pediatric age

Etiology	Pathophysiology	Examples
CHDs	Pressure overload	Aortic stenosis, aortic coarctation
	Volume overload	Left-to-right shunt
		Aortic or mitral regurgitation
	Pressure and volume overload	Hypoplastic left heart syndrome
	Ischemia	Coronary arteries anomalies
CMPs	Systolic dysfunction and/or diastolic dysfunction	Dilated cardiomyopathies
		Hypertrophic cardiomyopathies
		Restrictive cardiomyopathies
Myocarditis	Systolic dysfunction	-
Arrhythmias	Low cardiac output	Tachyarrhythmias
		Congenital heart blocks
Other	Different mechanisms	Chemotherapy-induced dysfunction
		Severe anemia
		Sepsis

(eg, congenitally corrected I-transposition in older children), may develop acute decompensation of HF with poor perfusion and multiorgan dysfunction if the closure of duct leads to reduced cardiac output.[12–14] The HF syndrome may occur in the postoperative period following cardiopulmonary bypass surgery or in patients with left to right shunts leading to chronic volume overload.[15] However, the clinical manifestations of HF associated with CHD occur more frequently in later life, especially in adults with CHD.

Primary CMPs are the predominant cause of early onset HF among children with a structurally normal heart,[8,16] and it is calculated that about 60% of children who require HT have an underlying CMP. As stated before, DCM is the most common cause of HF among CMPs.[9] Most of the early onset CMPs have a hereditary substrate and can be caused by mutations in different genes, including cytoskeletal proteins, sarcomeric proteins, cell membrane proteins, and ion channels[17]; otherwise, they can fall into more complex genetic syndromes. Recently, advances in medical research have demonstrated a high prevalence of cardiac involvement in children affected by muscular dystrophies (such as Duchenne's or myotonic muscular dystrophy) or other neuromuscular diseases.[18] In addition to the aforementioned congenital causes of HF, cardiac dysfunction caused by chemotherapy has an increasing prevalence among pediatric patients, thanks to improved survival of pediatric cancer.[19] In particular, the administration of anthracyclines is a common cause of acute systolic dysfunction among children, although the extent of myocardial injury and functional involvement seems to be partially reversible among survivors.

Other rare forms of HF in pediatric age are associated with systemic disease, including inflammatory diseases, metabolic and endocrine disorders, and chronic kidney disease.

PATHOPHYSIOLOGY

HF represents a condition in which the primary insult (eg, ischemia, infection, tachycardia) results in a cascade of secondary response, aiming to be adaptive and designed to preserve the flow to the vital organs.[3] In particular, low cardiac output induces a reduced baroreceptor stimulation, leading to three major compensatory mechanisms that provide support when the myocardium becomes dysfunctional.[20] First, sympathetic nervous system activation leads to an increased release and a decreased uptake of epinephrine and norepinephrine, resulting in a significant improvement of heart rate, cardiac contractility, and vasoconstriction which can initially support mean arterial pressure and organ perfusion.[21] Second, the high level of catecholamines coupled with the reduced renal blood flow leads to renin release and consequently renin angiotensin aldosterone system (RAAS) stimulation.[21] The subsequent peripheral vasoconstriction is accompanied by increased sodium and water retention with a rise in preload and cardiac output.[22] However, if prolonged, this compensatory mechanism causes fibrosis, apoptosis, endothelial dysfunction, and intracellular calcium depletion, promoting pathologic myocardial remodeling and HF progression (**Fig. 1**).[23]

Finally, another pathway activated in the early stages of HF is the natriuretic peptide system (NPS). B-type natriuretic peptide (BNP) and atrial natriuretic peptide (ANP), produced in cardiomyocytes, are stored in ventricular and atrial granules, respectively. The BNP precursor, pro-BNP, is proteolytically processed to the biologically active form N-terminal pro-BNP. Their production, stimulated by cardiac wall stretch and volume overload, causes vasorelaxation, natriuresis, diuresis, and reduced expression of inflammatory factors, through the cyclic guanosine monophosphate activity.[24] ANP and BNP also reduce renin secretion and aldosterone production, counteracting cardiac remodeling, myocardial hypertrophy, and fibrosis. Elevated plasma levels of neuropeptides are positively correlated with disease severity, but their activity is not sufficient to stop pathology progression because of neprilysin action.[25] Indeed, neprilysin degrades neuropeptides and promotes their elimination. In addition, RAAS can depress NPS renal responsiveness and accelerate HF progression.[26]

In the last few years, clinical research has shown interest in pediatric HF, promoting new findings in adrenergic signaling cascade and identifying

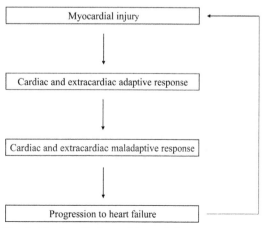

Fig. 1. Physiopathology of heart failure.

important differences between adult and children.[27,28] Specifically, β-adrenergic receptor expression, phosphorylation status of phospholamban, and expression of phosphatases are uniquely regulated in pediatric patients and may lead to a greater mitigation of adrenergic effects in children, impairing their responsiveness to HF medical therapy.[29]

DIAGNOSIS

The diagnosis of HF in pediatric age is challenging and requires a multiparametric approach because of the lack of specific symptoms and the difficulty to identify clinical signs. The clinical scenario of HF may vary depending on the age of presentation and can range from feeding difficulties, sinus tachycardia, cyanosis, and tachypnea in infants and young children to fatigue, exercise intolerance, and shortness of breath in older children and adolescents.[30] The severity of HF should be classified according to the Ross modified classification[31] or to the New York Heart Association (NYHA), in children younger and older than 6 years, respectively (**Table 2**).

Among pediatric patients, the caregivers should be educated to recognize a clinical deterioration requiring medical assistance; noteworthy, parents of children with CHD seem to be more prepared to recognize HF symptoms than parents of children affected by myocarditis or rapid-onset DCM, thus reflecting the benefit of parental medical education and better knowledge of the underlying disease.[30,31]

The clinical evaluation should assess the grade of congestion, and signs of peripheral edema, hepatomegaly, or a bulging anterior fontanel should be carefully evaluated. The 24-hour urine output should be calculated at least on daily basis and at shorter intervals in intensive patients. Noteworthy, diuresis should be adjusted for body weight in pediatric population. Body weight should be periodically recorded to identify a poor growth or a rapid weight gain, reflecting fluid retention.

Noninvasive investigations represent the first diagnostic tool in patients with suspected or definite HF.

Electrocardiography

A 12-lead electrocardiogram (ECG) often represents the first noninvasive screening, nonetheless it has low sensitivity and specificity. In acutely decompensated HF, the most common presentation is sinus tachycardia, whereas in chronic HF patients, an abnormal ECG can offer useful clues to orient diagnosis. Therefore, the finding of new-onset repolarization abnormalities should raise the suspicion of myocarditis, while conduction disturbances seem more prevalent among children with CHDs or CMPs.[32,33]

Echocardiography

Echocardiography provides information about left ventricular ejection fraction (LVEF), diastolic function, chamber volumes, and wall thickness and provides useful information about valve morphology and function. Moreover, it can identify signs of congestion as pleural or pericardial effusion. The origin and proximal course of coronary arteries can be studied, to exclude coronary arteries' aneurysms, commonly found in Kawasaki disease. The measurement of cardiovascular structure should be expressed as Z-scores to take account for the effect of body size. New techniques, as myocardial speckle tracking and global longitudinal strain (GLS), seem to help in differential diagnosis of HF and to guide management and therapy; nonetheless, data about the role of GLS in pediatric population are lacking, and further studies are needed.[34]

Table 2
Classification of heart failure in children

Class	Modified Ross Classification	NYHA Classification
I	Asymptomatic	Asymptomatic
II	Mild tachypnea or diaphoresis with feeding in infants Dyspnea on exertion in older children	Mild or moderate limitations of physical activity
III	Marked tachypnea or diaphoresis with feeding in infants Prolonged feeding times with growth failure Marked dyspnea on exertion in older children	Marked limitation of physical activity
IV	Symptoms such as tachypnea, retractions, grunting, or diaphoresis at rest	Symptoms at rest

Chest Radiography

Chest radiography is recommended in children with suspected HF, to assess heart size and signs of pulmonary congestion. Furthermore, its role is essential in the differential diagnosis of acute respiratory distress and to exclude pulmonary comorbidities.[35]

Laboratory Investigations

Laboratory investigations are useful to assess the severity of HF and to recognize other concomitant conditions. Natriuretic peptides (pro-BNP and NT-pro-BNP) seem to represent the most important parameter and closely correlate with NYHA/Ross classification and left ventricular filling pressures. The finding of low NT-pro-BNP levels has high negative predictive value in excluding the diagnosis of HF; their plasma concentration can be used as a marker both in acute and chronic HF.

In acutely decompensated HF patients, arterial blood gas analysis can be useful to quantify serum lactates, thus evaluating peripheral perfusion, whereas the finding of metabolic alkalosis can identify volume depletion, which is common after diuretic treatment. Electrolyte status can guide treatment in children with acutely decompensated HF. Indeed, hypokalemia and elevated serum creatinine are commonly observed during diuretic treatment. Complete blood count is mandatory in pediatric patients with HF, and the presence of anemia should be systematically excluded, as a significative reduction in hemoglobin levels requires a compensatory increase in heart rate to provide peripheral organ perfusion, thus worsening HF symptoms and poor oxygen delivery. Leukocytosis and inflammatory markers, such as elevated C-reactive protein serum levels, should be assessed to exclude an underlying sepsis.[28]

Cardiac Magnetic Resonance

Cardiac magnetic resonance (CMR) has spread as a new multiparametric imaging technique in pediatric cardiology as it offers a unique anatomic characterization. CMR is the gold standard for volume quantification and tissue characterization and is useful for surgical planning in children affected by CHD. Late gadolinium enhancement can be useful to assess myocardial fibrosis, thus providing a useful tool for risk stratification (**Fig. 2**).[36] The need for anesthesia to perform the examination and high heart rates commonly found in infants can represent possible limitations to the use of CMR in current clinical practice.

Cardiac Catheterization

Cardiac catheterization can be performed in pediatric patients to assess cardiac output, pulmonary pressures, and pulmonary vascular resistance and is indicated in patients being evaluated for HT or mechanical circulatory support, especially when there is high clinical probability of pulmonary hypertension and its reversibility should be assessed before HT. Less commonly, invasive catheterization may be considered to adjust medical therapy in patients who remain symptomatic despite

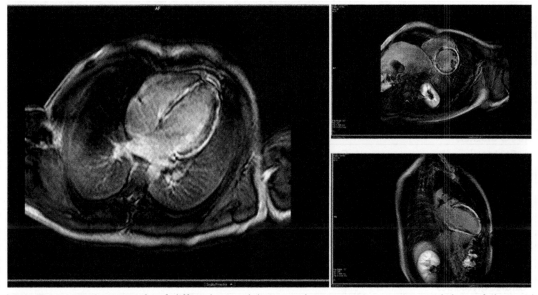

Fig. 2. Representative example of diffuse late gadolinium enhancement in a patient with heart failure with reduced ejection fraction.

optimal treatment, and whose hemodynamic status is unclear.[37]

Endomyocardial biopsy is an invasive procedure and may be considered to provide etiology and guide therapeutic management in selected clinical scenarios, as in children with suspected myocarditis, but it has a significant rate of complications and requires high-volume tertiary centers, with surgical standby.[38]

MEDICAL TREATMENT AND DEVICE THERAPY

The treatment of chronic HF aims to decrease pulmonary wedge pressure, increase cardiac output, improve symptomatic status and quality of life, and prevent disease progression. The treatment HF is largely dependent on etiology. For example, patients with large left-to-right shunt with pulmonary overcirculation or with severe symptomatic valvar regurgitation significantly benefit from early surgical treatment; thus, in these patient, chronic medical treatment is not recommended. Moreover, data on the treatment of patients with HF with preserved ejection fraction are scant. Indeed, the authors focus on the treatment of HF with reduced ejection fraction in children.

Similar to adult patients, HF with reduced ejection fraction in children is based on disease modifier drugs that counteract the overactivation of the neurohormonal systems (ie, beta-blocker, RAAS-blockers, mineralocorticoid antagonists) with the aim to prevent disease progression and reduce hospitalization and mortality, and on diuretics, that play an important role in reducing

congestion.[1] Dosages of drugs used in pediatric HF are reported in **Table 3**.

Diuretics

The use of diuretics, in particular, loop diuretics such as furosemide, is recommended in patients with HF with reduced ejection fraction and fluid retention to achieve a euvolemic state.[1] Diuretics interfere with the retention of sodium, stimulating the sodium excretion resulting in the reduction of filling pressure of the left ventricle and reduction in systemic and pulmonary congestion.

Diuretics in chronic HF have been showed to reduce worsening HF and rehospitalization for acute HF and to improve exercise tolerance.[39] The principal complications of diuretic treatment are electrolyte abnormalities (eg, hypokalemia, hyponatremia) and metabolic alkalosis, requiring close electrolyte balance monitoring, particularly during intravenous high-dose therapy.

Angiotensin Converting Enzyme Inhibitors and Angiotensin Receptor Antagonists

ACE inhibitors decrease afterload by antagonizing the RAAS and have been demonstrated to prevent, or even reverse, myocardial remodeling and disease progression.[40] ACE inhibitors are indicated both in patients with symptomatic HF or asymptomatic left ventricular dysfunction, and treatment should be started at low doses and uptitrated to the maximal tolerated dose.[1] Angiotensin receptor antagonists are indicated in patients who

Table 3
Dosages of drugs used in pediatric heart failure

Drugs	Routes of Administration	Doses
Diuretics		
Furosemide	Oral	1–2 mg/kg q6–12h
Furosemide	Intermittent bolus	0.5–2 mg/kg q6–12h
Furosemide	Continuous infusion	0.1–0.4 mg/kg/h
RAAS blockers		
Captopril	Oral	0.3–2 mg/kg q8h
Enalapril	Oral	0.05–0.25 mg/kg q12 h
Losartan	Oral	0.5–1.5 mg/kg/d
Beta-blockers		
Carvedilol	Oral	0.05 mg/kg/d q12 h
Metoprolol	Oral	0.25 mg/kg/d q12 h
Mineralocorticoid antagonists		
Spironolactone	Oral	0.5–1.5 mg/kg q12 h
Cardiac glycosides		
Digoxin	Oral	5–10 µg/kg/d

would benefit from RAAS blockade but are intolerant of ACE inhibitors.

Beta-Blockers

Beta-blockers antagonize the effect of chronic sympathetic myocardial activation and have been demonstrated to improve symptoms, survival, and ventricular remodeling both in adults and in children with HF.[41] Beta-blockers should be considered in symptomatic HF or asymptomatic left ventricular dysfunction, and the treatment should be started at low doses and uptitrated to the maximal tolerated dose.[1]

Mineralocorticoid Antagonists

Aldosterone antagonists play an important role in attenuating the development of aldosterone-induced myocardial fibrosis and catecholamine release.[42] They should be considered in children with symptomatic left ventricular dysfunction.[1]

Digoxin

Digitalis has been the mainstay of chronic HF treatment for centuries. However, in the last few decades, several studies showed that digoxin does improve symptoms but not improve survival.[43] Thus, the indications for the use of digoxin in pediatric HF are unclear. Similar to adult guidelines, it is reasonable to use digoxin in children with severe left ventricular dysfunction who remain symptomatic despite optimal medical treatment.

Angiotensin Receptor Neprilysin Inhibitor

Sacubitril/valsartan, the first angiotensin receptor neprilysin inhibitor, provides simultaneous blockade of the RAAS system, with the inhibition of angiotensin II type-I receptor and inhibition of neprilysin, responsible for an increased level of physiologically active natriuretic peptides, resulting in enhancement of natriuretic, diuretic, and vasodilators action. In adult patients with HF with reduced ejection fraction, sacubitril/valsartan was superior to enalapril in reducing the risk of death and hospitalization for HF. A multicenter study aiming to compare the effectiveness and safety of sacubitril/valsartan in pediatric patients (PANORAMA-HF [Prospective trial to assess the Angiotensin Receptor Blocker Neprilysin Inhibitor LCZ696 vs ACEi for Medical treatment of Pediatric HF]; NCT02678312) is still ongoing.

Device Therapy

Two main devices are used in patients with HF: the implantable converter defibrillator (ICD) and cardiac resynchronization therapy (CRT).

There are few data on the use of ICD in pediatric age. Although not proven, possible indications of ICD in children are aborted cardiac arrest or a previous episode of ventricular tachycardiac determining hemodynamic instability; severe left ventricular dysfunction (ie, LVEF<35%); unexplained syncope in surgically repaired CHDs.[44,45]

Studies in adult patients demonstrated that CRT results in improvement in quality of life, functional class, ejection fraction, and prognosis. However, the knowledge base for CRT in children is scant. Some small cohort studies showed possible beneficial effects also in children; however, the incidence of side effect is significant. Thus, the indications for CRT are still unclear, and their potential risk-benefit ratio remained to be determined.

MECHANIC CIRCULATORY SUPPORT

The role of pediatric mechanic circulatory support (MCS) has been assessed as an alternative treatment in patients in whom heart transplant could not be performed. Recent studies[46] have demonstrated a 50% reduction of mortality in pediatric patients receiving ventricular assistance device (VAD) support. In particular, MCS was found to be an independent predictor of survival, whereas weight less than 10 kg, CHD diagnosis, extracorporeal membrane oxygenation (ECMO), mechanical ventilation, and renal dysfunction were all independent predictors of mortality on the waitlist. Subgroup analysis[47] demonstrated that benefit was higher among children older than 11 years: This could likely reflect current stage of device implantation, with third-generation VADs used in older children and ECMO or pulsatile devices as the only available option for smaller children.

Indications

Although the main indication for pediatric MCS is bridge to transplantation, in almost 6% of the cases, it is used as bridge to recovery, and rarely (2%) as destination therapy.[48] Comparing patients bridged to transplantation with VAD and those who were candidates to standard medical therapy alone, no difference was found in the posttransplantation survival, rate of infection, and graft rejection.[49] Nonetheless, in the cohort of patients who needed MCS, the proportion of patients who had needed mechanical ventilation or inotropic support was significantly higher, along with renal and hepatic dysfunction. According to the PediMACS registry, glomerular filtration rate normalized in almost 67% of the patients undergoing MCS[50]; noteworthy, pretransplant renal disfunction is an independent predictor of survival.

MCS can may be considered as a destination therapy in some specific pediatric cohorts, such as patients affected by Duchenne's muscular dystrophy,[51] cancer patients, or in complex CHD with severe organ damage and contraindication to heart transplant. In the acute setting, MCS can be offered to patients with advanced heart failure or cardiogenic shock with evidence of refractoriness to medical therapy; timing of MCS should be carefully evaluated as multiple studies have corroborated better outcomes in patients without evidence of end-stage organ injury.[52] Thus, MCS should be considered in patients with early organ dysfunction. Contraindications to MCS include active infection and irreversible end-stage organ dysfunction.[53] MCS should be carefully evaluated for the risk of futility in patients with moderate organ failure, severe diastolic dysfunction with thick heart chambers, significant aortic regurgitation, or intracardiac shunts which could affect forward stroke volume and require additional interventions.

The need for respiratory support, the planned duration of MCS, and body surface area are the main parameters to be considered while evaluating the type of MCS. In patients with acute collapse or need for biventricular pulmonary support, ECMO is the first-line option.

ECMO is commonly implanted in case of failure to wean from cardiopulmonary bypass, after cardiac arrest and in early graft failure after HT.[54] Venoarterial extracorporeal membrane oxygenation (VA-ECMO) can be deployed with central or peripheral cannulation and allows rapid biventricular support. Nonetheless it is a short-term device, requires highly intensive care management, and due to long tubing, it triggers intense inflammatory response. Afterload is increased in recipients of a VA-ECMO, thus atrial septostomy or left atrial venting are often required to decompress left ventricle. VA-ECMO can support cardiopulmonary function until decannulation, in case of cardiopulmonary recovery or for withdrawal of support in case of multiorgan failure. In patients who recover from pulmonary disease, it allows insertion of longer term cardiac support. Despite its flexibility, ECMO carries a high rate of complication, as bleeding, systemic embolism, neurologic injury and infection, and rates of complication significantly increase after 2 weeks from implantation, requiring transition to longer term VADs.[55]

Short-term MCS (less than 14 days) can be used in patients with acute myocarditis, in acute post-transplant graft failure, or in case of unknown diagnosis/patients with unknown neurologic status. Long-term support (more than 14 days) is indicated in patients with chronic HF due to CMP or refractory CHD.

HEART TRANSPLANTATION

HT is the gold standard for children with advanced HF, nonetheless the number of suitable donors has not increased for decades, leading to prolonged waitlist times and increased mortality rates.[56] According to the 20th International Society of Heart and Lung Transplantation (ISHLT) Pediatric Heart Transplantation Report,[56] the annual number of heart transplants in children has increased from 414 reported in 2000 to 614 in 2015, and it is estimated that roughly 300 children are listed annually for HT due to DCM.[57] Furthermore, data from the registry showed a survival after transplantation of 91% and 81% at 1 and 5 years, respectively.[56] Age at transplantation and diagnosis modify the prognosis of patients with HT. Infants carry a high risk of short-term mortality but are relatively protected from later complication, whereas adolescents show lower short-term mortality but increased long-term mortality. Moreover, there is a significantly higher rate of mortality for patients with CHDs than for those transplanted for CMPs.[56]

HT is indicated in patients with end-stage HF because of CMPs, myocarditis, or previously repaired CDHs; postcardiotomy HF; life-threatening arrhythmias refractory to medical therapy; complex CHD with no option for surgical palliation; unresectable cardiac tumors causing ventricular dysfunction or obstruction; and unresectable ventricular diverticula.

SUMMARY

Pediatric HF is a complex clinical syndrome with heterogeneous etiology and clinical manifestations. Diagnosis is based on a multiparametric approach and is required to initiate early a specific treatment. Special management should be performed in patients with advanced HF, such as continuous inotropic therapy, mechanical circulatory support, or HT.

CLINICS CARE POINTS

- The clinical scenario of HF may vary depending on the age of presentation and its severity should be classified according to the Ross modified classification or to the New York Heart Association (NYHA), in children younger and older than 6 years, respectively.

- The treatment of HF with reduced ejection fraction in children is based on disease modifier drugs that counteract the overactivation of the neurohormonal systems (i.e., beta-blockers, RAAS blockers, mineralocorticoid antagonists) with the aim to prevent disease progression and reduce hospitalization and mortality, and on diuretics that play an important role in reducing congestion.

- HT is indicated: in patients with end-stage HF because of CMPs, myocarditis, or previously repaired CDHs; postcardiotomy HF; lifethreatening arrhythmias refractory to medical therapy; complex CHD with no option for surgical palliation; unresectable cardiac tumors causing ventricular dysfunction or obstruction; and unresectable ventricular diverticula.

DISCLOSURE

The authors have nothing to disclose.

REFERENCES

1. Kirk R, Dipchand AI, Rosenthal DN, et al. The International Society for Heart and Lung Transplantation Guidelines for the management of pediatric heart failure: Executive summary. [Corrected]. J Heart Lung Transplant 2014;33(9):888–909.
2. Ponikowski P, Voors AA, Anker SD, et al. 2016 ESC Guidelines for the diagnosis and treatment of acute and chronic heart failure: The Task Force for the diagnosis and treatment of acute and chronic heart failure of the European Society of Cardiology (ESC) Developed with the special contribution of the Heart Failure Association (HFA) of the ESC. Eur Heart J 2016;37(27):2129–200.
3. Fedak PW, Verma S, Weisel RD, et al. Cardiac remodeling and failure: from molecules to man (Part III). Cardiovasc Pathol 2005;14(3):109–19.
4. Crespo-Leiro MG, Metra M, Lund LH, et al. Advanced heart failure: a position statement of the Heart Failure Association of the European Society of Cardiology. Eur J Heart Fail 2018;20(11):1505–35.
5. Rossano JW, Kim JJ, Decker JA, et al. Prevalence, morbidity, and mortality of heart failure-related hospitalizations in children in the United States: a population-based study. J Card Fail 2012;18(6):459–70.
6. Shaddy RE, George AT, Jaecklin T, et al. Systematic Literature Review on the Incidence and Prevalence of Heart Failure in Children and Adolescents. Pediatr Cardiol 2018;39(3):415–36.
7. Alvarez JA, Orav EJ, Wilkinson JD, et al. Competing risks for death and cardiac transplantation in children with dilated cardiomyopathy: results from the pediatric cardiomyopathy registry. Circulation 2011;124:814–23.
8. Nugent AW, Daubeney PE, Chondros P, et al. The epidemiology of childhood cardiomyopathy in Australia. N Engl J Med 2003;348:1639–46.
9. Andrew RE, Fenton MJ, Ridout DA, et al. New-onset heart failure due to heart muscle disease in childhood: A prospective study in United Kingdom and Ireland. Circulation 2008;117:79–84.
10. Nandi D, Rossano JW. Epidemiology and cost of heart failure in children. Cardiol Young 2015;25(8):1460–8.
11. Massin MM, Astadicko I, Dessy H. Epidemiology of heart failure in a tertiary pediatric center. Clin Cardiol 2008;31:388–91.
12. Boucek MM, Aurora P, Edwards LB, et al. Registry of the International Society for Heart and Lung Transplantation: tenth official pediatric heart transplantation report–2007. J Heart Lung Transplant 2007;26:796–807.
13. Hosseinpour AR, Cullen S, Tsang VT. Transplantation for adults with congenital heart disease. Eur J Cardiothorac Surg 2006;30:508–14.
14. Lamour JM, Addonizio LJ, Galantowicz ME, et al. Outcome after orthotopic cardiac transplantation in adults with congenital heart disease. Circulation 1999;100:II200–5.
15. Webster G, Zhang J, Rosenthal D. Comparison of the epidemiology and co-morbidities of heart failure in the pediatric and adult populations: A retrospective, cross-sectional study. BMC Cardiovasc Disord 2006;6:23.
16. Lipshultz SE, Sleeper LA, Towbin JA, et al. The incidence of pediatric cardiomyopathy in two regions of the United States. N Engl J Med 2003;348:1647–55.
17. Nakano SJ, Miyamoto SD, Price JF, et al. Pediatric Heart Failure: An Evolving Public Health Concern. J Pediatr 2020;218:217–21.
18. Passamano L, Taglia A, Palladino A, et al. Improvement of survival in Duchenne Muscular Dystrophy: retrospective analysis of 835 patients. Acta Myol 2012;31(2):121–5.
19. Jemal A, Ward EM, Johnson CJ, et al. Annual Report to the Nation on the Status of Cancer, 1975-2014, Featuring Survival. J Natl Cancer Inst 2017;109(9):djx030.
20. Francis GS, McDonald KM, Cohn JN. Neurohumoral activation in preclinical heart failure. Remodeling and the potential for intervention. Circulation 1993;87(5 Suppl):IV90–I96.
21. Chaggar PS, Malkin CJ, Shaw SM, et al. Neuroendocrine effects on the heart and targets for therapeutic manipulation in heart failure. Cardiovasc Ther 2009;27(3):187–93.
22. Ames MK, Atkins CE, Pitt B. The renin-angiotensin-aldosterone system and its suppression. J Vet Intern Med 2019;33(2):363–82. https://doi.org/10.1111/

jvim.15454 [Erratum appears in J Vet Intern Med 2019;33(5):2551].

23. Sipido KR, Eisner D. Something old, something new: changing views on the cellular mechanisms of heart failure. Cardiovasc Res 2005;68(2):167–74.

24. Grépin C, Dagnino L, Robitaille L, et al. A hormone-encoding gene identifies a pathway for cardiac but not skeletal muscle gene transcription. Mol Cell Biol 1994;14(5):3115–29.

25. Volpe M, Carnovali M, Mastromarino V. The natriuretic peptides system in the pathophysiology of heart failure: from molecular basis to treatment. Clin Sci (Lond) 2016;130(2):57–77.

26. Braunwald E. The path to an angiotensin receptor antagonist-neprilysin inhibitor in the treatment of heart failure. J Am Coll Cardiol 2015;65(10):1029–41.

27. Hinton RB, Ware SM. Heart Failure in Pediatric Patients With Congenital Heart Disease. Circ Res 2017;120(6):978–94.

28. Masarone D, Valente F, Rubino M, et al. Pediatric Heart Failure: A Practical Guide to Diagnosis and Management. Pediatr Neonatol 2017;58(4):303–12.

29. Miyamoto SD, Stauffer BL, Nakano S, et al. Beta-adrenergic adaptation in paediatric idiopathic dilated cardiomyopathy. Eur Heart J 2014;35(1):33–41.

30. Kantor PF, Lougheed J, Dancea A, et al. Presentation, diagnosis, and medical management of heart failure in children: Canadian Cardiovascular Society guidelines. Can J Cardiol 2013;29(12):1535–52.

31. Ross RD, Bollinger RO, Pinsky WW. Grading the severity of congestive heart failure in infants. Pediatr Cardiol 1992;13:72e5.

32. O'Connor M, Mc Daniel N, Brady WJ. The pediatric electrocardiogram Part III: congenital heart disease and other cardiac syndromes. Am J Emerg Med 2008;26:497e503.

33. Bergmann KR, Kharbanda A, Haveman L. Myocarditis And Pericarditis In The Pediatric Patient: Validated Management Strategies. Pediatr Emerg Med Pract 2015;12(7):1–22 [quiz: 23].

34. Marwick TH, Shah SJ, Thomas JD. Myocardial Strain in the Assessment of Patients With Heart Failure: A Review. JAMA Cardiol 2019;4(3):287–94.

35. Satou GM, Lacro RV, Chung T, et al. Heart size on chest x-ray as a predictor of cardiac enlargement by echocardiography in children. Pediatr Cardiol 2001;22:218e22.

36. Mitchell FM, Prasad SK, Greil GF, et al. Cardiovascular magnetic resonance: Diagnostic utility and specific considerations in the pediatric population. World J Clin Pediatr 2016;5(1):1–15.

37. Feltes TF, Bacha E, Beekman RH 3rd, et al. Indications for cardiac catheterization and intervention in pediatric cardiac disease: a scientific statement from the American Heart Association. Circulation 2011;123(22):2607–52.

38. Webber SA, Boyle GJ, Jaffe R, et al. Role of right ventricular endomyocardial biopsy in infants and children with suspected or possible myocarditis. Br Heart J 1994;72:360e3.

39. Felker GM, Ellison DH, Mullens W, et al. Diuretic Therapy for Patients With Heart Failure: JACC State-of-the-Art Review. J Am Coll Cardiol 2020;75(10):1178–95.

40. Lewis AB, Chabot M. The effect of treatment with angiotensin-converting enzyme inhibitors on survival of pediatric patients with dilated cardiomyopathy. Pediatr Cardiol 1993;14:9–12.

41. Packer M, Coats AJ, Fowler MB, et al. Effect of carvedilol on survival in severe chronic heart failure. N Engl J Med 2001;344:1651–8.

42. Zannad F, Alla F, Dousset B, et al. Limitation of excessive extracellular matrix turnover may contribute to survival benefit of spironolactone therapy in patients with congestive heart failure: insights from the randomized aldactone evaluation study (RALES). Rales Investigators. Circulation 2000;102(22):2700–6.

43. Hood WB Jr, Dans AL, Guyatt GH, et al. Digitalis for treatment of congestive heart failure in patients in sinus rhythm. Cochrane Database Syst Rev 2004;2:CD002901.

44. Griksaitis MJ, Rosengarten JA, Gnanapragasam JP, et al. Implantable cardioverter defibrillator therapy in paediatric practice: a single-centre UK experience with focus on subcutaneous defibrillation. Europace 2013;15(4):523–30.

45. Rhee EK, Canter CE, Basile S, et al. Sudden death prior to pediatric heart transplantation: would implantable defibrillators improve outcome? J Heart Lung Transplant 2007;26(5):447–52.

46. Zafar F, Castleberry C, Khan MS, et al. Pediatric heart transplant waiting list mortality in the era of ventricular assist devices. J Heart Lung Transplant 2015;34(1):82–8.

47. Law SP, Oron AP, Kemna MS, et al. Comparison of transplant waitlist outcomes for pediatric candidates supported by ventricular assist devices versus medical therapy. Pediatr Crit Care Med 2018;19(5):442–50.

48. Blume ED, VanderPluym C, Lorts A, et al. Second annual Pediatric Interagency Registry for Mechanical Circulatory Support (Pedimacs) report: Pre-implant characteristics and outcomes. J Heart Lung Transplant 2018;37(1):38–45.

49. Sutcliffe DL, Pruitt E, Cantor RS, et al. Post-transplant outcomes in pediatric ventricular assist device patients: A PediMACS–Pediatric Heart Transplant Study linkage analysis. J Heart Lung Transplant 2018;37(6):715–22.

50. Schumacher KR, Almond C, Singh TP, et al. Predicting graft loss by 1 Year in pediatric heart transplantation candidates: An analysis of the Pediatric Heart

Transplant Study database. Circulation 2015; 131(10):890–8.

51. Amodeo A, Adorisio R. Left ventricular assist device in Duchenne Cardiomyopathy: Can we change the natural history of cardiac disease? Int J Cardiol 2012;161(3):e43.

52. Potapov EV, Stiller B, Hetzer R. Ventricular assist devices in children: Current achievements and future perspectives. Pediatr Transplant 2007;11(3):241–55.

53. Wilmot I, Lorts A, Morales D. Pediatric mechanical circulatory support. Korean J Thorac Cardiovasc Surg 2013;46(6):391–401.

54. Duncan BW, Ibrahim AE, Hraska V, et al. Use of rapid-deployment extracorporeal membrane oxygenation for the resuscitation of pediatric patients with heart disease after cardiac arrest. J Thorac Cardiovasc Surg 1998;116(2):305–11.

55. Wehman B, Stafford KA, Bittle GJ, et al. Modern outcomes of mechanical circulatory support as a bridge to pediatric heart transplantation. Ann Thorac Surg 2016;101(6):2321–7.

56. Rossano JW, Cherikh WS, Chambers DC, et al. The Registry of the International Society for Heart and Lung Transplantation: Twentieth Pediatric Heart Transplantation Report-2017; Focus Theme: Allograft ischemic time. J Heart Lung Transplant 2017; 36(10):1060–9.

57. Norozi K, Wessel A, Alpers V, et al. Incidence and Risk Distribution of Heart Failure in Adolescents and Adults With Congenital Heart Disease After Cardiac Surgery. Am J Cardiol 2006;97(8):1238–43.

Advanced Heart Failure in a Special Population
Heart Failure with Preserved Ejection Fraction

Simone Longhi, MD, PhD[a],*, Giulia Saturi, MD[a,b],
Angelo Giuseppe Caponetti, MD[a,b], Christian Gagliardi, MD, PhD[a],
Elena Biagini, MD PhD[a]

KEYWORDS

• HFpEF • Preserved • HF • Diastolic dysfunction

KEY POINTS

- According to main major society guidelines, heart failure with preserved ejection fraction (HFpEF) can be defined as the presence of signs and symptoms of heart failure associated with left ventricular ejection fraction greater than or equal to 50%, increased levels of natriuretic peptides, and relevant structural heart abnormalities such as diastolic dysfunction, left atrial enlargement, and/or left ventricular hypertrophy.
- Diagnostic algorithms, including several clinical and instrumental tools (H2FPEF or Heart Failure Association PEFF scores) have been developed in order to guide physicians to reach the diagnosis of HFpEF, although additional evaluations can be necessary in case of intermediate scores.
- HFpEF has a poor prognosis, with a mortality ranging from 20% to 29% at 1 year and from 53% to 74% at 5 years.
- Medical treatments have not yet been shown to reduce both cardiovascular and all-cause mortality, but upcoming data about tailored therapies, in some specific phenotypes of HFpEF, could provide interesting answers about these unmet (so far) research questions.

INTRODUCTION

Heart failure with preserved ejection fraction (HFpEF) is a complex clinical syndrome that has emerged in the last decades as a huge concern for life expectancy and for global health care.[1] The insidious nature of this disease is related to its high incidence and prevalence (ranging from 1% to 14% in Western countries)[1] along with a challenging diagnosis and a lack of therapies clearly related to an improvement of prognosis. This article summarizes the current knowledge about HFpEF, focusing on its definitions, diagnosis, natural history, and therapy.

DEFINITION

The classic physiologic and hemodynamic definition of heart failure (HF) by Dr Braunwald and Grossman[2] is "the heart's inability to meet the body's metabolic demands, or to do so at the expense of increased filling pressures." The current (2016) European Society of Cardiology (ESC) guidelines for the diagnosis and treatment of acute and chronic HF define it as a "clinical syndrome characterized by typical symptoms that may be accompanied by signs caused by a structural or functional cardiac abnormality, resulting in a reduced cardiac output and/or

[a] Cardiology Unit, St. Orsola Hospital, IRCCS Azienda Ospedaliero-Universitaria di Bologna, Via Massarenti 9, Bologna 40138, Italy; [b] Department of Experimental, Diagnostic and Specialty Medicine (DIMES), University of Bologna, Italy
* Corresponding author.
E-mail address: simone.longhi@aosp.bo.it

Heart Failure Clin 17 (2021) 685–695
https://doi.org/10.1016/j.hfc.2021.05.012
1551-7136/21/© 2021 Elsevier Inc. All rights reserved.

heartfailure.theclinics.com

increased intracardiac pressures at rest or during stress."[3]

The current classification is based on the measurement of left ventricular ejection fraction (LVEF) and identifies 3 different conditions: HF with reduced ejection fraction (HFrEF; ie, LVEF<40%), HF with midrange ejection fraction (LVEF40%–49%), and HF with preserved ejection fraction (LVEF $\geq$ 50%). The use of LVEF as the sole classification criterion is weak, and clinicians treating HF are becoming aware that there are different phenotypes, each with its own definition, diagnosis, and therapy grouped under the heart-failure umbrella.

Major society guidelines give different definitions of HFpEF (**Table 1**). The American College of Cardiology (ACC)/American Heart Association (AHA) in 2013 defined HFpEF as the presence of symptoms of HF (New York Heart Association II–IV) with an LVEF greater than or equal to 50%, after excluding noncardiac causes of exercise intolerance.[4] The Heart Failure Society of America (HFSA) in 2010 defined HFpEF as the presence of typical symptoms and signs, echocardiographic signs of diastolic dysfunction, left ventricular (LV) hypertrophy or left atrial (LA) enlargement, and previous hospitalization for cardiovascular causes.[5]

Following the 2016 ESC guidelines, HFpEF is a clinical syndrome that could be diagnosed in the presence of signs and symptoms of HF, LVEF greater than or equal to 50%, increased levels of natriuretic peptides (NPs), and at least 1 additional criterion between relevant structural heart disease or diastolic dysfunction.[3]

DIAGNOSIS

There is no a unique parameter that can rule the diagnosis in or out, but the work-up must be multi-parametric, including clinical evaluation, laboratory data, echocardiographic assessment, and direct hemodynamic measurements at rest and during exercise.

In recent years, new diagnostic algorithms have also been proposed to help clinicians in this complex setting.

Symptoms and Signs

Dyspnea and asthenia are the most common manifestations of HF, but they are often nonspecific. It is possible to distinguish 2 different clinical presentations: rest congestion (hospitalized patients), characterized by classic signs of volume overload at physical examination; and exercise intolerance related to exertional dyspnea (euvolemic patients in the early stages of the disease or in patients treated with diuretics). These symptoms could severely limit life quality, but they can be multifactorial and physical examination may be normal.[6]

Table 1
Definitions of heart failure with preserved ejection fraction

	HFSA	ACC/AHA	ESC
Reference	Lindelfeld et al, 2010[77]	Yancy et al, 2013[4]	Ponikowsky et al, 2016[3]
Year	2010	2013	2016
Symptoms	+	+	+
Signs	+	—	+/−
LVEF (%)	≥50	≥50	≥50
Natriuretic Peptides	—	—	+
Echocardiography	Diastolic dysfunction, left ventricular hypertrophy, left atrial enlargement (without atrial fibrillation)	—	Diastolic dysfunction (without left ventricular dilation), left ventricular hypertrophy, left atrial enlargement
Catheter	—	—	Pulmonary capillary wedge pressure ≥15 mm Hg
Hospital Admission for Cardiovascular Cause	+	—	—

Abbreviations: ACC, American College of Cardiology; AHA, American Heart Association; ESC, European Society of Cardiology; HFSA, Heart Failure Society of America.

Biomarkers

Increased plasma levels of brain NP (BNP) and N-terminal pro-BNP (NT-proBNP) indirectly reflect increased filling pressure.[7]

ECS guidelines in 2016 established that increased serum levels of NPs in nonacute setting (BNP>35 pg/mL and/or NT-proBNP>125 pg/mL) are mandatory for the diagnosis of HFpEF. These cutoffs have high negative predictive value (NPV; 95%–99%), but they can be abnormal in the presence of atrial fibrillation (AF), tachycardia, ischemia, aging, and renal failure.[8] In stable symptomatic patients with invasively confirmed HFpEF, NPs levels could be below the diagnostic thresholds in up to 20% of the population, especially in obese patients.[9,10]

Echocardiogram

The echocardiogram is a noninvasive, widely available diagnostic tool, essential in the context of HF. The HFpEF phenotype is suggested by the presence of nondilated LV, with a normal ejection fraction, concentric remodeling or hypertrophy, and LA enlargement with diastolic dysfunction, although these characteristics are neither specific nor sensitive for HFpEF.[11] Echocardiographic evaluation in this setting should be multiparametric and includes LV systolic and diastolic function, right ventricular (RV) structure and function, and estimation of pulmonary arterial pressure. If rest evaluation is inconclusive, stress echocardiography should be performed.

Left ventricular systolic function

LVEF estimates LV global function. Despite a preserved LVEF ($\geq$50%), more sensitive tools, such as tissue Doppler imaging (TDI), deformation analysis, LV stroke volume index, and cardiac output, might show subclinical systolic dysfunction with different prevalence accordingly to the technique used (40%–65% of patients with HFpEF).[12,13]

Left ventricular diastolic function

Impaired LV diastolic relaxation and increased diastolic stiffness lead to high filling pressures at rest with a limited cardiac performance during exercise.[14]

Functional evaluation includes the peak velocity of mitral inflow during early diastole (E wave), the early diastolic velocity of mitral annular motion (e' wave) at TDI, and the E/e' velocity ratio.[15] The e' velocity is primarily determined by LV diastolic filling pressure and reflects preload conditions.[16] The normality cutoff is 7 cm/s for the septal e' and 10 cm/s for the lateral e', but, being influenced by aging, different cutoffs have been proposed for patients more than 75 years old (septal e' <5 cm/s, lateral e' <7 cm/s).[17] The E/e' velocity ratio reflects the mean pulmonary capillary wedge pressure (PCWP) and correlates with LV stiffness and fibrosis. It is less dependent on age and preload than e' velocity, but it is influenced by LV hypertrophy.[17] The normal cut off currently used is E/e' less than 14.[18]

More recently, new diagnostic tools have been proposed, such as atrial strain, studied in the research context but not yet widely used in the clinical setting.[19]

The LA volume index is a marker of LA remodeling and indirectly correlates to LV filling pressure. The upper limit in healthy people is 34 mL/m^2 in sinus rhythm and 40 mL/m^2 in AF.[20,21]

LV geometry is well classified using relative wall thickness (RWT) and LV mass index (LVMI), describing 4 different patterns. Concentric remodeling (normal LVMI, RWT>0.42) and concentric hypertrophy (increased LVMI, RWT>0.42) are typical features in patients with HFpEF.[22]

Right ventricular function and pulmonary arterial pressure

The following measures can reflect RV systolic function: tricuspid annular plane systolic excursion (abnormal, <17 mm), TDI tricuspid lateral annular systolic velocity (s' wave, with abnormal velocity <9.5 cm/s), fractional area change (abnormal, <35%), and systolic pulmonary artery pressure (sPAP). The increase of sPAP and RV dysfunction are predictors of mortality in HFpEF.[23]

Stress test echocardiography

Exercise or pharmacologic stress echocardiography is a well-known tool in some kinds of valvular and ischemic heart disease but, more recently, it has gained diagnostic application in HFpEF.[9,24]

During exercise, in healthy people, enhanced LV relaxation prevents LV filling pressure from increasing. In contrast, in patients with HFpEF, impaired diastolic relaxation and LV stiffness lead to an inadequate increase of stroke volume, with abnormal increase of LV filling pressure and sPAP.[25]

The 2 parameters better studied and used in stress echocardiography are E/e' ratio and sPAP, which correlate with 2 hemodynamic parameters, PCWP and mean pulmonary artery pressure (mPAP) respectively.[26]

Exercise echocardiography should be considered abnormal if average E/e' ratio at peak stress increases to greater than or equal to 15, with or without a peak tricuspid regurgitant jet (TR) velocity greater than 3.4 m/s.[27,28]

Heart Catheterization

Invasive hemodynamic assessment, with left and right heart catheterization, at rest and during exercise remains the gold standard for the definition of HFpEF.[29] LV end-diastolic pressure (LVDP) greater than or equal to 12 mm Hg indicates an increase of filling pressure. Moreover, the end-diastolic pressure-volume relationship describes well the LV compliance and stiffness.[14]

Resting PCWP greater than or equal to 15 mm Hg with a normal LV end-diastolic volume index confirms a definite diagnosis of HFpEF. However, volume depletion or intensification diuretic treatment may mask the underlying condition with normalization of hemodynamic parameters at rest.

During supine exercise, in healthy people, cutoffs for peak PCWP and LV end-diastolic pressure are greater than or equal to 20 to 23 mm Hg and greater than or equal to 25 mm Hg respectively.[30]

A sharp increase of PCWP is a typical hemodynamic response to exercise in patients with HFpEF[31] and it helps in stratifying risk.[32]

Exercise Tests

In selected patients, a cardiopulmonary exercise test with spiroergometry may be performed. It provides objective evidence of limitation in functional capacity and discriminates cardiac and noncardiac causes of dyspnea. Peak oxygen consumption (Vo$_2$ max) and ventilatory efficiency (VE/Vco$_2$) with values, respectively, less than or equal to 20 mL/kg/min and greater than or equal to 30 indicate cardiogenic exercise intolerance.[33]

Diagnostic Algorithms

Two different recent diagnostic algorithms have been proposed, integrating clinical data with noninvasive and invasive diagnostic tools to help clinicians with the diagnosis of HFpEF. Both algorithms are designed to exclude or confirm HFpEF diagnosis for low and high scores respectively, but they require additional evaluations for intermediate scores.

- A group of researchers from Mayo Clinic have recently developed and validated a score that could estimate the likelihood of HFpEF among patients with unexplained dyspnea to guide further testing: the H2FPEF score.[34] This score includes 6 variables: obesity, AF, age greater than 60 years, treatment with greater than or equal to 2 antihypertensives, echocardiographic E/e' ratio greater than 9, and echocardiographic sPAP greater than 35 mm Hg, with different points assigned to each variable for a total of 9 points. This approach aims to establish the likelihood of the disease: low scores (0 or 1) rule out the disease, higher scores (5–9) could establish the diagnosis with reasonably high confidence, and intermediate scores (2–5) identify patients for whom additional testing is needed.

- A recent consensus document from the Heart Failure Association (HFA) of the ESC has proposed a different stepwise diagnostic process.[7] Step 1 (pretest assessment) includes assessment of symptoms and signs, laboratory tests, electrocardiogram, and echocardiogram. HFpEF can be suspected in the absence of other manifest noncardiac causes of exertional dyspnea if there is a normal LVEF, no significant heart valve disease or cardiac ischemia, and at least 1 typical risk factor (age>70 years, overweight, metabolic syndrome or diabetes mellitus, deconditioning, hypertension, AF, electrocardiogram abnormalities and increased NP levels). Step 2 (echocardiography and NP score) combines major and minor criteria (functional, morphologic, and biomarkers) into a diagnostic score (HFA PEFF score). A score greater than or equal to 5 points indicates a definite diagnosis of HFpEF; less than or equal to 1 point rules out HFpEF. An intermediate score (2–4 points) leads to step 3 (functional testing) with stress echocardiogram or invasive hemodynamic test. Step 4 (final cause) looks for a specific cause of HFpEF or alternative causes.

Therefore, the definition and diagnosis of HFpEF in patients with unexplained dyspnea remain a clinical challenge in the absence of a unique diagnostic algorithm universally recognized and applied, and a step approach is recommended to reach the correct diagnosis (Fig. 1).

CAUSAL DIAGNOSIS

As discussed earlier, it is crucial to get investigate the intricate and multistep diagnostic pathway of HFpEF to identify a potential specific pathophysiologic process causing the clinical phenotype. Many cardiovascular conditions (eg, valvular heart disease, ischemic heart disease, pericardial disease, primary cardiomyopathy) share with the typical pure form of HFpEF some hemodynamic parameters, although with typical red flags and distinctive features, as summarized in Fig. 2. Also, high-output states such as anemia or thyroid disease, and fluid overload from kidney or liver disorder, can mimic HFpEF, but currently most experts agree to not include those cardiac or extracardiac conditions in the category of HFpEF.[6]

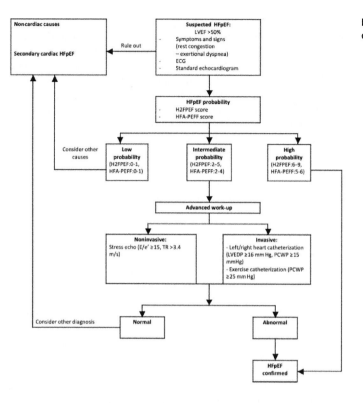

Fig. 1. Diagnostic algorithm. LVEDP, LV end-diastolic pressure.

The identification of an underlying disease could have a severe impact in terms of beneficial therapy. For example, cardiac amyloidosis (CA) is a disorder caused by extracellular deposition of misfolded proteins whose precursors can originate, as known, from a plasma cell dyscrasia (amyloid light-chain [AL] amyloidosis) or from abnormal disaggregation of a protein called transthyretin (TTR) in the presence or absence of a TTR gene mutation. The prevalence of CA is widespread, and it now represents a well-known cause of hospitalization for HF, especially with normal or mildly reduced ejection fraction. González-López and colleagues,[35] in a prospective study enrolling 120 patients with HFpEF and maximum wall thickness greater than or equal to 12 mm, revealed that 13% of subjects had a significant cardiac uptake at bone scan scintigraphy. Recognizing the cause becomes especially critical when dealing with CA, because the therapy for AL amyloidosis is

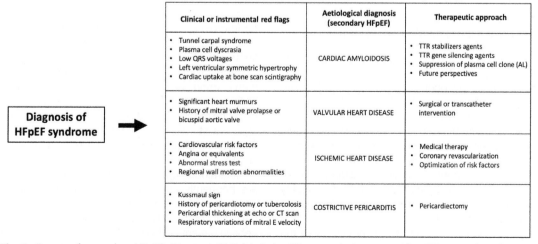

Fig. 2. Causes of secondary HFpEF. AL, amyloid light chain; CT, computed tomography; TTR, transthyretin.

mainly based on the suppression of the plasma cell clone in the bone marrow, whereas, for TTR-related amyloidosis (ATTR), many drugs are emerging as possible weapons against the progression of the disease. First, the ATTR-ACT (The Transthyretin Amyloidosis Cardiomyopathy Clinical Trial) study, a multicenter, double-blind, placebo-controlled, phase 3 trial, showed that the use of tafamidis, a TTR stabilizer, was associated with a lower rate of death and cardiovascular-related hospitalizations in patients affected by ATTR.[36] Given these promising therapies, it is now recommended to exclude the underlying presence of CA in patients with HFpEF, especially in older patients or those who have features of hypertrophic or restrictive cardiomyopathy.[37] For possible causal diagnosis in HFpEF, a dilemma exists in determining whether conditions such as coronary artery disease (CAD) or heart valve disease play a central pathophysiologic role or whether they act as bystanders in standard HFpEF. A retrospective analysis conducted on 376 patients admitted to hospital for HFpEF showed the presence of angiographic CAD in 68% of the cohort; symptoms of angina and heart failure were similar in patients with and without CAD, although the presence of CAD represented an independent risk factor for death.[38] Regarding valvular heart disease, mild or moderate mitral regurgitation (MR) is frequently detected in patients with HFpEF, and it is usually considered an innocent bystander. However, it has been recently shown that these patients display worse biventricular function and more altered pulmonary hemodynamics.[39] In addition, a moderate MR at rest can increase after exercise, sometimes explaining exertional symptoms[40]; these dynamic changes of MR carry well-established prognostic importance in HFrEF, whereas their impact on the natural history of HFpEF is unclear.

NATURAL HISTORY AND OUTCOMES

The natural history of HFpEF is controversial. Several epidemiologic and observational studies have shown the poor prognosis of HFpEF, with mortality ranging from 20% to 29% at 1 year and from 53% to 74% at 5 years.[41–44] Other noncardiovascular comorbidities, such as diabetes, chronic kidney disease, and cerebrovascular disorders, or the concomitant presence of RV dysfunction, affect survival.[45–47] In contrast, large clinical trials have reported lower mortality (4%–5% at 1 year), probably because of a more stringent selection of patients with less comorbidity.[48,49]

Regarding the long-standing dilemma about the comparison between HFrEF and HFpEF prognosis,

2 meta-analyses including 73,597 and 24,501 patients from 31 and 17 studies respectively, have shown a significantly lower risk of death in HFpEF, even without taking randomized clinical trials into account.[50,51] By the way, some other small observational studies have shown similar hospitalization rates or subjective quality of life between HFpEF and HFrEF.[52,53] One of the most uncontroversial aspects of these conditions is that HF, and in particular HFpEF, itself carries a heightened risk of all-cause and cardiovascular mortality.[54,55]

In recent years, many researchers have speculated about the existence of different phenotypes within the wide spectrum of HFpEF, affecting the prognosis of these patients and, in some cases, the response to specific therapies.[56] Some of the most exciting data come from latent class analyses of large clinical trials conducted in this regard. Cohen and colleagues[58] identified 3 HFpEF phenogroups based on standard clinical or instrumental features and multiple biomarkers measured from frozen plasma among participants of the TOPCAT trial.[57] The third phenogroup (which included patients with obesity, diabetes, chronic kidney disease, concentric LV hypertrophy, high renin level, biomarkers of tumor necrosis factor-alpha–mediated inflammation, liver fibrosis, and tissue remodeling) showed the highest risk of cardiovascular death, HF hospitalization, or aborted cardiac arrest (hazard ratio [HR], 3.44; 95% confidence interval [CI], 2.79–4.24) but also a more pronounced prognostic benefit from spironolactone therapy.[58]

MANAGEMENT AND THERAPY

In patients with HFpEF, medical treatments have not yet been shown to reduce both cardiovascular and all-cause mortality[4] but can alleviate symptoms and improve well-being.[52]

The guidelines recommend the use of diuretics for improving symptoms and signs of HF regardless of LVEF.[3,4,59,60] Titration of loop diuretic in patients with HFpEF reduces hospitalization.[61] In the CHAMPION trial, hemodynamic-guided medical management of diuretic in patients with HF and LVEF greater than or equal to 40% resulted in a lower hospitalization rate than standard HF management strategies.[52] Therefore, diuretics can be considered pillars of the current management of HFpEF.

Mineralocorticoid receptor antagonists (MRAs) are frequently associated with diuretics, despite a lack of evidence of improving survival. The TOPCAT trial compared spironolactone (MRA) and placebo in patients with HFpEF (LVEF $\geq$ 45%) without a significant reduction in the primary end point (death from cardiovascular causes, aborted cardiac arrest, or hospitalizations for HF) between the groups even if a reduction in the secondary end point of HF hospitalizations favored spironolactone (HR, 0.83; CI, 0.69–0.99; P = .04).[57] Post hoc analyses showed a significant reduction of the primary end point among American but not in Russian and Georgian patients (HR, 0.82; CI, 069–0.98; P = .03).[62] Nevertheless, the standard management of patients with HFpEF provides MRAs for their diuretic and antihypertensive properties, for modifying serum levels of the biomarker of collagen deposition and cardiac remodeling.[63]

Three randomized controlled trials conducted in patients with HFpEF treated with angiotensin II receptor blockers and angiotensin-converting enzyme inhibitors versus placebo failed to improve the primary outcomes (composite of cardiovascular death or HF/cardiovascular hospitalization): candesartan in CHARM-Preserved,[64] perindopril in PEP-CHF,[49] and irbesartan in I-PRESERVE.[65] Moreover, there is inconsistent evidence for an improvement in symptoms in these patients.[4] In the CHARM-Preserved study, candesartan reduced hospitalizations for HF compared with placebo (nonpredefined end point),[64] and this is the rationale for using this medical treatment in patients with HFpEF.

Sacubitril/valsartan, with the double action of angiotensin receptor blocker and neprilysin inhibitor, has natriuretic and diuretic properties and provides better control of blood pressure. In the PARAMOUNT study, sacubitril/valsartan reduced NT-proBNP value and LA size compared with valsartan in patients with HFpEF[66] and was the prerequisite for the PARAGON-HF trial. In this 3-phase trial,[67] sacubitril/valsartan did not show a significant reduction in the primary outcome (cardiovascular mortality and hospitalizations for HF); a benefit was evident in the subgroup of patients with an LVEF less than or equal to 57% and in women. Moreover, in patients enrolled within 30 days from a previous hospitalization, sacubitril/valsartan had a relative risk reduction in recurrent clinical events compared with patients never hospitalized, identifying a group of patients with HFpEF who might be particularly responsive to the treatment.[68]

The J-DHF and the ELANDD study evaluated the role of β-blockers compared with placebo, but neither showed a clinical benefit in the risk of death or hospitalization.[69,70] In patients with HFrEF, HFpEF, or HF with midrange ejection fraction, nebivolol reduced the combined end point of death or cardiovascular hospitalization,[71] with no significant interaction between treatment effect and baseline LVEF.

No clear clinical benefit has been shown in treating HFpEF with calcium channel blockers[4] and digoxin. The DIG-PEF study did not reduce mortality or incidence of hospitalization for HF in patients with LVEF greater than 45% and concomitant treatment with digoxin.[72]

There is no role for ivabradine in the routine treatment of HFpEF. This drug was tested in the EDIFY trial without reducing the E/e' ratio, NT-proBNP levels, or improving the walking test performance.[73]

The results of the RELAX study do not suggest the routine use of phosphodiesterases-5 inhibitors in HFpEF. In this randomized, placebo-controlled, multicenter clinical trial, long-term phosphodiesterases-5 inhibitors had no effect on maximal or submaximal exercise capacity, clinical status, quality of life, LV remodeling, diastolic function parameters, or pulmonary artery systolic pressure.[74]

In addition to medical therapy, exercise is strongly recommended in all patients with HFpEF: it improves peak oxygen consumption, diastolic function, and quality of life.[75]

Moreover, in the near future, data from clinical trials on gliflozins (dapagliflozin and empagliflozin), soluble guanylate cyclase activators (vericiguat), prostanoids (iloprost), antifibrotic drugs (pirfenidone), and intravenous iron (FAIR-HFpEF)[76] will become available, bringing new knowledge of the complex scenario of HFpEF therapy.

SUMMARY

HFpEF is a complex clinical syndrome that requires a multistep diagnostic pathway and a critical interpretation of the whole clinical framework. Prognosis is still poor, and medical therapy has not yet shown a significant benefit, although upcoming data about more tailored therapies could provide interesting answers about this controversial disease.

CLINICS CARE POINTS

- Instrumental and laboratory tests can reveal hemodynamic features related to HFpEF, but it is essential to investigate a potential underlying causal diagnosis (eg, CA, ischemic heart disease).

- Normal LVEF ($\geq$50%) does not always mean normal systolic function: many advanced imaging techniques, such as tissue Doppler or speckle tracking, can detect a subclinical systolic dysfunction.

- Although no medical therapy carries a strong prognostic impact in HFpEF, sacubitril/valsartan has shown in the PARAGON-HF trial a significant reduction of primary end point (hospitalizations for heart failure and death from cardiovascular causes) in prespecified subgroups: women and patients with ejection fraction less than 57% (median value of the study).

DISCLOSURE

The authors have nothing to disclose.

REFERENCES

1. Borlaug BA. Evaluation and management of heart failure with preserved ejection fraction. Nat Rev Cardiol 2020;17(9):559–73.
2. Braunwald E, Grossman W. Clinical aspects of heart failure. In: Braunwald E, editor. Heart disease: a textbook of cardiovascular medicine. 4th edition. Saunders; 1992. p. 444–63.
3. Ponikowski P, Voors AA, Anker SD, et al. 2016 ESC Guidelines for the diagnosis and treatment of acute and chronic heart failure. Eur Heart J 2016;37(27): 2129–2200m.
4. Yancy CW, Jessup M, Bozkurt B, et al. 2013 ACCF/ AHA guideline for the management of heart failure: Executive summary: A report of the American college of cardiology foundation/american heart association task force on practice guidelines. J Am Coll Cardiol 2013;62(16):1495–539.
5. Heart Failure Society of America. HFSA 2010 Comprehensive Heart Failure Practice Guideline. J Card Fail 2010;16(6):e1.
6. Ho JE, Redfield MM, Lewis GD, et al. Deliberating the Diagnostic Dilemma of Heart Failure with Preserved Ejection Fraction. Circulation 2020;1770–80. https://doi.org/10.1161/CIRCULATIONAHA.119. 041818.
7. Pieske B, Tschöpe C, De Boer RA, et al. How to diagnose heart failure with preserved ejection fraction: The HFA-PEFF diagnostic algorithm: A consensus recommendation from the Heart Failure Association (HFA) of the European Society of Cardiology (ESC). Eur Heart J 2019;40(40):3297–317.
8. Roberts E, Ludman AJ, Dworzynski K, et al. The diagnostic accuracy of the natriuretic peptides in heart failure: Systematic review and diagnostic meta-analysis in the acute care setting. BMJ 2015; 350. https://doi.org/10.1136/bmj.h910.
9. Obokata M, Kane GC, Reddy YNV, et al. Role of Diastolic Stress Testing in the Evaluation for Heart Failure with Preserved Ejection Fraction: A Simultaneous Invasive-Echocardiographic Study. Circulation 2017;135(9):825–38.
10. Buckley LF, Canada JM, Del Buono MG, et al. Low NT-proBNP levels in overweight and obese patients do not rule out a diagnosis of heart failure with preserved ejection fraction. ESC Hear Fail 2018;5(2): 372–8.
11. Wan SH, Vogel MW, Chen HH. Pre-clinical diastolic dysfunction. J Am Coll Cardiol 2014;63(5):407–16.
12. Kraigher-Krainer E, Shah AM, Gupta DK, et al. Impaired systolic function by strain imaging in heart failure with preserved ejection fraction. J Am Coll Cardiol 2014;63(5):447–56.
13. Wang J, Khoury DS, Yue Y, et al. Preserved left ventricular twist and circumferential deformation, but depressed longitudinal and radial deformation in patients with diastolic heart failure. Eur Heart J 2008; 29(10):1283–9.
14. Zile MR, Baicu CF, Gaasch WH. Diastolic Heart Failure — Abnormalities in Active Relaxation and Passive Stiffness of the Left Ventricle. N Engl J Med 2004;350(19):1953–9.
15. Nagueh SF, Smiseth OA, Appleton CP, et al. Recommendations for the Evaluation of Left Ventricular Diastolic Function by Echocardiography: An Update from the American Society of Echocardiography and the European Association of Cardiovascular Imaging. J Am Soc Echocardiogr 2016;29(4):277–314.
16. Opdahl A, Remme EW, Helle-Valle T, et al. Determinants of left ventricular early-diastolic lengthening velocity independent contributions from left ventricular relaxation, restoring forces, and lengthening load. Circulation 2009;119(19):2578–86.
17. Shah AM, Claggett B, Kitzman D, et al. Contemporary Assessment of Left Ventricular Diastolic Function in Older Adults: The Atherosclerosis Risk in Communities Study. Circulation 2017;135(5): 426–39.
18. Mitter SS, Shah SJ, Thomas JD. A Test in Context: E/ A and E/e′ to Assess Diastolic Dysfunction and LV Filling Pressure. J Am Coll Cardiol 2017;69(11): 1451–64.
19. Donal E, Galli E, Schnell F. Left Atrial Strain: A Must or a Plus for Routine Clinical Practice? Circ Cardiovasc Imaging 2017;10(10). https://doi.org/10.1161/ CIRCIMAGING.117.007023.
20. Kou S, Caballero L, Dulgheru R, et al. Echocardiographic reference ranges for normal cardiac chamber size: Results from the NORRE study. Eur Heart J Cardiovasc Imaging 2014;15(6):680–90.
21. Melenovsky V, Hwang SJ, Redfield MM, et al. Left atrial remodelling and function in advanced heart failure with preserved or reduced ejection fraction. Circ Hear Fail 2015;8(2):295–303.
22. Shah AM, Claggett B, Sweitzer NK, et al. Cardiac structure and function and prognosis in heart failure

with preserved ejection fraction. Circ Hear Fail 2014; 7(5):740–51.

23. Gorter TM, van Veldhuisen DJ, Bauersachs J, et al. Right heart dysfunction and failure in heart failure with preserved ejection fraction: mechanisms and management. Position statement on behalf of the Heart Failure Association of the European Society of Cardiology. Eur J Heart Fail 2018;20(1):16–37.

24. Lancellotti P, Pellikka PA, Budts W, et al. The clinical use of stress echocardiography in non-ischaemic heart disease: recommendations from the European Association of Cardiovascular Imaging and the American Society of Echocardiography. Eur Heart J Cardiovasc Imaging 2016;17(11):1191–229.

25. Holland DJ, Prasad SB, Marwick TH. Contribution of exercise echocardiography to the diagnosis of heart failure with preserved ejection fraction (HFpEF). Heart 2010;96(13):1024–8.

26. Erdei T, Smiseth OA, Marino P, et al. A systematic review of diastolic stress tests in heart failure with preserved ejection fraction, with proposals from the EU-FP7 MEDIA study group. Eur J Heart Fail 2014;16(12):1345–61.

27. Burgess MI, Jenkins C, Sharman JE, et al. Diastolic Stress Echocardiography: Hemodynamic Validation and Clinical Significance of Estimation of Ventricular Filling Pressure With Exercise. J Am Coll Cardiol 2006;47(9):1891–900.

28. Belyavskiy E, Morris DA, Url-Michitsch M, et al. Diastolic stress test echocardiography in patients with suspected heart failure with preserved ejection fraction: a pilot study. ESC Hear Fail 2019;6(1):146–53.

29. Borlaug BA, Kass DA. Invasive Hemodynamic Assessment in Heart Failure. Heart Fail Clin 2009; 5(2):217–28.

30. Thadani U, Parker JO. Hemodynamics at rest and during supine and sitting bicycle exercise in normal subjects. Am J Cardiol 1978;41(1):52–9.

31. Maeder MT, Thompson BR, Brunner-La Rocca HP, et al. Hemodynamic basis of exercise limitation in patients with heart failure and normal ejection fraction. J Am Coll Cardiol 2010;56(11):855–63.

32. Dorfs S, Zeh W, Hochholzer W, et al. Pulmonary capillary wedge pressure during exercise and long-term mortality in patients with suspected heart failure with preserved ejection fraction. Eur Heart J 2014;35(44):3103–12.

33. Malhotra R, Bakken K, D'Elia E, et al. Cardiopulmonary Exercise Testing in Heart Failure. JACC Hear Fail 2016;4(8):607–16.

34. Reddy YNV, Carter RE, Obokata M, et al. A simple, evidence-based approach to help guide diagnosis of heart failure with preserved ejection fraction. Circulation 2018;138(9):861–70.

35. González-López E, Gallego-Delgado M, Guzzo-Merello G, et al. Wild-type transthyretin amyloidosis as a cause of heart failure with preserved ejection fraction. Eur Heart J 2015;36(38):2585–94.

36. Maurer MS, Schwartz JH, Gundapaneni B, et al. Tafamidis Treatment for Patients with Transthyretin Amyloid Cardiomyopathy. N Engl J Med 2018;379(11): 1007–16.

37. Seferovic PM, Ponikowski P, Anker SD, et al. Clinical practice update on heart failure 2019: pharmacotherapy, procedures, devices and patient management. An expert consensus meeting report of the Heart Failure Association of the European Society of Cardiology. Eur J Heart Fail 2019;21(10): 1169–86.

38. Hwang SJ, Melenovsky V, Borlaug BA. Implications of coronary artery disease in heart failure with preserved ejection fraction. J Am Coll Cardiol 2014. https://doi.org/10.1016/j.jacc.2014.03.034.

39. Tamargo M, Obokata M, Reddy YNV, et al. Functional mitral regurgitation and left atrial myopathy in heart failure with preserved ejection fraction. Eur J Heart Fail 2020;22(3):489–98.

40. Bertrand PB, Schwammenthal E, Levine RA, et al. Exercise Dynamics in Secondary Mitral Regurgitation: Pathophysiology and Therapeutic Implications. Circulation 2017;135(3):297–314.

41. Pérez de Isla L, Cañadas V, Contreras L, et al. Diastolic heart failure in the elderly: In-hospital and long-term outcome after the first episode. Int J Cardiol 2009;134(2):265–70.

42. Tribouilloy C, Rusinaru D, Mahjoub H, et al. Prognosis of heart failure with preserved ejection fraction: A 5 year prospective population-based study. Eur Heart J 2008;29(3):339–47.

43. Owan TE, Hodge DO, Herges RM, et al. Trends in Prevalence and Outcome of Heart Failure with Preserved Ejection Fraction. N Engl J Med 2006; 355(3):251–9.

44. Bhatia RS, Tu JV, Lee DS, et al. Outcome of Heart Failure with Preserved Ejection Fraction in a Population-Based Study. N Engl J Med 2006; 355(3):260–9.

45. Murad K, Goff DC, Morgan TM, et al. Burden of Comorbidities and Functional and Cognitive Impairments in Elderly Patients at the Initial Diagnosis of Heart Failure and Their Impact on Total Mortality. The Cardiovascular Health Study. JACC Hear Fail 2015;3(7):542–50.

46. Paulus WJ, Tschöpe C. A novel paradigm for heart failure with preserved ejection fraction: Comorbidities drive myocardial dysfunction and remodeling through coronary microvascular endothelial inflammation. J Am Coll Cardiol 2013;62(4):263–71.

47. Aschauer S, Zotter-Tufaro C, Duca F, et al. Modes of death in patients with heart failure and preserved ejection fraction. Int J Cardiol 2017;228: 422–6.

48. Savill P. Spironolactone in heart failure with preserved ejection fraction. Practitioner 2014; 258(1774):10.

49. Cleland JGF, Tendera M, Adamus J, et al. The perindopril in elderly people with chronic heart failure (PEP-CHF) study. Eur Heart J 2006;27(19): 2338–45.

50. Somaratne JB, Berry C, McMurray JJV, et al. The prognostic significance of heart failure with preserved left ventricular ejection fraction: A literature-based meta-analysis. Eur J Heart Fail 2009;11(9): 855–62.

51. Jones NR, Roalfe AK, Adoki I, et al. Survival of patients with chronic heart failure in the community: a systematic review and meta-analysis. Eur J Heart Fail 2019;21(11):1306–25.

52. Lewis EF, Lamas GA, O' Meara E, et al. Characterization of health-related quality of life in heart failure patients with preserved versus low ejection fraction in CHARM. Eur J Heart Fail 2007;9(1):83–91.

53. Loop MS, Van Dyke MK, Chen L, et al. Comparison of length of stay, 30-day mortality, and 30-day readmission rates in medicare patients with heart failure and with reduced versus preserved ejection fraction. Am J Cardiol 2016;118:79–85.

54. Campbell RT, Jhund PS, Castagno D, et al. What have we learned about patients with heart failure and preserved ejection fraction from DIG-PEF, CHARM-preserved, and I-PRESERVE? J Am Coll Cardiol 2012;60(23):2349–56.

55. Kitzman DW, Gardin JM, Gottdiener JS, et al. Importance of heart failure with preserved systolic function in patients $\geq$65 years of age. Am J Cardiol 2001; 87(4):413–9.

56. Kao DP, Lewsey JD, Anand IS, et al. Characterization of subgroups of heart failure patients with preserved ejection fraction with possible implications for prognosis and treatment response. Eur J Heart Fail 2015;17(9):925–35.

57. Pitt B, Pfeffer MA, Assmann SF, et al. Spironolactone for heart failure with preserved ejection fraction. N Engl J Med 2014. https://doi.org/10.1056/NEJMoa1313731.

58. Cohen JB, Schrauben SJ, Zhao L, et al. Clinical Phenogroups in Heart Failure With Preserved Ejection Fraction: Detailed Phenotypes, Prognosis, and Response to Spironolactone. JACC Hear Fail 2020; 8(3):172–84.

59. Faris RF, Flather M, Purcell H, et al. Diuretics for heart failure. Cochrane Database Syst Rev 2012;2: CD003838.

60. Faris R, Flather M, Purcell H, et al. Current evidence supporting the role of diuretics in heart failure: a meta analysis of randomised controlled trials. Int J Cardiol 2002;82:149–58.

61. Adamson PB, Abraham WT, Bourge RC, et al. Wireless pulmonary artery pressure monitoring guides management to reduce decompensation in heart failure with preserved ejection fraction. Circ Heart Fail 2014;7(6):935–44.

62. Pfeffer MA, Claggett B, Assmann SF, et al. Regional variation in patients and outcomes in the Treatment of Preserved Cardiac Function Heart Failure With an Aldosterone Antagonist (TOPCAT) trial. Circulation 2015;131(1):34–42.

63. Ravassa S, Trippel T, Bach D, et al. Biomarker-based phenotyping of myocardial fibrosis identifies patients with heart failure with preserved ejection fraction resistant to the beneficial effects of spironolactone: results from the Aldo-DHF trial. Eur J Heart Fail 2018;20(9):1290–9.

64. Yusuf S, Pfeffer MA, Swedberg K, et al. Effects of candesartan in patients with chronic heart failure and preserved left-ventricular ejection fraction: the CHARM-preserved trial. Lancet 2003. https://doi.org/10.1016/S0140-6736(03)14285-7.

65. Massie BM, Carson PE, McMurray JJ, et al. Irbesartan in patients with heart failure and preserved ejection fraction. N Engl J Med 2008. https://doi.org/10.1056/NEJMoa0805450.

66. Solomon SD, Zile M, Pieske B, et al. The angiotensin receptor neprilysin inhibitor LCZ696 in heart failure with preserved ejection fraction: a phase 2 double-blind randomised controlled trial. Lancet 2012; 380(9851):1387–95.

67. Solomon SD, McMurray JJV, Anand IS, et al. Angiotensin–neprilysin inhibition in heart failure with preserved ejection fraction. N Engl J Med 2019. https://doi.org/10.1056/NEJMoa1908655.

68. Vaduganathan M, Claggett BL, Desai AS, et al. Prior heart failure hospitalization, clinical outcomes, and response to Sacubitril/valsartan compared with valsartan in HFpEF. J Am Coll Cardiol 2020; 75:245–54.

69. Conraads VM, Metra M, Kamp O, et al. Effects of the long-term administration of nebivolol on the clinical symptoms, exercise capacity, and left ventricular function of patients with diastolic dysfunction: results of the ELANDD study. Eur J Heart Fail 2012. https://doi.org/10.1093/eurjhf/hfr161.

70. Yamamoto K, Origasa H, Hori M. Effects of carvedilol on heart failure with preserved ejection fraction: the Japanese Diastolic Heart Failure Study (J-DHF). Eur J Heart Fail 2013. https://doi.org/10.1093/eurjhf/hfs141.

71. Flather MD, Shibata MC, Coats AJS, et al. SENIORS Investigators. Randomized trial to determine the effect of nebivolol on mortality and cardiovascular hospital admission in elderly patients with heart failure (SENIORS). Eur Heart J 2005;26:215–25.

72. Ahmed A, Rich MW, Fleg JL, et al. Effects of digoxin on morbidity and mortality in diastolic heart failure: the ancillary digitalis investigation group trial. Circulation 2006;114(5):397–403.

73. Komajda M, Isnard R, Cohen-Solal A, et al. Effect of ivabradine in patients with heart failure with preserved ejection fraction: the EDIFY randomized placebo-controlled trial. Eur J Heart Fail 2017. https://doi.org/10.1002/ejhf.876.

74. Redfield MM, Chen HH, Borlaug BA, et al. Effect of phosphodiesterase-5 inhibition on exercise capacity and clinical status in heart failure with preserved ejection fraction: a randomized clinical trial. JAMA 2013;309(12):1268–77.

75. Pandey A, Parashar A, Kumbhani D, et al. Exercise Training in Patients with Heart Failure and Preserved Ejection Fraction: A Meta-analysis of Randomized Control Trials. Circ Heart Fail 2015; 8(1):33–40.

76. Del Buono MG, Iannaccone G, Scacciavillani R, et al. Heart failure with preserved ejection fraction diagnosis and treatment: An updated review of the evidence. Prog Cardiovasc Dis 2020;63(5): 570–84.

77. Lindenfeld J, Albert NM, Boehmer JP, et al. HFSA 2010 Comprehensive Heart Failure Practice Guideline. J Card Fail 2010 Jun;16(6):e1–194.

Treatment of Advanced Heart Failure—Focus on Transplantation and Durable Mechanical Circulatory Support
What Does the Future Hold?

Federica Guidetti, MD[a],*, Mattia Arrigo, MD[b], Michelle Frank, MD[a], Fran Mikulicic, MD[a], Mateusz Sokolski, MD[c], Raed Aser, MD[d], Markus J. Wilhelm, MD[d], Andreas J. Flammer, MD[a], Frank Ruschitzka, MD[a], Stephan Winnik, MD, PhD[a]

KEYWORDS

- Advanced heart failure • Mechanical circulatory support • Heart transplantation
- Hemocompatibility • RVAD • TAH • DCD donors • Xenotransplantation

KEY POINTS

- The prevalence of heart failure (HF) is estimated at 1% to 2% of the general adult population in developed countries. Improved survival rates with medical and device therapy notwithstanding, patients with advanced HF experience a 5-year mortality exceeding 50%.
- Patients progressing to advanced HF on optimal medical therapy should be evaluated for heart transplantation (HTx) and/or long-term mechanical circulatory support (LTMCS). If both options are not desired or contraindicated, palliative care should be offered.
- The advanced HF team plays a pivotal role in providing the best treatment and allocating resources: young patients should be prioritized for HTx, and LTMCS should be reserved for good candidates at the right time.

BACKGROUND

Heart failure (HF) has become a substantial public health problem, affecting 2% of the adult population. The number of hospital admissions related to HF has tripled since the 1990s.[1] Modern HF treatment, including pharmacologic and device therapy, has led to strikingly improved survival rates of patients with HF with reduced left ventricular ejection fraction (HFrEF).[2]

However, despite optimal medical treatment, 1% to 10% of the overall HF population still progresses to advanced HF, which is associated with a 5-year mortality exceeding 50%.[3,4]

With the advent of recent outcome trials with sacubitril/valsartan and sodium-glucose cotransporter-2 inhibitors in patients with HFrEF, the therapeutic armamentarium has been further expanded. However, because of the poor representation of patients with advanced HF in these

Funded by: SWISS2021.
a Department of Cardiology, University Hospital of Zürich, Rämistrasse 100, Zürich 8091, Switzerland; b Department of Internal Medicine, Triemli Hospital Zürich, Birmensdorferstrasse 497, 8063 Zürich, Switzerland; c Department of Heart Diseases, Wroclaw Medical University, Borowska 213, 50-556 Wroclaw, Poland; d Department of Cardiac Surgery, University Hospital of Zürich, Rämistrasse 100, Zürich 8091, Switzerland
* Corresponding author. Department of Cardiology, University Hospital of Zürich, Rämistrasse 100, Zürich 8091, Switzerland.
E-mail address: federica.guidetti@usz.ch

trials (around 1% of patients with New York Heart Association class IV in DAPA-HF and PARADIGM-HF) and the frequent intolerance of medical therapy in patients with severely symptomatic HF, studies specifically in this population (as, eg, the LIFE trial) will shed further light on the efficacy of these therapies in advanced HF.[5] Further studies are also required to define the role of vericiguat in patients with advanced HF. The VICTORIA trial showed that the treatment effect on the primary outcome was consistent across most prespecified subgroups, except in patients with the highest NT-proBNP levels.[6] High expectations exist for the introduction of omecamtiv mecarbil, into clinical practice, which is an orally administered inotropic therapy, capable of reducing cardiovascular mortality and HF events among ambulatory or hospitalized patients with HFrEF, including those with moderate or severe HF symptoms, reduced ejection fraction, low systolic blood pressure, and reduced renal function.[7] These and other medical approaches are discussed in the respective articles in this issue by Iacovello and colleagues and Masarone and colleagues.

Once medical management is insufficient, advanced therapies need to be evaluated. For these patients, heart transplantation (HTx) is considered the gold-standard therapy. Survival rates after HTx, reaching up to 87% at 1 year and up to 57% at 10 years, are excellent.[8] However, the imbalance between the growing numbers of advanced HF patients and the scarcity of donor organs, along with the high prevalence of contraindications to HTx, hampers this therapeutic option for many patients. In recent years, novel strategies to increase the number of donor hearts or to provide alternatives to HTx, such as left ventricular assist devices (LVADs), have emerged.[9] This review aims to provide an overview of current practice, recent advances, and future developments in the treatment of advanced HF. To avoid overlap with other articles of this article series, the authors focus on long-term mechanical circulatory support (LTMCS) and HTx (**Table 1**).

Heart Transplantation

Although HTx has never been compared with medical therapy in a randomized trial, survival rates after HTx (80% at 1 year, 50% at 10 years) are markedly higher compared with those reported in registries of patients on medical therapy.[8,10] Despite great recent improvements in survival of patients receiving LTMCS instead of or as bridge to HTx, the incidence of complications associated with LTMCS remains high and negatively affects outcome, quality of life (QoL), and health care

cost.[11] Therefore, current guidelines recommend HTx as gold standard for advanced HF patients in the absence of contraindications.[12,13] After a period of stagnation, the global number of HTx has started to grow slightly again.[14] However, this positive trend, which is primarily explained by the opium crisis and the consequent increase of drug intoxication donors, has remained confined to the United States.[15] Accordingly, because of the increasing prevalence of advanced HF, especially in Europe, tremendous scarcity of donor organs is still being encountered.

Donation after circulatory death heart transplantation

To address the shortage of donor organs, heart donation after circulatory death (DCD) in addition to donation after brain death (DBD) has been revisited in HTx (**Fig. 1**). This possibility has been restricted to the Maastricht III donor category: these are cases of catastrophic brain injury that do not meet the DBD criteria, but in which, after the withdrawal of life-supporting therapies (WLST), a cardiac arrest is expected. One of the chief concerns of DCD is the difficulty to quantify the so-called warm ischemia time (WIT = time from WLST to organ reperfusion) responsible for cardiac injury and consecutive primary graft failure. Another major concern is the inability to perform a functional assessment of the asystolic heart. Following a series of positive preclinical studies and successful animal DCD transplantations, an American group reported the successful transplantation of 3 DCD pediatric hearts using a *direct procurement and cold storage technique* in 2008.[16–18] To minimize WIT, donors and recipients were located at the same hospital, donors were cannulated antemortem, heparinization was performed, and the obligatory standard observation period before declaration of death after asystole ("stand-off period") was reduced from 3 minutes to 75 seconds.

In most countries, antemortem treatment is not allowed for ethical reasons; the legally defined observation period is generally longer (2–20 minutes), and colocation of donor and recipient is often not feasible. Therefore, the use of an ex situ perfusion machine, already successfully used in DBD donors, was tested in a porcine DCD model.[19] Use of an ex situ perfusion machine led to better heart preservation compared with cold storage, and, for the first time, allowed indirect assessment of the DCD heart by lactate measurements of the perfusion solution. In addition, ex situ perfusion allowed DCD-organ transfer from different hospitals. In 2015, an Australian group reported the first 3 successful DCD-HTx with a direct

Table 1
Unmet needs and future directions in advanced heart failure

Unmet Needs in Advanced HF	Future Directions
Safety, tolerability, efficacy of new HF drugs	Randomized trials in patients with advanced HF
Increase contractility without increasing adverse events	Omecantiv
Scarcity of donor organs	Development of DCD donation Improvement in ex situ perfusion techniques Xenotransplantation
Biventricular dysfunction in patients ineligible for transplantation requiring MCS	TAH Syncardia 70cc as destination therapy Implantable biventricular assist device (technology yet to be developed)
Biventricular dysfunction in BTT patients requiring MCS	CARMAT TAH, BiVACOR TAH Implantable biventricular assist device (technology yet to be developed)
Prediction of RV dysfunction after LVAD-implantation	Randomized trials to define parameters and scores
Acute post/intraoperatively RV dysfunction after LVAD Implantation	Further development of temporary RVAD
Driveline infections	Wireless energy transfer
Hemocompatibility-related adverse events	Improvement device technology, development of biocompatible inner surfaces Tailored antithrombotic management New antithrombotic strategy: low-intensity novel anticoagulation protocols (no aspirin?)

distant procurement and ex situ heart perfusion using the TransMedics Organ Care System (Andover, MA, USA). After WLST resulting in asystole and subsequent "stand-off" period of 2 to 5 minutes, the donors were declared deceased and transferred to the operating room.[20] After administration of cardioplegia and direct organ procurement, the organ was connected to the Organ Care System. During the ex situ preservation, donor organ function was continuously, indirectly evaluated using aortic pressure, coronary flow, and arteriovenous lactate concentration.

In 2016, the Papworth group in the United Kingdom first established a new DCD protocol based on *in situ normothermic regional perfusion followed by ex situ perfusion*, as well as used the Organ Care System.[21] After a 5-minute "stand-off period," death was declared, and the patient was transferred to the operating room. The cerebral circulation was excluded (clamping of the supra-aortic circulation), and the perfusion to the potentially transplantable organs was restored using a centrifugal pump and oxygenator, allowing a complete functional donor organ assessment using echocardiography and Swan-Ganz measurements before organ procurement. Reestablishment of a beating heart and circulation after the declaration of death remains a matter of an intense ethical debate.

All 3 methods described here (see **Fig. 1**) are currently in use in the few centers worldwide running a DCD-HTx program. Their results are very promising, showing the same length of in-hospital stay as well as a comparable short-term outcome as in DBD-HTx.[20,22] Importantly, long-term follow-up of these patients is not yet available and will shed further light on this promising approach.

DCD-HTx holds the potential to increase the number of donor organs in a relevant fashion. During the study period of the 2 protagonists in the field, overall HTx activity increased by 33% in Papworth and by 45% in Sydney. Some predict a 56% to 81% increase of possible HTx by adopting strict DCD-HTx donor selection criteria and including also older patients aged 51 to 60 years, respectively.[23] When comparing the 2 most widely used methods of DCD heart retrieval (distant procurement and ex situ perfusion vs normothermic regional perfusion + ex situ perfusion), there are advantages and disadvantages of either technique, although their clinical outcome appears similar to date.[22] The main advantages of in situ normothermic regional perfusion are earlier

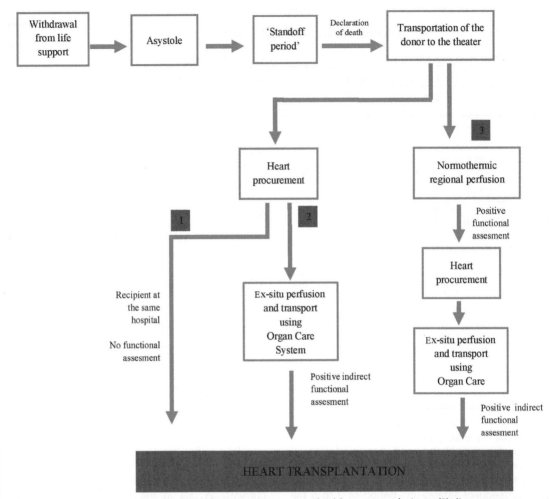

Fig. 1. DCD-HTx: 3 available methods: (1) direct procurement and cold storage technique; (2) distant procurement and ex situ perfusion; (3) normothermic regional perfusion + ex situ perfusion.

reperfusion and the possibility of standard functional in situ assessment. The latter may allow expanding the DCD donor pool, as the functional organ assessment may loosen restrictions related to donor age or WIT. The main drawbacks of in situ normothermic regional perfusion are ethical concerns with respect to incalculable reperfusion of the central nervous system, the need for high-technological expertise, and the human and economic resources required for its realization. Distant procurement and ex situ perfusion are less demanding to perform but until now were limited by indirect organ assessment.

To further expand DCD-HTx programs, many challenges will need to be tackled:

a. Provision of a strong scientific justification for allowing antemortem interventions (heparinization, extracorporeal membrane oxygenation cannulation)

b. Acceptance of the shortest "stand-off" time to reduce WIT
c. Subscription of a unified approach of DCD donor management considering ethical and technical issues
d. Definition of the best retrieval techniques
e. Development and use of the best possible perfusion solutions
f. Reduction of the costs and increase in resources
g. Improvement of the ex situ perfusion technology

Ex situ perfusion of donor hearts
The ex situ perfusion has played a key role in recent years, especially by enabling the use of DCD hearts and by allowing longer time intervals between organ procurement and implantation, thereby allowing the safe application of extended-criteria DBD donation. Only 1 model of

ex situ organ perfusion is currently approved; however, many systems are being evaluated in preclinical studies. Much hope is pinned on testing new models that allow functional and viability assessment of the ex situ beating heart.[24] Such models hold the potential to reduce myocardial damage and perform immunomodulation by the use of smart perfusion solutions.[25] Ex situ perfusion also represents an important opportunity to study biochemical markers that could be used as indicators of organ quality and as predictors of primary graft dysfunction in the future. Allowing for longer extracorporeal times, allografts may be shared over a larger geographic area, thereby improving donor-recipient matching and further increasing the donor pool. Further investigations are required to confirm these potential benefits and their impact on outcome and costs.

Organ donor systems

Moreover, a transition from an "opt-in" organ donor system to an "opt-out" policy (ie, deceased patients are considered to have agreed to be an organ donor unless they have recorded a decision not to donate) has repetitively been discussed in several countries worldwide. Data comparing these 2 models have shown conflicting results. Shepherd and colleagues[26] demonstrated that "opt-out" countries have higher rates of kidney and liver transplantation activity from more deceased organ donors compared with "opt-in" countries. In contrast, Arshad and colleagues[27] documented no difference comparing these 2 systems. This discrepancy does not demonstrate the uselessness of the opt-out strategy but rather that other barriers to organ donation must be addressed, even in settings where consent for donation is presumed. Indeed, the optimal increase in organ donation rates is achieved only with the optimal interplay of legislation changes, adequate funding, education, medical training, and the development of novel strategies of donor selection and organ procurement to overcome current obstacles.

Xenotransplantation

Furthermore, another possibility to increase the number of donor organs is xenotransplantation. Animals (ie, pigs) might become a readily, virtually unlimited, functioning organ source for human HTx. Critical limitations to the clinical use of xenotransplantation are related to immunologic and infectious issues.[28] The hyperacute rejection owing to the presence of human anti-pig antibodies directed against 3 pig-carbohydrates (antigens) and the activation of the coagulation cascade as well as the complement system

leading to delayed xenograft rejection represent the most relevant problems.[29] Using gene knockout technology made it possible to produce porcine organs that do not express the respective antigens and, thereby, contributes to overcome the problem of hyperacute rejection.[30] Using clustered regularly interspaced short palindromic repeats–based technology, it was further possible to eliminate the porcine endogenous retrovirus, which may cause infections in the recipients.[31,32] It was recently shown that genetically modified porcine hearts were successfully transplanted into primates using a modified preservation and immunosuppression protocol with an excellent 90-day survival rate and without signs of rejection.[33] If these strategies can be further developed, future clinical trials in humans may show whether xenotransplantation will provide an effective alternative. Meanwhile, basic research will further explore the mechanisms of rejection in xenotransplantation and to improve tolerance and clinical outcome.

Long-Term Mechanical Circulatory Support

During the last 50 years, technological developments have improved 2-year survival after LVAD implantation from 23% using the first-generation pulsatile-flow LVAD to 81% using the contemporary LVADs. Improved outcomes in association with the HF epidemic and donor organ scarcity have led to an increase in the use of LVADs as bridge to transplantation (BTT) or as destination therapy (DT). Importantly, only a minority of the LVAD recipients starting on a BTT strategy will undergo HTx because of the increasing donor organ shortage and long waiting times, making the line between BTT and DT even more blurred.[34]

Despite substantial advances in the field of mechanical circulatory support (MCS), postimplantation morbidity (including infection, bleeding, neurologic dysfunction, and right ventricular [RV] failure) remains high. Indeed, nearly one-third of patients are readmitted within 30 days after LVAD implantation.[35] Similarly, the cumulative number of rehospitalizations per 100 patients is 59 at 3 months and 218 at 1 year.[36] In addition to the impact on survival and QoL, the economic challenge created by adverse events (AEs) is huge. The ability to reduce the incidence of these AEs will be crucial to further establish the role of LVAD as a cost-effective alternative to HTx for the treatment of advanced HF. Notably, the incidence of AEs depends not only on the technological evolution of devices and its clinical management but also on proper timing for LVAD implantation. INTERMACS profiles 1 to 3 are associated with increased mortality and AEs after implantation, which is related to biventricular dysfunction, irreversible peripheral organ damage, infection, and the need of stabilization with a temporary MCS. Early LVAD implantation (ie, at a less severe INTERMACS profile), especially in patients with a low likelihood to receive HTx, might be an applicable solution to improve outcome after implantation. The analysis of the ROADMAP study revealed potential benefits for LVAD compared with optimal medical management in patients in INTERMACS profile 4.[37] Patients in INTERMACS profile 5 to 7 should be followed carefully and repetitively to recognize disease progression.

Infections: wireless power transmission

Infections are the most common cause of hospitalization among patients with LVAD (37%).[38] They occur usually in the first 3 months after implantation and constitute a relevant burden in the management of LVAD patients. Patient frailty and LVAD-related impairment of cellular immunity are relevant risk factors. These factors explain why non-LVAD-related infections are the most common infections in this population. Among LVAD-related infections, driveline infections are the most frequent ones. In this context, several device companies are currently developing a wireless power delivery system for future LVADs in order to avoid bacterial entry through a driveline exit site. The first human attempts using transcutaneous energy transfer systems and coplanar energy transfer have not succeeded, but the road is marked.[39–41] Although further technological development is still required to allow wireless energy transfer and it is not clear when LVADs will become fully wireless, its impact on outcome and QoL will be immediate.

Biventricular and right ventricular dysfunction—biventricular support and total artificial heart

RV dysfunction represents one of the most critical challenges in the treatment of advanced HF patients (**Fig. 2**).[42] RV dysfunction impairs renal and hepatic function, thus further limiting efficacy of medical, interventional, and surgical treatment options in this patient population. Accordingly, patients with RV dysfunction need to be evaluated timely for HTx or LTMCS and/or (temporary and or durable) RV support, taking into account the waiting time for HTx and the difficulty of dealing with an LTMCS in the case of acute or rapid deterioration. In patients with a clinical indication for LTMCS, RV dysfunction can be either evident in the form of severe RV dysfunction contraindicating

LVAD implantation itself (eg, in arrhythmogenic RV cardiomyopathy) or in the form of a light/moderate RV dysfunction before LVAD implantation with worsening and clinical manifestation only after LVAD implantation. Generally, it is important to recognize that patients requiring biventricular support are a different population from those who undergo univentricular support. These patients are generally sicker and suffer from more profound multiple organ dysfunctions. That explains why once biventricular support is required, the survival is uniformly poorer compared with patients receiving LVAD support, regardless of the chosen device system.[43]

In patients with *manifested severe biventricular dysfunction* requiring MCS, surgeons have access to *total artificial heart* (TAH) or *paracorporeal-BiVAD* (EXCOR; Berlin Heart, Berlin, Germany) systems. The pneumatic pulsatile Syncardia TAH (Tucson, AZ, USA) has been historically the only TAH with Food and Drug Administration approval for clinical use in patients eligible for HTx. In the largest analysis of patients receiving a Syncardia 70cc, Arabia and colleagues[44] reported an overall 3-, 6-, and 12-month survival of 73%, 62%, and 53%, respectively. The use of a TAH versus an EXCOR remains controversial, with most of the studies showing no difference.[45,46] In the absence of randomized trials comparing these 2 strategies, the decision about which type of device should be implanted is taken based on the center and surgeon preference and experience. However, it is important to point out that, although the approval of the Syncardia 50cc has made possible the extension of the use of a TAH in patients with lower body mass index, the EXCOR system can be implanted in a much wider range of body sizes, including pediatric patients. Furthermore, actually, both of these options are restricted to the BTT indication. An ongoing trial (SynCardia 70cc Temporary Total Artificial Heart for Destination Therapy, NCT02232659) evaluates whether the Syncardia 70cc could be an option also in patients with biventricular dysfunction who are not eligible for HTx, potentially allowing to treat patients with biventricular dysfunction who are not eligible for transplantation. Nevertheless, Syncardia and EXCOR are based on a decades-old technology, which limits their use mainly because of AEs and impact on the QoL. Very recently, a new TAH device (CARMAT TAH, CARMAT SA, Vélizy-Villacoublay, France) received European Conformity approval. The implanted device replaces the 2 ventricles and 4 valves with biocompatible blood-contacting materials and provides a pulsatile blood flow, adapted to the patient's activities by autoregulation. In the PIVOTAL study, the

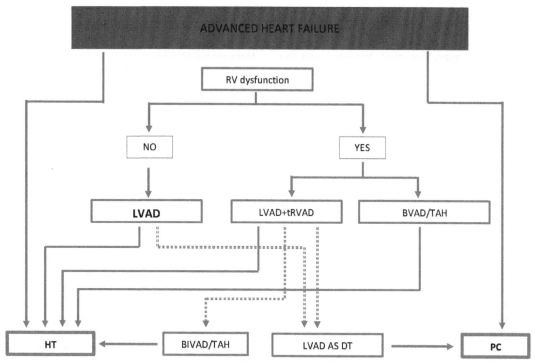

Fig. 2. The central role of RV dysfunction in patients with advanced HF evaluated for MCS. BVAD, biventricular assist device; HT, heart transplantation; PC, palliative care; tRVAD, temporary right ventricular assist device.

CARMAT TAH has demonstrated a 70% 6-month survival with an encouraging hemocompatibility profile in BTT patients with biventricular dysfunction.[47] Another new device, the BiVACOR TAH (BiVACOR Inc, Houston, TX, USA), using a magnetic levitation technology that can generate continuous or pulsatile flow, is currently under clinical investigation.[48] The research for a long-term heart replacement continues with designs in the form of the Rein Heart TAH (ReinHart, Aachen, Germany), the CCFTAH (Cleveland, OH, USA), the Oregon Heart TAH (Portland, OR, USA), the Helical Flow TAH (Tokyo, Japan), and a hybrid CF-TAH (Philadelphia, PA, USA).[49–51]

Importantly, clinically relevant RV dysfunction requiring RV support (right ventricular assist device [RVAD]) may unexpectedly develop in 9% to 42% of patients undergoing LVAD implantation, either acutely intraoperatively or postoperatively or months to years after LVAD implantation.[52,53] This wide range of reported RV failure is due to the lack of a universal definition of post-LVAD RV failure as well as frequent underdiagnosis. Acute severe RV dysfunction requiring RVAD is the greatest risk factor for early death in LVAD recipients,[54] especially when it occurs unplanned or later after LVAD implantation.[55] Unlike other AEs, the incidences of which

have been reduced with technological advances, the occurrence of RV dysfunction has remained stable even with the latest generation of devices.[56] Probably this is due to the poor comprehension of the cause of RV failure and the still impaired ability to precisely diagnose or even predict RV failure.[57] Indeed, in the absence of validated scores, each center has developed its own algorithm to predict RV dysfunction, making data comparison across studies and strategies difficult. If severe RV dysfunction acutely manifests intraoperatively, an RVAD is commonly implanted as soon as possible. Treating physicians can choose between surgical (Centri-Mag; Abbott, Chicago, IL, USA), tandem with ProTek (LivaNova PLC, London, UK), or percutaneous temporary devices like Impella RP (Abiomed, Inc, Danvers, MA, USA). Surgical devices have the advantage of allowing greater support in terms of flow at the cost of a more complex, invasive removal procedure. Percutaneous devices are easier to implant and to remove but have limited durability and restrict patient mobility. To date, no trials are comparing these devices. Therefore, the choice is based on expected recovery time and center experience and preference. Research is focusing on temporary RVAD devices, which allow both early mobilization and percutaneous removal in order to offer intermediate support for up to 30 days. In the future, the ability to identify patients with RV dysfunction who have recovery potential, together with the technical advancements of temporary RVADs, could pave the way for the possibility to plan simultaneous LVAD and temporary RVAD implantation for temporary RV support in the early, most critical postoperative period. This strategy was already proposed by Loforte and colleagues[58] and warrants further investigation. Another option that has been investigated is the combination of 2 LVAD pumps in 1 patient as a biventricular support system. The most significant advantage of this strategy is that it can be started as left ventricular support, and only if RV failure occurs during the operation, a second permanent device in the right position can be implanted. The first multicenter experience with HeartMate3 as biventricular support has shown a 55% survival rate at 21 months.[59]

In patients at risk of RV failure, every effort must be made to optimize the preoperative, intraoperative, and postoperative status via reduction of preload, afterload, and RV contractility support.[42] Of note, rapid and adequate decongestion with intravenous loop diuretics remains one of the mainstays of therapy. Although inotropic therapy may be used as a bridging strategy, and in particular, inodilators may conceptually provide clinical benefit in this patient group, they have failed to improve outcome in randomized clinical trials.

With many durable and temporary biventricular systems under development, randomized controlled trials are required to establish parameters and/or a predictive score for permanent and temporary RV dysfunction that can guide the choice between LVAD ± RVAD versus BIVAD/TAH. The ongoing EuroEchoVAD Study (NCT03552679) aims to investigate the evolution of RV function before and after LVAD implantation, using novel echocardiographic quantification methods (2-, 3-dimensional, and multiplane echocardiography) in combination with comprehensive hemodynamic, laboratory, and clinical parameters, in order to enhance the prediction of RV failure as well as to define its optimal management.

Computed tomography virtual implantation

Given the many possibilities of MCS devices but also in order to extend their use to patients with more complex anatomy (congenital heart disease, restrictive cardiomyopathy), computed tomography virtual implantation may offer great support in the future.[60] Such an approach may allow testing several surgical approaches for device placement and optimal device size before the patient arrives in the operating theater.

Hemocompatibility

The magnetic levitation of the pump rotor in the latest LVAD HeartMate3 (Abbott) has led to a significant improvement in hemocompatibility-related adverse events (HRAE). Pump thrombosis and nondisabling stroke, that is, pump-related embolic events, have become very rare using this latest technology. Further improvements in HRAEs will depend on advances in device engineering (reduction of device-related shear stress, development of materials with high biocompatibility, and potentially increased pump pulsatility) in combination with further advances in antithrombotic clinical management. Despite impressive technological improvements, hemocompatibility remains one of the major clinical challenges in LVAD therapy, even with the latest-generation LVADs. Novel approaches to antithrombotic treatment are currently under investigation. The ongoing ARIES HeartMate 3 Pump IDE Study (NCT04069156) raises high expectations. This noninferiority trial will answer the question of whether daily aspirin 100 mg can be omitted without negatively affecting the composite end point of survival free of nonsurgical major HRAE after 12 months. Moreover, following the positive results of the MAGENTUM 1 study (international normalized ratio 1.5–1.7 in selected LVAD patients on aspirin), another ongoing trial (Anti-Thrombotic Monotherapy with the HM3 LVAS; NCT03704220) aims to assess the safety of a complete discontinuation of anticoagulation in a selected patient population.[61] At the same time, much research is focusing on biomarkers as well as clinical patient characteristics in order to predict the individual thrombotic and hemorrhagic risk.[62,63] These studies have the potential to individually tailor antithrombotic therapy in each patient. Although experience with direct oral anticoagulants (DOACs) in LVAD patients has been unfavorable so far, data for the latest pump are lacking.[64] Future studies using DOAC in patients with HeartMate3 (Abbott) are in the pipeline.

Miniaturization, less-invasive implantation, and telemetric monitoring

The evolution of LVAD technology has been accompanied by a reduction in the device size, which has allowed intrapericardial implantation with lower perioperative risk and improved QoL for patients. The efficacy of the smallest LVAD to date, the novel Miniaturized Ventricular Assist Device (MVAD; HeartWare Inc, Framingham, MA, USA), is currently under investigation

(NCT01831544). The MVAD is an axial-flow pump that can generate a full cardiac output despite being a third of the size of its predecessor still in use, the HVAD device.[65]

Concomitantly to the miniaturization of the devices, minimally invasive operative techniques have been developed. The LATERAL trial has recently demonstrated that the thoracotomy approach for implanting the HVAD in a BTT setting was safe and effective, thereby providing a successful alternative to median sternotomy in selected patients.[66] This evolution toward less invasive surgical implantation offers the advantage of reducing perioperative/postoperative complications, which, in addition, holds great promise to reduce the incidence of postoperative right heart failure. This development may open LVAD therapy to a wider field of patients in future.

Another new technology, telemonitoring, as implanted in the Heart Assist 5 (Reliant Heart Inc, Houston, TX, USA), may offer a promising tool to improve long-term patient management during follow-up.[67] Specifically, monitoring of pump flow may allow early detection of complications like pump thrombosis or outlet obstruction as well as better volume management.

CLINICS CARE POINTS

- The prevalence of heart failure and the number of patients with end-stage disease are increasing worldwide.

- Donor organ shortage needs to be addressed not only by raising public awareness of the importance of organ donation but also by increasing investments, education, and driving novel developments, like donation after circulatory death, ex situ organ perfusion, and even xenotransplantation.

- As there is a long way to go, it can be expected that also in the coming years donor organ demand will continue to exceed supply.

- With a focus on optimizing resources, the role of the advanced heart failure team is pivotal in smart patient selection, for both heart transplantation and durable mechanical circulatory support therapy.

- For those with contraindications to heart transplantation and those too sick to survive long waiting times, long-term mechanical circulatory support is a valuable option. Novel developments in the near future hold great promise to make this therapy safely available to a broader patient population.

- Also in this context, a crucial task of the HF specialist will be patient selection, that is, selection of those patients with the lowest risk/benefit ratio. This ratio can be expected to shift in a favorable way as a result of ongoing developments, both in device technology and implantation procedures and in patient management.

- Nonetheless, randomized clinical trials will be inevitable to prove the benefit before extended indications for long-term mechanical circulatory support will become reality.

- Improvements in clinical management derived both from years of experience and from ongoing trials to adopt an individually tailored antithrombotic therapy can be expected to lead to a further reduction in morbidity and mortality of patients on long-term mechanical circulatory support.

- Importantly, none of these developments will release us from our duty to individualize decisions based on patient preference after careful patient education on the individual risks and benefits of either way, including palliation.

- With an increasingly complex therapeutic approach, the role of an *advanced heart failure team* of heart failure specialists, cardiac surgeons, cardiac anesthesiologists, and other specialists depending on the individual patient's comorbidities takes on greater significance than ever before.

DISCLOSURE

A.J. Flammer: fees from Alnylam, Amgen, AstraZeneca, Bayer, Boehringer Ingelheim, Bristol Myers Squibb, Fresenius, Imedos Systems, Medtronic, MSD, Mundipharma, Novartis, Pierre Fabre, Pfizer, Roche, Schwabe Pharma. Vifor, and Zoll, as well as grant support by Novartis, AstraZeneca, and Berlin Heart unrelated to this article. S. Winnik: educational grant support and/or travel support and/or consulting/speaker fees from Abbott, Bayer, Boehringer-Ingelheim, Boston-Scientific, Cardinal Health, Daichi-Sankyo, Fehling Instruments, and Servier. F. Ruschitzka: related to the present work: none. Outside the submitted work: the Department of Cardiology (University Hospital of Zurich/University of Zurich) reports research, educational, and/or travel grants from Abbott, Amgen, AstraZeneca, Bayer, B. Braun, Biosense Webster, Biosensors Europe AG, Biotronik, BMS, Boehringer Ingelheim, Boston Scientific, Bracco, Cardinal Health Switzerland, Daiichi, Diatools, AG, Edwards Lifesciences, Guidant Europe NV (BS),

Hamilton Health Sciences, Kaneka Corporation, Labormedizi-nisches Zentrum, Medtronic, MSD, Mundipharma Medical Company, Novartis, Novo Nordisk, Orion, Pfizer, Quin-tiles Switzerland Sarl, Sanofi, Sarstedt AG, Servier, SIS Medical, SSS International Clinical Research, Terumo Deutschland, V-Wave, Vascular Medical, Vifor, Wissens Plus, and ZOLL. F. Ruschitzka has not received personal payments by pharmaceutical companies or device manufacturers in the last 3 years (remuneration for the time spent in activities, such as participation in steering committee member of clinical trials, were made directly to the University of Zurich). F. Ruschitzka is an unpaid member of the Pfizer Research Award selection committee in Switzerland. The research and educational grants do not impact on F. Ruschitzka's personal remuneration. M.J. Wilhelm: travel fees and speaker honoraria from Berlin Heart.

REFERENCES

1. Arrigo M, Jessup M, Mullens W, et al. Acute heart failure. Nat Rev Dis Primers 2020;6(1):16.
2. McMurray JJ. CONSENSUS to EMPHASIS: the overwhelming evidence which makes blockade of the renin-angiotensin-aldosterone system the cornerstone of therapy for systolic heart failure. Eur J Heart Fail 2011;13(9):929–36.
3. Xanthakis V, Enserro DM, Larson MG, et al. Prevalence, neurohormonal correlates, and prognosis of heart failure stages in the community. JACC Heart Fail 2016;4(10):808–15.
4. Mamas MA, Sperrin M, Watson MC, et al. Do patients have worse outcomes in heart failure than in cancer? A primary care-based cohort study with 10-year follow-up in Scotland. Eur J Heart Fail 2017;19(9):1095–104.
5. Mann DL, Greene SJ, Givertz MM, et al. Sacubitril/valsartan in advanced heart failure with reduced ejection fraction: rationale and design of the LIFE Trial. JACC Heart Fail 2020;8(10):789–99.
6. Armstrong PW, Pieske B, Anstrom KJ, et al. Vericiguat in patients with heart failure and reduced ejection fraction. N Engl J Med 2020;382(20): 1883–93.
7. Teerlink JR, Diaz R, Felker GM, et al. Cardiac myosin activation with omecamtiv mecarbil in systolic heart failure. N Engl J Med 2020;384(2):105–16.
8. Khush KK, Cherikh WS, Chambers DC, et al. The International Thoracic Organ Transplant Registry of the International Society for Heart and Lung Transplantation: Thirty-fifth Adult Heart Transplantation Report-2018; focus theme: multiorgan transplantation. J Heart Lung Transplant 2018;37(10): 1155–68.

9. Crespo-Leiro MG, Metra M, Lund LH, et al. Advanced heart failure: a position statement of the Heart Failure Association of the European Society of Cardiology. Eur J Heart Fail 2018;20(11): 1505–35.
10. Crespo-Leiro MG, Anker SD, Maggioni AP, et al. European Society of Cardiology Heart Failure Long-Term Registry (ESC-HF-LT): 1-year follow-up outcomes and differences across regions. Eur J Heart Fail 2016;18(6):613–25.
11. Adams EE, Wrightson ML. Quality of life with an LVAD: a misunderstood concept. Heart Lung 2018; 47(3):177–83.
12. Mehra MR, Canter CE, Hannan MM, et al. The 2016 International Society for Heart Lung Transplantation listing criteria for heart transplantation: a 10-year update. J Heart Lung Transplant 2016; 35(1):1–23.
13. Ponikowski P, Voors AA, Anker SD, et al. 2016 ESC Guidelines for the diagnosis and treatment of acute and chronic heart failure: the Task Force for the Diagnosis and Treatment of Acute and Chronic Heart Failure of the European Society of Cardiology (ESC) developed with the special contribution of the Heart Failure Association (HFA) of the ESC. Eur Heart J 2016;37(27):2129–200.
14. Lund LH, Khush KK, Cherikh WS, et al. The Registry of the International Society for Heart and Lung Transplantation: Thirty-fourth Adult Heart Transplantation Report-2017; focus theme: allograft ischemic time. J Heart Lung Transplant 2017;36(10):1037–46.
15. Mehra MR, Jarcho JA, Cherikh W, et al. The drug-intoxication epidemic and solid-organ transplantation. N Engl J Med 2018;378(20):1943–5.
16. White CW, Lillico R, Sandha J, et al. Physiologic changes in the heart following cessation of mechanical ventilation in a porcine model of donation after circulatory death: implications for cardiac transplantation. Am J Transplant 2016;16(3):783–93.
17. Ali AA, White P, Xiang B, et al. Hearts from DCD donors display acceptable biventricular function after heart transplantation in pigs. Am J Transplant 2011;11(8):1621–32.
18. Boucek MM, Mashburn C, Dunn SM, et al. Pediatric heart transplantation after declaration of cardiocirculatory death. N Engl J Med 2008;359(7):709–14.
19. Iyer A, Gao L, Doyle A, et al. Normothermic ex vivo perfusion provides superior organ preservation and enables viability assessment of hearts from DCD donors. Am J Transplant 2015;15(2):371–80.
20. Chew HC, Iyer A, Connellan M, et al. Outcomes of donation after circulatory death heart transplantation in Australia. J Am Coll Cardiol 2019;73(12):1447–59.
21. Messer S, Page A, Axell R, et al. Outcome after heart transplantation from donation after circulatory-determined death donors. J Heart Lung Transplant 2017;36(12):1311–8.

22. Messer S, Cernic S, Page A, et al. A 5-year single-center early experience of heart transplantation from donation after circulatory-determined death donors. J Heart Lung Transplant 2020;39(12):1463–75.

23. Messer S, Page A, Rushton S, et al. The potential of heart transplantation from donation after circulatory death donors within the United Kingdom. J Heart Lung Transplant 2019;38(8):872–4.

24. Hatami S, White CW, Ondrus M, et al. Normothermic ex situ heart perfusion in working mode: assessment of cardiac function and metabolism. J Vis Exp 2019; 143. https://doi.org/10.3791/58430.

25. Korkmaz-Icoz S, Li S, Huttner R, et al. Hypothermic perfusion of donor heart with a preservation solution supplemented by mesenchymal stem cells. J Heart Lung Transplant 2019;38(3):315–26.

26. Shepherd L, O'Carroll RE, Ferguson E. An international comparison of deceased and living organ donation/transplant rates in opt-in and opt-out systems: a panel study. BMC Med 2014;12:131.

27. Arshad A, Anderson B, Sharif A. Comparison of organ donation and transplantation rates between opt-out and opt-in systems. Kidney Int 2019;95(6): 1453–60.

28. Pierson RN 3rd, Fishman JA, Lewis GD, et al. Progress toward cardiac xenotransplantation. Circulation 2020;142(14):1389–98.

29. Cooper DK, Good AH, Koren E, et al. Identification of alpha-galactosyl and other carbohydrate epitopes that are bound by human anti-pig antibodies: relevance to discordant xenografting in man. Transpl Immunol 1993;1(3):198–205.

30. Azimzadeh AM, Kelishadi SS, Ezzelarab MB, et al. Early graft failure of GalTKO pig organs in baboons is reduced by expression of a human complement pathway-regulatory protein. Xenotransplantation 2015;22(4):310–6.

31. Niu D, Wei HJ, Lin L, et al. Inactivation of porcine endogenous retrovirus in pigs using CRISPR-Cas9. Science 2017;357(6357):1303–7.

32. Fishman JA, Scobie L, Takeuchi Y. Xenotransplantation-associated infectious risk: a WHO consultation. Xenotransplantation 2012;19(2):72–81.

33. Langin M, Mayr T, Reichart B, et al. Consistent success in life-supporting porcine cardiac xenotransplantation. Nature 2018;564(7736):430–3.

34. Zimpfer D, Gustafsson F, Potapov E, et al. Two-year outcome after implantation of a full magnetically levitated left ventricular assist device: results from the ELEVATE Registry. Eur Heart J 2020;41(39):3801–9.

35. Agrawal S, Garg L, Shah M, et al. Thirty-day readmissions after left ventricular assist device implantation in the United States: insights from the Nationwide Readmissions Database. Circ Heart Fail 2018;11(3):e004628.

36. Teuteberg JJ, Cleveland JC Jr, Cowger J, et al. The Society of Thoracic Surgeons Intermacs 2019 Annual Report: the changing landscape of devices and indications. Ann Thorac Surg 2020;109(3):649–60.

37. Shah KB, Starling RC, Rogers JG, et al. Left ventricular assist devices versus medical management in ambulatory heart failure patients: an analysis of INTERMACS profiles 4 and 5 to 7 from the ROADMAP study. J Heart Lung Transplant 2018;37(6):706–14.

38. Hannan MM, Xie R, Cowger J, et al. Epidemiology of infection in mechanical circulatory support: a global analysis from the ISHLT Mechanically Assisted Circulatory Support Registry. J Heart Lung Transplant 2019;38(4):364–73.

39. Mehta SM, Pae WE Jr, Rosenberg G, et al. The LionHeart LVD-2000: a completely implanted left ventricular assist device for chronic circulatory support. Ann Thorac Surg 2001;71(3 Suppl):S156–61 [discussion: S183–4].

40. Dowling RD, Gray LA Jr, Etoch SW, et al. Initial experience with the AbioCor implantable replacement heart system. J Thorac Cardiovasc Surg 2004; 127(1):131–41.

41. Pya Y, Maly J, Bekbossynova M, et al. First human use of a wireless coplanar energy transfer coupled with a continuous-flow left ventricular assist device. J Heart Lung Transplant 2019;38(4):339–43.

42. Arrigo M, Huber LC, Winnik S, et al. Right ventricular failure: pathophysiology, diagnosis and treatment. Card Fail Rev 2019;5(3):140–6.

43. Cleveland JC Jr, Naftel DC, Reece TB, et al. Survival after biventricular assist device implantation: an analysis of the Interagency Registry for Mechanically Assisted Circulatory Support database. J Heart Lung Transplant 2011;30(8):862–9.

44. Arabia FA, Cantor RS, Koehl DA, et al. Interagency registry for mechanically assisted circulatory support report on the total artificial heart. J Heart Lung Transplant 2018;37(11):1304–12.

45. Nguyen A, Pozzi M, Mastroianni C, et al. Bridge to transplantation using paracorporeal biventricular assist devices or the Syncardia temporary total artificial heart: is there a difference? J Cardiovasc Surg (Torino) 2015;56(3):493–502.

46. Cheng A, Trivedi JR, Van Berkel VH, et al. Comparison of total artificial heart and biventricular assist device support as bridge-to-transplantation. J Card Surg 2016;31(10):648–53.

47. Netuka I, Pya Y, Bekbossynova M, et al. Initial bridge to transplant experience with a bioprosthetic autoregulated artificial heart. J Heart Lung Transplant 2020;39(12):1491–3.

48. Emmanuel S, Watson A, Connellan M, et al. First in Man Anatomical Fitting Study of the BiVACOR Total Artificial Heart. J Heart Lung Transplant 2020;39(4, Supplement):S189.

49. Pelletier B, Spiliopoulos S, Finocchiaro T, et al. System overview of the fully implantable destination

therapy–ReinHeart-total artificial heart. Eur J Cardio-thorac Surg 2015;47(1):80–6.

50. Glynn J, Song H, Hull B, et al. The OregonHeart Total Artificial Heart: design and performance on a mock circulatory loop. Artif Organs 2017;41(10):904–10.

51. Fox C, Chopski S, Murad N, et al. Hybrid continuous-flow total artificial heart. Artif Organs 2018;42(5):500–9.

52. Miller LW, Pagani FD, Russell SD, et al. Use of a continuous-flow device in patients awaiting heart transplantation. N Engl J Med 2007;357(9):885–96.

53. Pagani FD, Miller LW, Russell SD, et al. Extended mechanical circulatory support with a continuous-flow rotary left ventricular assist device. J Am Coll Cardiol 2009;54(4):312–21.

54. Kirklin JK, Pagani FD, Kormos RL, et al. Eighth annual INTERMACS report: special focus on framing the impact of adverse events. J Heart Lung Trans-plant 2017;36(10):1080–6.

55. Fitzpatrick JR 3rd, Frederick JR, Hiesinger W, et al. Early planned institution of biventricular mechanical circulatory support results in improved outcomes compared with delayed conversion of a left ventric-ular assist device to a biventricular assist device. J Thorac Cardiovasc Surg 2009;137(4):971–7.

56. Mehra MR, Uriel N, Naka Y, et al. A fully magnetically levitated left ventricular assist device - final report. N Engl J Med 2019;380(17):1618–27.

57. Soliman OII, Akin S, Muslem R, et al. Derivation and validation of a novel right-sided heart failure model after implantation of continuous flow left ventricular assist devices: the EUROMACS (European Registry for Patients with Mechanical Circulatory Support) Right-Sided Heart Failure Risk Score. Circulation 2018;137(9):891–906.

58. Loforte A, Stepanenko A, Potapov EV, et al. Tempo-rary right ventricular mechanical support in high-risk left ventricular assist device recipients versus per-manent biventricular or total artificial heart support. Artif Organs 2013;37(6):523–30.

59. Lavee J, Mulzer J, Krabatsch T, et al. An interna-tional multicenter experience of biventricular sup-port with HeartMate 3 ventricular assist systems. J Heart Lung Transplant 2018;37(12):1399–402.

60. Moore RA, Lorts A, Madueme PC, et al. Virtual im-plantation of the 50cc SynCardia total artificial heart. J Heart Lung Transplant 2016;35(6):824–7.

61. Netuka I, Ivak P, Tucanova Z, et al. Evaluation of low-intensity anti-coagulation with a fully magnetically levitated centrifugal-flow circulatory pump-the MA-GENTUM 1 study. J Heart Lung Transplant 2018; 37(5):579–86.

62. Bansal A, Uriel N, Colombo PC, et al. Effects of a fully magnetically levitated centrifugal-flow or axial-flow left ventricular assist device on von Willebrand factor: a prospective multicenter clinical trial. J Heart Lung Transplant 2019;38(8):806–16.

63. Patel SR, Madan S, Saeed O, et al. Association of Nasal Mucosal Vascular Alterations, gastrointestinal arteriovenous malformations, and bleeding in pa-tients with continuous-flow left ventricular assist de-vices. JACC Heart Fail 2016;4(12):962–70.

64. Andreas M, Moayedifar R, Wieselthaler G, et al. Increased thromboembolic events with dabigatran compared with vitamin K antagonism in left ventric-ular assist device patients: a randomized controlled pilot trial. Circ Heart Fail 2017;10(5):e003709.

65. Cheung A, Chorpenning K, Tamez D, et al. Design concepts and preclinical results of a miniaturized HeartWare Platform: the MVAD system. Innovations (Phila). 2015;10(3):151–6.

66. McGee E Jr, Danter M, Strueber M, et al. Evaluation of a lateral thoracotomy implant approach for a centrifugal-flow left ventricular assist device: the LATERAL clinical trial. J Heart Lung Transplant 2019;38(4):344–51.

67. Hohmann S, Veltmann C, Duncker D, et al. Initial experience with telemonitoring in left ventricular assist device patients. J Thorac Dis 2019;11(Suppl 6):S853–63.

UNITED STATES POSTAL SERVICE®

Statement of Ownership, Management, and Circulation
(All Periodicals Publications Except Requester Publications)

1. Publication Title	2. Publication Number	3. Filing Date
HEART FAILURE CLINICS	025 – 055	9/18/2021

4. Issue Frequency	5. Number of Issues Published Annually	6. Annual Subscription Price
JAN, APR, JUL, OCT	4	$277.00

7. Complete Mailing Address of Known Office of Publication (Not printer) (Street, city, county, state, and ZIP+4®)

ELSEVIER INC.
230 Park Avenue, Suite 800
New York, NY 10169

Contact Person: Malathi Samayan
Telephone (Include area code): 91-44-4299-4507

8. Complete Mailing Address of Headquarters or General Business Office of Publisher (Not printer)

ELSEVIER INC.
230 Park Avenue, Suite 800
New York, NY 10169

9. Full Names and Complete Mailing Addresses of Publisher, Editor, and Managing Editor (Do not leave blank)

Publisher (Name and complete mailing address)

DOLORES MELONI, ELSEVIER INC.
1600 JOHN F KENNEDY BLVD. SUITE 1800
PHILADELPHIA, PA 19103-2899

Editor (Name and complete mailing address)

JOANNA COLLETT, ELSEVIER INC.
1600 JOHN F KENNEDY BLVD. SUITE 1800
PHILADELPHIA, PA 19103-2899

Managing Editor (Name and complete mailing address)

PATRICK MANLEY, ELSEVIER INC.
1600 JOHN F KENNEDY BLVD. SUITE 1800
PHILADELPHIA, PA 19103-2899

10. Owner (Do not leave blank. If the publication is owned by a corporation, give the name and address of the corporation immediately followed by the names and addresses of all stockholders owning or holding 1 percent or more of the total amount of stock. If not owned by a corporation, give the names and addresses of the individual owners. If owned by a partnership or other unincorporated firm, give its name and address as well as those of each individual owner. If the publication is published by a nonprofit organization, give its name and address.)

Full Name	Complete Mailing Address
WHOLLY OWNED SUBSIDIARY OF REED/ELSEVIER, US HOLDINGS	1600 JOHN F KENNEDY BLVD. SUITE 1800 PHILADELPHIA, PA 19103-2899

11. Known Bondholders, Mortgagees, and Other Security Holders Owning or Holding 1 Percent or More of Total Amount of Bonds, Mortgages, or Other Securities. If none, check box. ▶ ☐ None

Full Name	Complete Mailing Address
N/A	

12. Tax Status (For completion by nonprofit organizations authorized to mail at nonprofit rates) (Check one)
The purpose, function, and nonprofit status of this organization and the exempt status for federal income tax purposes:
☒ Has Not Changed During Preceding 12 Months
☐ Has Changed During Preceding 12 Months (Publisher must submit explanation of change with this statement)

PS Form 3526, July 2014 (Page 1 of 4 (see instructions page 4)) PSN: 7530-01-000-9931   PRIVACY NOTICE: See our privacy policy on www.usps.com

---

13. Publication Title	14. Issue Date for Circulation Data Below
HEART FAILURE CLINICS	JULY 2021

15. Extent and Nature of Circulation			Average No. Copies Each Issue During Preceding 12 Months	No. Copies of Single Issue Published Nearest to Filing Date
a. Total Number of Copies (Net press run)			36	31
b. Paid Circulation (By Mail and Outside the Mail)	(1)	Mailed Outside-County Paid Subscriptions Stated on PS Form 3541 (Include paid distribution above nominal rate, advertiser's proof copies, and exchange copies)	18	16
	(2)	Mailed In-County Paid Subscriptions Stated on PS Form 3541 (Include paid distribution above nominal rate, advertiser's proof copies, and exchange copies)	0	0
	(3)	Paid Distribution Outside the Mails Including Sales Through Dealers and Carriers, Street Vendors, Counter Sales, and Other Paid Distribution Outside USPS®	10	9
	(4)	Paid Distribution by Other Classes of Mail Through the USPS (e.g., First-Class Mail®)	0	0
c. Total Paid Distribution (Sum of 15b (1), (2), (3), and (4))		▶	28	25
d. Free or Nominal Rate Distribution (By Mail and Outside the Mail)	(1)	Free or Nominal Rate Outside-County Copies included on PS Form 3541	8	6
	(2)	Free or Nominal Rate In-County Copies Included on PS Form 3541	0	0
	(3)	Free or Nominal Rate Copies Mailed at Other Classes Through the USPS (e.g., First-Class Mail)	0	0
	(4)	Free or Nominal Rate Distribution Outside the Mail (Carriers or other means)	0	0
e. Total Free or Nominal Rate Distribution (Sum of 15d (1), (2), (3) and (4))		▶	8	6
f. Total Distribution (Sum of 15c and 15e)		▶	36	31
g. Copies not Distributed (See Instructions to Publishers #4 (page #3))		▶	0	0
h. Total (Sum of 15f and g)		▶	36	31
i. Percent Paid (15c divided by 15f times 100)			77.77%	80.64%

* If you are claiming electronic copies, go to line 16 on page 3. If you are not claiming electronic copies, skip to line 17 on page 3.

16. Electronic Copy Circulation		Average No. Copies Each Issue During Preceding 12 Months	No. Copies of Single Issue Published Nearest to Filing Date
a. Paid Electronic Copies	▶		
b. Total Paid Print Copies (Line 15c) + Paid Electronic Copies (Line 16a)	▶		
c. Total Print Distribution (Line 15f) + Paid Electronic Copies (Line 16a)	▶		
d. Percent Paid (Both Print & Electronic Copies) (16b divided by 16c × 100)	▶		

☒ I certify that 50% of all my distributed copies (electronic and print) are paid above a nominal price.

17. Publication of Statement of Ownership

☒ If the publication is a general publication, publication of this statement is required. Will be printed in the OCTOBER 2021 issue of this publication.   ☐ Publication not required.

18. Signature and Title of Editor, Publisher, Business Manager, or Owner	Date
Malathi Samayan - Distribution Controller *Malathi Samayan*	9/18/2021

I certify that all information furnished on this form is true and complete. I understand that anyone who furnishes false or misleading information on this form or who omits material or information requested on the form may be subject to criminal sanctions (including fines and imprisonment) and/or civil sanctions (including civil penalties).

PS Form 3526, July 2014 (Page 2 of 4)   PRIVACY NOTICE: See our privacy policy on www.usps.com

Printed and bound by CPI Group (UK) Ltd, Croydon, CR0 4YY

03/10/2024

01040365-0019